Topics in Palliative Care
Volume 2

Series Editors
Russell K. Portenoy, M.D.
Eduardo Bruera, M.D.

TOPICS
IN
PALLIATIVE
CARE
Volume 2

Edited by

Eduardo Bruera
Grey Nuns Community Health Center
University of Alberta
Edmonton, Alberta

Russell K. Portenoy
Beth Israel Medical Center
New York, New York

New York   Oxford
OXFORD UNIVERSITY PRESS
1998

Oxford University Press

Oxford New York
Athens Auckland Bangkok Bogota Bombay Buenos Aires
Calcutta Cape Town Dar es Salaam Delhi Florence Hong Kong
Istanbul Karachi Kuala Lumpur Madras Madrid Melbourne
Mexico City Nairobi Paris Singapore Taipei Tokyo Toronto Warsaw

and associated companies in
Berlin Ibadan

Published by Oxford University Press, Inc.,
198 Madison Avenue, New York, New York 10016

Oxford is a registered trademark of Oxford University Press

Library of Congress Cataloging-in-Publication Data
Topics in palliative care / edited by Eduardo Bruera, Russell K. Portenoy.
p. cm.—(Topics in palliative care: v. 2)
Includes bibliographical references and index.
ISBN 0-19-510245-2
1. Cancer—Palliative treatment.
I. Portenoy, Russell K.
II. Bruera, Eduardo.
III. Series.
[DNLM: 1. Palliative Care. 2. Neoplasms—drug therapy. 3. Pain—drug therapy.
WB 310 T674 1997] RC271.P33T664 1997
616.99′406—dc20 DNLM/DLC for Library of Congress 96-22250

1 3 5 7 9 8 6 4 2

Printed in the United States of America
on acid-free paper

To our wives,
Susan and Maria,
whose love and support
make our work possible.

Preface to the Series

Palliative Care, a series devoted to research and practice in palliative care, was created to address the growing need to disseminate new information about this rapidly evolving field.

Palliative care is an interdisciplinary therapeutic model for the management of patients with incurable, progressive illness. In this model, the family is considered the unit of care. The clinical purview includes those factors—physical, psychological, social, and spiritual—that contribute to suffering, undermine quality of life, and prevent a death with comfort and dignity. The definition promulgated by the World Health Organization exemplifies this perspective.[*]

> Palliative care is the active total care of patients whose disease is not responsive to curative treatment. Control of pain, of other symptoms, and of psychological, social and spiritual problems is paramount. The goal of palliative care is the achievement of the best possible quality of life for patients and their families.

Palliative care is a fundamental part of clinical practice, the "parallel universe" to therapies directed at cure or prolongation of life. All clinicians who treat patients with chronic life-threatening diseases are engaged in palliative care, continually attempting to manage complex symptomatology and functional disturbances.

The need for specialized palliative care services may arise at any point during the illness. Symptom control and psychological adaptation are the usual concerns during the period of active disease-oriented therapies. Toward the end of life, however, needs intensify and broaden. Psychosocial distress or family distress, spiritual or existential concerns, advance care planning, and ethical concerns, among many other issues, may be considered by the various disciplines that coalesce in the delivery of optimal care. Clinicians who specialize in palliative care perceive their role as similar to those of specialists in other disciplines of medicine: referring patients to other primary caregivers when appropriate, acting as primary caregivers (as members of the team) when the challenges of the case warrant this involvement, and teaching and conducting research in the field of palliative care.

[*]World Health Organization. Technical Report Series 804, Cancer Pain and Palliative Care. Geneva: World Health Organization, 1990:11.

With recognition of palliative care as an essential element in medical care and as an area of specialization, there is a need for information about the approaches used by specialists from many disciplines in managing the varied problems that fall under the purview of this model. The scientific foundation of palliative care is also advancing, and similarly, methods are needed to highlight for practitioners at the bedside the findings of empirical research. Topics in Palliative Care has been designed to meet the need for enhanced communication in this changing field.

To highlight the diversity of concerns in palliative care, each volume of Topics in Palliative Care is divided into sections that address a range of issues. Various sections address aspects of symptom control, psychosocial functioning, spiritual or existential concerns, ethics, and other topics. The chapters in each section review the area and focus on a small number of salient issues for analysis. The authors present and evaluate existing data, provide a context drawn from both the clinic and research, and integrate knowledge in a manner that is both practical and readable.

We are grateful to the many contributors for their excellent work and their timeliness. We also thank our publisher, who has expressed great faith in the project. Such strong support has buttressed our desire to create an educational forum that may enhance palliative care in the clinical setting and drive its growth as a discipline.

Edmonton, Alberta   E. B.
New York, N.Y.   R.K.P.

Contents

III   Asthenia

IV   Psychological Issues in the Caregiver

Contributors

H. RICHARD ALEXANDER, M.D.
Senior Investigator, Surgery Branch
National Cancer Institute
National Institutes of Health
Bethesda, Maryland, USA

EDUARDO BRUERA, M.D.
Director, Palliative Care Program
Grey Nuns Community Health Centre
Edmonton, Alberta, Canada

HARVEY MAX CHOCHINOV, M.D.
Psychiatric Consultant
Manitoba Treatment & Research
  Foundation
Winnipeg, Manitoba, Canada

JAMES F. CLEARY, M.D.
Assistant Professor of Medicine
Department of Oncology
Medical Director, Palliative Medicine
  Service
University of Wisconsin
Madison, Wisconsin, USA

TESS CRAMOND, M.D.
Director, Pain Relief Service
Royal Brisbane Hospital
Herston, Queensland, Australia

ROBIN L. FAINSINGER, M.D.
Director, Palliative Care Program
Royal Alexandria Hospital
Edmonton, Alberta, Canada

DAVID J. HEWITT, M.D.
Department of Neurology
Emory University Medical Center
Atlanta, Georgia, USA

IRENE HIGGINSON, M.D.
Palliative Care Research Group
Health Services Research
London School of Hygiene & Tropical
  Medicine
London, England

ALEJANDRO R. JADAD, M.D.
Department of Clinical Epidemiology
  & Biostatistics
McMaster University
Hamilton, Ontario, Canada

CATHERINE JENKINS, M.D.
Regional Palliative Care Program
Grey Nuns Community Health Centre
Edmonton, Alberta, Canada

LAURENCE KATZ, M.D.
Department of Psychiatry
University of Manitoba
Winnipeg, Manitoba, Canada

CHARLES LOPRINZI, M.D.
Professor & Chair, Medical Oncology
Mayo Clinic
Rochester, Minnesota, USA

MATTHEW LOSCALZO, A.C.S.W.
Director, Oncology Social Work
Johns Hopkins Oncology Center
Research Associate, Johns Hopkins
  University School of Medicine
Baltimore, Maryland, USA

GRACE MA, M.D.
Department of Surgery
New York University
New York, New York, USA

NEIL MACDONALD, M.D.
Director, Cancer Ethics Programme
Center for Bioethics
Clinical Research Institute of Montreal
Professor, Oncology,
McGill University
Montreal, Quebec, Canada

DWIGHT E. MOULIN, M.D.
Associate Professor
Department of Clinical Neurological
  Sciences & Oncology
University of Western Ontario
The London Health Sciences Center
London, Ontario, Canada

HANS NEUENSCHWANDER, M.D.
Internal Medicine/Oncology Hospice
Lugano Ticino, Switzerland

RUSSELL K. PORTENOY, M.D.
Chairman, Department of Pain
  Medicine and Palliative Care
Beth Israel Medical Center
New York, New York, USA

MARY L.S. VACHON, R.N., PH.D.
Consultant, Psychological Oncology
Coordinator, Palliative Care
Sunnybrook Health Science Center
Toronto Sunnybrook Regional
  Cancer Center
Toronto, Ontario, Canada

JAMES R. ZABORA, M.S.W.
Director of Patient & Family Services
The Johns Hopkins Oncology Center
Research Associate, The Johns Hopkins
  University School of Medicine
Baltimore, Maryland, USA

I

NEUROPATHIC PAIN

Introduction: Neuropathic Pain: From Unresolved Questions to Clinical Practice

RUSSELL K. PORTENOY

There is a remarkable degree of agreement in the clinical community about the syndromes generally denoted by the term "neuropathic pain." This agreement is remarkable because neuropathic pain is not a discrete physiologically measurable phenomenon, but rather, a construct based on a constellation of clinical observations. In labeling a pain neuropathic, the clinician is inferring that the pain is probably sustained by aberrant somatosensory processes in the peripheral or central nervous systems. These processes are believed to be different from those that sustain pain caused by ongoing tissue injury, or so-called nociceptive pain.

This categorization by inferred pathophysiology has attained clinical acceptance because it is useful to clinicians in the evaluation and treatment of patients with chronic pain. If pain has neuropathic features, such as a dysesthetic (unfamiliar, bizarre) quality, a lesion in the nervous system will be sought. The finding of a responsible lesion may suggest options for primary therapy, such as decompression of an entrapped peripheral nerve. If neuropathic features are associated with focal autonomic dysregulation or trophic changes, the lesion is often labeled a reflex sympathetic dystrophy (complex regional pain syndrome type I) or causalgia (complex regional pain syndrome type II).[1] These diagnoses, in turn, raise the possibility that the pain is sympathetically maintained and suggest a trial of a specific intervention, sympathetic blockade, that would not otherwise be considered. Finally, the diagnosis of neuropathic pain may suggest the potential utility of numerous adjuvant analgesics, such as anticonvulsants or oral local anesthetics, which are currently administered specifically for pain of this type.[2]

Given the utility of inferred pathophysiology in the clinical setting, the lack of empirical foundation for the neuropathic construct is astonishing. Although diagnostic criteria for specific neuropathic pain syndromes have been elaborated,[1] there are no clear criteria for the diagnosis of neuropathic pain in general. The variability in the symptoms, signs, and syndromes labeled as neuropathic is very large and the development of criteria would be challenging. Whereas some pains associated with neural injury are burning and stabbing in quality, others are aching and throbbing. Pains may be intermittent or continuous, and mild or severe. Pain may fluctuate independent of any identifiable precipitating or palliative factors, or change dramatically with specific events. Pains may or may not be associated with neurological deficits, and a careful evaluation may or may not reveal an overt site of injury to the nervous system.

This type of uncertainty extends to existing information about basic mechanisms. Injury to neural structures in experimental models has been associated with a diverse array of aberrant somatosensory processes that could be involved in the persistence of pain in humans with neural injury.[3] Many of these mechanisms have been identified in experimental models of nociceptive pain (injury to soft tissue, for example), which has led some to doubt the validity of the neuropathic–nociceptive dichotomy.[4]

It is reasonable to postulate that specific types, or groups, of mechanisms may occur in identified neuropathic pain syndromes. For example, a core group of mechanisms may be associated fundamentally with pain following injury to the central nervous system. It is also reasonable to hypothesize that identical mechanisms occur in syndromes that are clinically distinct. If a specific mechanism underlies a particular type of pain, such as a lancinating dysesthesia or a burning dysesthesia, then the overlap among mechanisms may explain the observation that different neuropathic pain syndromes are often described in similar terms by patients. None of the these links between phenomenology and pathophysiology have been established in humans, however, and the large variability among neuropathic pain syndromes does not yet have a mechanistic interpretation.

Thus, different clinicians may or may not agree that the presentation of a pain warrants the label "neuropathic." Even if experienced clinicians would agree, there can be no independent verification of a neuropathic pathophysiology in the clinical setting. Although a syndromic diagnosis (such as central pain, reflex sympathetic dystrophy, or pain of peripheral neuropathy) may be possible and lends some additional specificity to the label, neither the neuropathic pain construct nor the syndrome diagnosis establishes the actual mechanisms responsible for the pain. Indeed, the notion that some set of mechanisms distinguishes neuropathic from nociceptive pain is reasonable on the basis of clinical observations, but there has been no confirmation that a constellation of "neuropathic mechanisms" actually exists. If such mechanisms do exist, they are very likely to be complex and highly variable, both within and across pain syndromes. The construct of neuropathic pain is, therefore, grossly simplistic.

Yet, clinicians find this limited construct useful. There is great promise that research into the pain pathophysiology may be able to elucidate the range of mechanisms responsible for particular types of pain or specific pain syndromes. In the future, clinical assessment, or some combination of clinical and laboratory (such as electrophysiologic or sensory testing) evaluation, may allow valid inferences about specific mechanisms. The broad construct of inferred pathophysiology will still be used, but the global label of neuropathic pain may become superannuated by precise designations that indicate the mechanisms that are probably operating in the individual patient. This information will provide an opportunity for clinical trials of specific interventions targeted to these mechanisms. Ultimately, the trial-and-error approach to the management of neuropathic pain depicted in this section will be supplanted by specific therapies selected on the basis of accurate inferences about the actual mechanisms underlying the pain.

References

1. Merskey H, Bogduk N, eds. *Classification of Chronic Pain: Descriptions of Chronic Pain Syndromes and Definitions of Pain Terms*, 2nd ed. Seattle: IASP Press; 1994.
2. Portenoy RK. Adjuvant analgesics in pain management. In: Doyle D, Hanks GW, MacDonald N, eds. *Oxford Textbook of Palliative Medicine*. Oxford: Oxford University Press; 1998:361–390.
3. Elliott KJ. Taxonomy and mechanisms of neuropathic pain. *Semin Neurol* 1994; 14:195–205.
4. Devor M, Basbaum AI, Bennett GJ, et al. Group report: mechanisms of neuropathic pain following peripheral injury. In: Basbaum AI, Besson J-M eds. *Towards a New Pharmacotherapy of Pain*. Chichester: John Wiley & Sons; 1991:417–440.

1

Neuropathic Cancer Pain: Syndromes and Clinical Controversies

DWIGHT E. MOULIN

Neuropathic cancer pain can be due to direct tumor infiltration of neural structures or to secondary effects produced by treatments of the underlying neoplasm. Neuropathic pain due to the former etiology is present in 20%–30% of patients attending specialized cancer pain centers, and pain due to the latter occurs in about 10% of attendees.[1-3]

Although patients with neuropathic pain due to tumor infiltration clinically resemble those with neuropathic pain arising from nonmalignant causes, there are important differences between these populations. Neuropathic cancer pain is almost always accompanied by other pain syndromes, including bone pain and visceral pain.[3] Tumor infiltration usually implies progressive incurable disease, inevitably leading to loss of motor, sensory, and autonomic function. Relentless disability that is obvious to the patient and the physician, and the knowledge that the disease process is ultimately fatal, adds a major suffering component to the pain syndrome that must be addressed.[4] Finally, the dynamics of progressive nerve injury attributable to tumor infiltration may impact on the pathophysiology of neuropathic pain in a way that is not present following monophasic nerve injury (e.g., trauma), and this also has implications for treatment.

This review describes the clinical characteristics of cancer-related neuropathic pain. It focuses on the range of pain syndromes encountered in this population, the varied treatment strategies, and ongoing controversies based on the underlying pathophysiologic mechanisms.

Clinical Features and Mechanisms of Neuropathic Pain

Damage to a peripheral nerve due to trauma or some other nonmalignant disease process may simply produce a sensory deficit in the territory of the involved nerve. However, tumor infiltration of nerve almost always results in a characteristic pain syndrome with distinctive symptoms and signs. The pathophysiologic basis of these symptoms and signs involves peripheral and central generators of pain that are set in motion by nerve injury.[5]

Clinical features

There are three cardinal symptoms of neuropathic pain that are present to variable degrees in most patients. These sensations usually arise from the territory of the injured nerve but can radiate into adjacent normally innervated areas. The first is constant, burning dysesthetic pain. This is often associated with aching or cramp-like pain in the deep tissues. This spontaneous pain is sometimes described as if the involved area were "on fire." Dysesthetic pain can also take the form of a severe pressure-like sensation, as if the involved limb were about to explode.

The second major symptom of neuropathic pain is paroxysmal pain. This pain is usually fleeting and intense, shock-like, or lancinating. It can be spontaneous or evoked by movement or tactile stimulation.

The third symptom is the aberrant perception of pain in response to what is normally an innocuous stimulus (allodynia). The contact of clothing or a gentle breeze across the skin may produce unbearable pain. The aberrant perception of ice as intense heat is especially pathognomic of neuropathic pain.

The physical signs of neuropathic pain involve hyperpathic or exaggerated responses to various stimuli and evidence of autonomic instability. Hyperalgesia is characterized by an intensely painful response to modest irritation, such as a pinprick. Sometimes a single mechanical stimulus, such as light touch, will not evoke any sensation. However, repeated or sustained stimulation of this type may build into an explosive pain over several seconds that radiates beyond the territory of the injured nerve. These features illustrate temporal and spatial summation of the stimulus.

Autonomic dysregulation sometimes accompanies nerve injury (also known as causalgia or complex regional pain syndrome type II) or neuropathic pain following soft tissue injury (also known as reflex sympathetic dystrophy or complex regional pain syndrome type I). The involved limb becomes edematous and shows vasomotor and sweating abnormalities. There may also be local trophic changes: the skin becomes thin and shiny with loss of subcutaneous tissue, the nails grow coarse and brittle, and the bone becomes osteoporotic. The potential for a salutary response to interruption of sympathetic efferent activity has led to the designation *sympathetically maintained pain* to describe a subgroup of these patients.[6] Although sympathetic activity may play a role in some neuropathic cancer pain syndromes, the autonomic and trophic changes may be difficult to discern because of limb swelling due to venous and lymphatic obstruction and the poor nutritional status of the patient. Edema may also confound the assessment of neuropathic pain by making the limb feel tight and stiff.

Peripheral generators of neuropathic pain

Nerve injury can generate pain in a number of ways. Distortion or compression of peripheral nerve may produce nerve sheath pain by irritating the small primary afferents (nervi nervorum) that innervate nerve trunks.[7] Axonal injury generates nerve sprouts, which are sources of ectopic impulse formation.[8] If advancing nerve sprouts become trapped in scar tissue, they form neuromas that are similarly active.[9] Dorsal root ganglion cells and local patches of demyelination along the axon also become sources of ectopic discharge.[10,11] In addition to firing spontaneously, these sites are sensitive to mechanical stimulation, which can produce prolonged discharges over seconds, minutes, or even hours.[12,13] The Tinel's sign evoked by tapping along an injured nerve demonstrates the mechanosensitivity of regenerating axons. Axonal sprouts and neuromas are also highly sensitive to circulating and locally released catecholamines.[14–16] The recent finding of increased alpha-adrenoceptor responsiveness in the limbs of patients with reflex sympathetic dystrophy[17] provides a further rationale for sympathetic blockade in selected patients with neuropathic pain and autonomic instability.[18] Finally, injured nerves are capable of cross-excitation or ephaptic transmission.[19,20] Direct electrical coupling between axons has pathophysiological significance in hemifacial spasm and, perhaps, in trigeminal neuralgia.[21,22]

The fact that there are several potential generators of pain may explain the failure of any single treatment modality to provide relief. Local anesthetic blockade or neurectomy proximal to the site of nerve injury may provide only transient relief because there is an ectopic pacemaker in the dorsal root ganglion or central mechanisms have developed (see below). Although phenytoin and carbamazepine inhibit spontaneous activity in experimental neuromas,[23,24] these drugs frequently fail to control burning dysesthetic pain following nerve transection.[25,26] The only type of neuropathic pain that seems to have a clear pathophysiologic substrate is the lancinating pain associated with demyelination of the nerve root entry zone. Anticonvulsants, such as carbamazepine, consistently provide sustained relief from trigeminal neuralgia and painful tonic spasms in the setting of multiple sclerosis.[27]

Central generators of pain

The common failure of rhizotomy to control some neuropathic pain syndromes[28] indicates that central generators of pain are important. Central mechanisms are also necessary to explain allodynia and hyperpathia that appear to be due to aberrant somatosensory processing.

Central or deafferentation pain can be initiated by a lesion in the central nervous system (e.g., thalamic injury) or peripheral nervous system. Cancer-related peripheral nerve lesions can generate central pain through several mechanisms. A brief but massive afferent barrage from a peripheral generator of pain can trigger sustained changes in the excitability of dorsal horn neurons.[29] Studies in animals, for example, demonstrate that constrictive ligatures around sciatic nerves produce massive ongoing afferent volleys that result in hyperexcitability of the dorsal horn.[30] Progressive tumor infiltration of a peripheral nerve trunk or plexus in cancer patients likely produces similar afferent activity and central changes.

Nerve transections such as rhizotomy can result in denervation hypersensitivity of the dorsal horn, thalamus, and primary somatosensory cortex.[31,32] Dorsal horn neurons that are deafferented lose pre- and postsynaptic inhibition, become spontaneously active, and expand their receptive fields.[29] Allodynia and hyperpathic phenomena such as temporal and spatial summation can be explained by convergence of low-threshold sensory afferents on sensitized wide dynamic-range dorsal horn neurons.[33] This mechanism has also been invoked to explain the striking allodynia seen in reflex sympathetic dystrophy.[34]

Malignant Neuropathic Pain Syndromes

A large number of neuropathic cancer pain syndromes have been identified (Table 1.1).[35] Since pain is a common presenting symptom of neurologic involvement, recognition of these pain syndromes is important in defining appropriate treatment and prognosis.

Pain syndromes associated with direct tumor involvement

Cranial neuralgias
Classic trigeminal neuralgia may be the presenting symptom of middle and posterior fossa tumors[36] and glossopharyngeal neuralgia associated with syncope can occur with head and neck malignancies. For the latter syndrome, severe pain in the neck radiating into the ear may be the presenting symptom of a malignancy in the head and neck region.[37]

Leptomeningeal metastases
Diffuse infiltration of the subarachnoid space by metastatic tumor can involve the neuraxis at multiple levels.[38] Headache, confusion, and radicular pain in the low back and buttocks are common presenting symptoms. At least half the patients with leptomeningeal disease have cranial nerve abnormalities, including visual loss, ocular muscle and facial weakness, and impaired hearing. A similar proportion of patients have weakness and sensory loss in the lower extremities, often associated with bowel or bladder dysfunction. The diagnosis of leptomeningeal metastases is confirmed through cytological analysis of the cerebrospinal fluid. The extent of disease can be determined by magnetic resonance imaging (MRI) of the head and spinal cord, using gadolinium enhancement. Treatment includes steroids and radiation therapy to involved areas. Intraventricular or intrathecal chemotherapy is useful for leptomeningeal disease due to lymphomas or breast carcinoma.

Table 1.1. Neuropathic cancer pain syndromes

Associated with direct tumor involvement

Cranial neuralgias

Leptomeningeal metastases

Epidural spinal cord compression

Brachial and lumbosacral plexopathies

Peripheral nerve syndromes

Painful polyneuropathies

Associated with cancer therapy

Postsurgical pain syndromes

    Postmastectomy and postaxillary node dissection pain

    Post-thoracotomy pain

    Postradical neck dissection pain

    Phantom limb and stump pain

Postradiation pain syndromes

    Radiation fibrosis of the brachial plexus

    Radiation fibrosis of the lumbosacral plexus

    Radiation-induced peripheral nerve tumors

    Radiation myelopathy

Postchemotherapy pain syndromes

    Painful peripheral neuropathy

Acute herpetic and postherpetic neuralgia

Epidural spinal cord compression

Epidural spinal cord or cauda equina compression usually arises from a metastatic deposit to the vertebral body that spreads to the epidural space.[39] Pain is due to bone destruction, traction on epidural tissues, and nerve root compression. Local bone pain is the initial symptom in over 95% of patients and may be followed in days or weeks by radicular pain, which is frequently unilateral in the cervical or lumbosacral region and bilateral in the thoracic region. Interscapular pain may be referred from lower cervical disease and sacroiliac pain may be experienced from L1 vertebral body involvement. Recumbency aggravates the pain of metastatic epidural compression, but frequently relieves the pain of degenerative joint disease. Tumor progression into the spinal canal results in weakness, sensory loss, bowe or bladder dysfunction, and reflex abnormalities.

Because prognosis is determined primarily by the level of neurologic function at the beginning of treatment, early diagnosis of epidural disease is critical. Plain radiographs provide important guidelines for the presence of neoplasm in the epidural space. Greater than 50% collapse of the vertebral body is associated with an 87% risk of epidural disease and pedicle erosion carries a 31% risk.[40] Definitive imaging of the spinal cord and cauda equina can be obtained with myelography or MRI (Fig. 1.1). MRI is equal to myelography in detecting epidural disease and is less invasive.

Steroids and radiation therapy are the mainstays of treatment for epidural neoplasm. Surgery is indicated when a tissue diagnosis is required (unknown primary tumor), when there is neurologic deterioration despite radiation therapy, and in the setting of spinal instability.

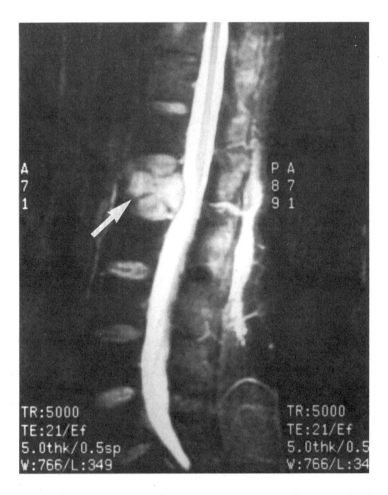

Figure 1.1. Mid-sagittal MRI of lumbar spine showing tumor infiltration and collapse of L$_1$ vertebral body (arrow) with encroachment on spinal canal.

Brachial plexopathy

Brachial plexopathy is responsible for 15% of the neurologic complications of cancer and occurs most frequently in patients with lymphoma, breast, and lung carcinomas.[35] Tumor can extend to the brachial plexus from adjacent lymph nodes or the lung apex. Pain is the most common presenting symptom and may precede neurologic signs by up to 9 months.[41] Aching shoulder and paraspinal pain is usually accompanied by burning, dysesthetic pain into the ulnar aspect of the forearm and the medial hand in lower brachial plexus distribution (C7, C8, T1). Neurologic signs including focal weakness, atrophy, and sensory loss follow the same distribution. Rapidly increasing pain, evidence of diffuse brachial plexus infiltration, or Horner's syndrome suggests tumor extension into the epidural space and are markers for incipient epidural spinal cord compression. Computerized tomographic (CT) scan or MRI usually shows a well circumscribed tumor mass (Fig. 1.2), which defines the radiation port prior to radiotherapy.

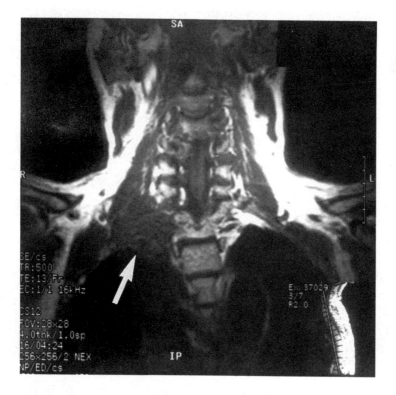

Figure 1.2. Coronal MRI of upper chest showing right Pancoast tumor adjacent to T_1 vertebral body (arrow). The tumor invades the lower brachial plexus.

Lumbrosacral plexopathy

The lumbosacral plexus can be infiltrated by extension from a primary tumor or spread from metastases in adjacent lymph nodes or bony pelvis. Rectal, cervical, and breast carcinomas, and lymphomas are the common primary tumors. Pain is the most frequent initial symptom. Leg weakness, sensory loss, reflex asymmetry, and leg edema develop weeks to months later.[42] Upper lumbar plexus involvement in the paravertebral psoas region usually refers pain to the groin and anterior thigh, whereas infiltration of the lumbosacral plexus deep in the pelvis or the presacral region produces pain in the perineum, buttock, and posterior thigh and leg. A pelvic and abdominal CT scan or MRI usually determines tumor extent (Fig. 1.3) and evidence of secondary complications such as hydronephrosis.

Peripheral nerve syndromes and painful neuropathies

Paravertebral or chest wall lesions can cause painful mononeuropathies. A metastatic deposit involving a proximal rib with the development of an intercostal neuralgia is a common example.

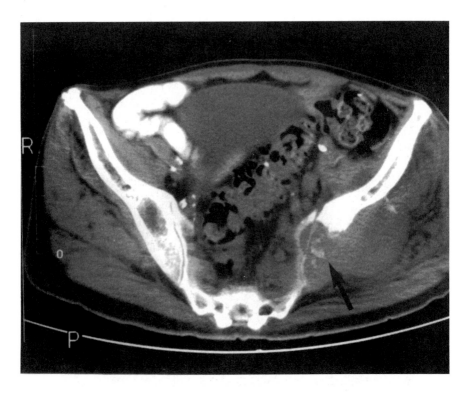

Figure 1.3. CT scan of the pelvis showing large metastatic tumor mass in the left gluteal muscle with destruction of the sacroiliac joint and extension into the pelvic side wall (arrow). The patient presented with a lumbosacral plexopathy .

Painful polyneuropathies in the setting of cancer usually reflect a paraneoplastic or remote effect of the underlying tumor.[43] Subacute sensory neuronopathy is a discrete paraneoplastic syndrome characterized by tingling and burning pain in the extremities, with superimposed shock-like pains. Examination reveals marked sensory ataxia and impairment of joint position sense, which is attributable to an inflammatory process involving the dorsal root ganglia. Sensory symptoms may antedate the clinical appearance of the neoplasm by several months and the neuropathy usually runs a course independent of the primary tumor. The most common underlying tumors are small-cell carcinoma of the lung and carcinoma of the breast and ovary. A painful distal sensory motor neuropathy may also occur as a paraneoplastic syndrome associated with diverse neoplasms.

Pain syndromes associated with cancer therapy

Postsurgical pain syndromes

Postmastectomy and postaxillary node dissection pain
Five to ten percent of women who undergo surgical procedures on the breast or adjacent lymph nodes develop chronic neuropathic pain. Postmastectomy pain has been classically associated with radical or modified radical mastectomy. The usual cause is a neuroma involving the intercostobrachial nerve (a cutaneous branch of T1–T2), which has been severed as a result of the surgical procedure.[44] Lumpectomy is less likely to cause this pain syndrome, especially if the intercostobrachial nerve is not involved. However, axillary node dissection is still routinely carried out as part of the staging procedure for breast carcinoma and frequently damages the intercostobrachial nerve.

Postmastectomy or postaxillary node dissection pain is characterized by burning, constricting pain in the anterior chest, axilla, and posterior upper arm in the area of sensory loss.[45] It may develop at any time from the immediate postoperative period until a year or more later. The character of the pain and its distribution is quite stereotyped and this syndrome is usually easily distinguished from recurrent disease.

Post-thoracotomy pain
Persistent or recurrent pain along the distribution of the incision following thoracotomy for lung carcinoma is commonly associated with recurrent tumor invading the chest wall.[46] Neuropathic pain without tumor recurrence, which is due to neuromas along the thoracotomy scar, does occur, but is rare. Plain chest radiographs are unlikely to provide a diagnosis and a CT scan of the chest with bone and soft tissue windows is indicated.

Postradical neck dissection pain
Injury to the cervical nerves and cervical plexus can produce neuropathic pain in the anterior neck and upper shoulder region. Escalating pain may reflect recur-

rent disease, which can be confirmed by repeated CT scans through the neck region.[47]

Phantom limb and stump pain

Phantom pain has a burning, lancinating quality and is much more likely if there was sustained pre-amputation limb pain.[48] The pain may initially increase and then gradually fade over time. Recurrence of pain in a phantom limb may be a harbinger of proximal recurrent disease. Stump pain occurs at the site of the surgical scar and results from the development of traumatic neuroma. Mechanical stimulation of the neuroma often reproduces the pain.

Postradiation pain syndromes

Radiation fibrosis of the brachial plexus

Radiation fibrosis may occur anywhere from 6 months to 20 years after radiation treatment. Most patients present with numbness and tingling, rather than pain, and then develop progressive weakness and lymphedema. Pain commonly occurs, but in contrast to tumor infiltration of the brachial plexus, is rarely severe. The assertion that radiation fibrosis tends to involve the upper plexus (C5–C6), whereas tumor infiltration involves the lower plexus (C8–T1),[49] has been disputed.[50–52] Both types of plexopathy commonly involve the lower plexus or the entire brachial plexus. The relative absence of pain, gradual deterioration, myokymic discharges on electromyography, and loss of normal tissue planes rather than a discrete mass on imaging studies are all strongly suggestive of radiation-induced injury to the brachial plexus.

Radiation fibrosis of the lumbosacral plexus

Radiation fibrosis is less common in the lumbosacral than in the brachial plexus and may become manifest up to 30 years after treatment.[53] Bilateral distal weakness with numbness and tingling are the usual presenting symptoms. Pain is eventually present in about half of patients but is rarely a major problem. Unilateral symptoms raise the possibility of a radiation-induced peripheral nerve tumor and this diagnosis should be pursued with a CT scan or MRI of the pelvis.

Postchemotherapy pain syndromes

Painful peripheral neuropathy

Vincristine, cisplatin, and procarbazine are most commonly associated with a painful neuropathy.[54] The pain is in glove and stocking distribution and usually improves slowly after chemotherapy has been stopped.

Acute herpetic and postherpetic neuralgia

Herpes zoster is caused by a reactivation of the varicella zoster virus, which is usually contracted in childhood. Reactivation in sensory ganglia is likely because of declining immunity with advancing age or an immunocompromised state. Herpes zoster occurs more frequently in previously irradiated dermatomes and in patients receiving chemotherapy.[55]

Postherpetic neuralgia is pain that follows resolution of acute zoster for some specified period, such as more than 1 month after lesion healing.[56] It is more common in older age groups. The development of herpes zoster at age 60 carries a 50% risk of postherpetic neuralgia, and at age 70, the risk is almost 75%. Herpes zoster and postherpetic neuralgia produce typical neuropathic pain. The natural history is generally favorable—only 20%–30% of patients have severe pain at 1 year[57,58] and some patients spontaneously become pain-free[56] even after this period. Severe chronic pain remains a problem for an unfortunate minority.

Neuropathic Cancer Pain—Management and Controversies

Management of neuropathic cancer pain is based largely on survey data and extrapolation from randomized controlled trials of nonmalignant neuropathic pain syndromes. Data derived from studies of nonmalignant neuropathic pain may not provide an accurate reflection of efficacy in the setting of cancer because rapidly progressive disease involving the peripheral nervous system may have a greater impact on central generators of pain.[59] Similarly, the feasibility of neurolytic procedures, such as rhizotomy, in cancer patients with a limited life expectancy should be an advantage, but this may be offset by a major component of central pain. Management of neuropathic cancer pain is therefore based on a variety of approaches without any clear guidelines as to the expected outcome.

The role of neuro-oncologic consultation

The role of a comprehensive neuro-oncologic evaluation of neuropathic cancer pain is not always appreciated. Because management is largely empiric, neurologic assessment prior to treatment is valuable when the disease process is not clearly defined. A review of admissions to an oncology service revealed that a neurologic diagnosis was made in almost half the patients.[60] A prospective survey of pain consultations in a major cancer center determined that new neurologic diagnoses were made in 36%, of patients half of whom received radiotherapy, surgery, or chemotherapy on the basis of these findings.[61]

The following clinical scenario illustrates how the neurologic diagnosis can influence treatment. A 56-year-old woman was treated with intracavitary and external radiation therapy for invasive carcinoma of the cervix and 1 year later presented with burning pain in the groin and anterior thighs. She had weakness in hip flexion bilaterally and was hyperalgesic to pinprick in the distribution of her pain. A pelvic CT scan and laparotomy showed no evidence of recurrent disease. Neurologic assessment indicated that her pain, weakness, and abberrant sensation were in upper lumbar distribution and she went on to have a CT scan of the abdomen which revealed markedly enlarged para-aortic nodes, reflecting retroperitoneal extension of her disease. She was treated with radiation therapy to the lumbar region, which provided significant palliation of her symptoms. This is a fairly common presentation of a neuropathic cancer pain syndrome where recognition of the mechanism of referred pain is crucial to patient management.

Pharmacologic approaches

Table 1.2 lists the medications that have shown efficacy in the management of neuropathic pain. Very few of these drugs have been subjected to randomized controlled trials in cancer patients with neuropathic pain.[62-65]

Antidepressants

Survey data suggest that antidepressants are well accepted in the management of cancer pain.[66] Although tricyclic antidepressants have traditionally been used for continuous dysesthetic pain, they may also be of value for lancinating neuropathic pain.[67] In addition to their analgesic effects, antidepressants may stimulate the appetite, provide night-time sedation, and counteract depression. The efficacy of tricyclic antidepressants for neuropathic pain can be inferred from randomized controlled trials involving diabetic neuropathy[67-69] and postherpetic neuralgia.[70-73]

The role of the selective serotonin uptake inhibitors in the management of neuropathic pain is controversial. Fluoxetine was not efficacious in the management of diabetic neuropathy,[74] independent of its antidepressant effects, but paroxetine was.[75] Venlafaxine and nefazodone are novel antidepressants which inhibit reuptake of both serotonin and norepinephrine with minimal anticholinergic and adrenergic blocking activity. There are anecdotal reports of analgesic activity with these drugs, but efficacy has not been established through randomized controlled trials.

Anticonvulsants and baclofen

The anticonvulsants have their greatest value in the management of lancinating neuropathic pain. Carbamazepine has shown a favorable result in diabetic neuropathy.[76,77] Clonazepam and valproate have also been advocated for lancinating neuropathic pain.[25,78] Newer anticonvulsants such as gabapentin appear promising in the management of neuropathic pain,[79] but controlled trials are lacking. Although baclofen is marketed for the treatment of spasticity, it has efficacy in trigeminal neuralgia[80] and is sometimes useful for other neuropathic pain syndromes.

Table 1.2. Pharmacologic agents used for neuropathic pain

Class	Example
Antidepressants	Amitriptyline
	Desipramine
	Paroxetine
	Venlafaxine
	Nefazodone
Anticonvulsants	Carbamazepine
	Phenytoin
	Clonazepam
	Valproate
	Gabapentin
Muscle relaxants	Baclofen
Local anesthetics	Lidocaine
	Mexiletine
	Flecainide
	Tocainide
Sympathetic blockers	Clonidine
	Phenoxybenzamine
	Prazosin
Topical agents	Capsaicin
	EMLA cream
	Lidocaine gel
Opioid analgesics	Morphine
	Fentanyl
	Methadone
NMDA antagonists	Ketamine

Local anesthetics
Systemic and oral local anesthetics produce membrane stabilization and can suppress ectopic neural pacemaker sites.[81] Since ectopic impulse formation is more sensitive to these agents than normal impulse conduction along the nerve,[82] abnormal firing may be reduced selectively and may outlast conventional conduction block.

Randomized controlled trials of intravenous lidocaine have shown significant benefit in postherpetic neuralgia[83] and diabetic neuropathy.[84] Another small study involving various pain syndromes showed pain relief from intravenous lidocaine that was maintained with oral mexiletine.[85] Two double-blind, randomized trials of intravenous lidocaine with limited sample size showed no benefit,[62,63] whereas a study of subcutaneous lidocaine infusion using a similar study design showed sustained pain relief in three patients.[64] There are inconsistent data regarding the efficacy of systemic local anesthetics in central pain syndromes. A single-blind, placebo-controlled study suggested benefit,[86] whereas a recent survey did not.[87]

A controlled trial of mexiletine demonstrated efficacy for painful diabetic neuropathy.[88] Another oral local anesthetic, tocainide, was found to be effective for trigeminal neuralgia,[89] but it has the potential for considerable toxicity and must be regarded as a second line agent. Anecdotally, oral flecainide has been useful for neuropathic cancer pain and may be substituted for mexiletine.

Sympathetic blockers

Clonidine is an alpha-2-adrenergic agonist with analgesic properties. Randomized controlled trials have shown benefit in postherpetic neuralgia[90] and diabetic neuropathy.[91] A large double-blind, placebo-controlled trial of epidural clonidine revealed significant pain relief in neuropathic cancer pain.[65] Phenoxybenzamine is an alpha-adrenergic antagonist that has been efficacious in causalgia,[92] although postural hypotension can be a significant problem.

Topical agents

Topical agents can have analgesic actions at the site of transdermal absorption. Capsaicin has the potential to relieve neuropathic pain by depleting local tissues of substance P. Although controlled trials have shown benefit in postherpetic neuralgia[93] and painful diabetic neuropathy,[94] clinical experience with capsaicin has been disappointing. A recent double-blind, placebo-controlled study of capsaicin cream in chronic distal painful polyneuropathy did not show any benefit.[95]

Some patients with postherpetic neuralgia respond to a eutectic mixture of local anesthetics (EMLA cream).[96] Similarly, 5% lidocaine gel has been reported to be efficacious in postherpetic neuralgia.[97]

Opioid analgesics

Considerable controversy surrounds the use of opioid analgesics for neuropathic cancer pain. Two reports were particularly influential in asserting the notion that neuropathic pain generally does not respond to opioids.[98,99] Some reported clinical experience does in fact suggest that neuropathic cancer pain responds less well to opioid analgesics than some forms of nociceptive pain.[2,100] Other clinical surveys indicate that neuropathic pain may respond well to opioid therapy.[101–103] A randomized controlled trial showed that patients with neuropathic pain obtain pain relief from intravenous morphine[83] and another trial revealed significant pain relief from intravenous fentanyl relative to diazepam and saline.[104] Methadone may be a useful agent for neuropathic pain, perhaps in part because of its N-methyl-D-aspartate (NMDA) antagonist properties.[105] A combined analysis of several controlled single-dose studies in cancer patients demonstrated that neuropathic pain responds to a standard opioid dose, but the response was less than that to nociceptive pain.[105a]

The crucial factor in this controversy is the balance between analgesia and opioid-induced side effects. Two studies involving patient-controlled analgesia suggest that a favorable balance between analgesia and side effects is less likely to occur among those with neuropathic pain than nociceptive pain.[106,107] A pharmacokinetic–pharmacodynamic analysis of brief opioid infusions suggests that neuropathic pain responds to opioid drugs in a classic dose-dependent fashion with a shift to the right in the dose–response curve.[108] Overall, the extant literature indicates that neuropathic pain does respond to opioids, but the doses required may increase the risk of side effects and this may have a negative impact on quality of life.

NMDA antagonists

N-methyl-D-aspartate agonists and receptors play a major role in the type of neuronal hyperexcitability of the dorsal horn that has been associated with neuropathic pain.[109] Ketamine is a commonly used intravenous anesthetic with NMDA receptor blocking activity.[110] Open trials of intravenous and subcutaneous ketamine have suggested benefit in phantom limb pain and postherpetic neuralgia.[111,112] Small double-blind, placebo-controlled trials of intravenous ketamine have also reported pain relief in postherpetic neuralgia[113] and a variety of chronic neuropathic pain syndromes,[114] although psychomimetic side effects can be intolerable.

Dextromethorphan, a common cough suppressant, is another NMDA receptor antagonist that has been studied in neuropathic pain states. A human experimental model involving painful electric shocks showed that dextromethorphan reduced temporal summation.[115] However, a double-blind randomized crossover trial of oral dextromethorphan in a variety of central and peripheral pain syndromes did not show any benefit.[116] Although the results to date have not been dramatic, novel NMDA antagonists with acceptable side-effect profiles hold great promise in the management of neuropathic pain.

Anesthetic approaches

Peripheral nerve blocks are best suited for patients with segmental pain in the chest or abdomen, who can undergo interruption of involved motor and sensory fibers without significant disability. The patient with somatic and neuropathic pain from a rib metastasis can be treated with a local anesthetic block to localize the lesion followed by a neurolytic procedure using phenol, alcohol, or cryoanalgesia.

Subarachnoid injection of a neurolytic agent can be used to control cancer pain that involves several spinal segments. Phenol 5% in glycerin has been recommended as the neurolytic agent of choice.[117] Phenol has local anesthetic as well as neurolytic properties and is painless to inject.

Subarachnoid neurolysis should be considered in cancer patients with advanced disease where loss of bladder function is no longer an issue. The goal of subarachnoid phenol is to produce a chemical dorsal rhizotomy. Sparing of motor fibers is more a function of positioning than any selective action on small myelinated or unmyelinated nerves.[117]

The results of subarachnoid phenol neurolysis for malignant neuropathic pain syndromes, such as lumbosacral plexopathy, are difficult to interpret because most patients are being treated for somatic bone pain as well as nerve injury. Temporary relief with a local anesthetic block, such as epidural bupivacaine, is not predictive of sustained relief following neurolysis.[117] Nevertheless, good relief of cancer pain (defined as complete pain relief for at least 1 month) has been reported in about 50% of patients undergoing phenol neurolysis, with complication rates in the range of 1%–14%.[118] The usual complications are bladder and bowel dysfunction and extremity weakness. Failure of this treatment modality may indicate that there is a central pain generator that has become independent of the peripheral nerve lesion.

Some patients with neuropathic pain as a result of cancer treatment (e.g., postmastectomy pain syndrome) respond to sympathetic blockade. The presence of sympathetically maintained pain may be determined with systemic alpha-adrenergic blockade with phentolamine,[119] although this has been disputed.[120,121] Patients with neuropathic pain on the basis of tumor infiltration are less likely to be candidates for sympathetic blockade because the nerve damage may include sympathetic fibers. Tumor infiltration of the brachial or lumbosacral plexus may produce a warm, dry, painful limb that is not going to respond to further attempts at sympatholysis.

Neurosurgical approaches

Central abnormalities of somatosensory processing extending as high as the thalamus and cortex explain the failure of neurolytic procedures, such as neurectomy, rhizotomy, and cordotomy, to provide long-term pain relief in neuropathic pain syndromes such as causalgia, phantom pain, and postherpetic neuralgia.[18,28,122] Neurolytic approaches are rarely considered in these conditions.

Percutaneous cervical cordotomy has a better track record for unilateral cancer pain below the shoulder level, although the results are again difficult to interpret because most reported series do not indicate the specific pain syndromes being treated. The success rate of percutaneous cordotomy (usually defined as complete pain relief until death) generally ranges from 61% to 89%, with mirror pain involving the opposite side of the body developing in 10%–15% of patients.[123] Permanent complications, which include hemiparesis and urinary retention, occur in 5%–10% of patients. A study confined to patients with Pancoast syndrome reported complete pain relief until death in 44% of 45 patients.[124] All of these patients had neurological signs of lower brachial plexus infiltration. Mirror pain developed in 31% of patients but was more amenable to control with analgesic drugs. Bilateral percutaneous cordotomy provides only a 50% success rate and the risk of complications including sleep apnea is higher.[123]

Summary

The presentation of neuropathic cancer pain poses important diagnostic and therapeutic challenges for clinicians. Although the symptoms and signs of neuropathic cancer pain are usually distinctive, the mechanisms of pain are complex because peripheral nerve injury results in central nervous system changes that play an important role in pain generation. Clinical assessment must be designed to identify the cause of the pain even if the mechanisms are not clear, so that appropriate treatment and prognosis can be provided. Management is largely empiric and involves a variety of adjuvant analgesics—none of which is likely to provide complete relief. Neuropathic pain is responsive to opioid analgesics, but this may be at the expense of side effects that impair quality of life. Percutaneous cordotomy may provide significant relief for patients with unilateral pain below the shoulder level. Management of neuropathic cancer pain is controversial because a favorable balance between analgesia and side effects is sometimes unachievable. Novel analgesics targeted at central generators of neuropathic pain hold promise for the future.

References

1. Foley KM. Pain syndromes in patients with cancer. In: Bonica JJ, Ventafridda V (eds). *Advances in Pain Research and Therapy.* Vol. 2. New York: Raven Press; 1979:59–75.
2. Moulin DE, Foley KM. A review of hospital-based pain service. In: Foley KM, Bonica JJ, Ventafridda V, eds. *Advances in Pain Research and Therapy.* Vol 16, and *Int Cong Cancer Pain.* New York: Raven Press; 1990:413–427.
3. Banning A, Sjøgren P, Henriksen H. Pain causes in 200 patients referred to a multidisciplinary cancer pain clinic. *Pain* 1991; 45:45–48.
4. Vachon MLS: Emotional problems in palliative medicine: patient, family, and professional. In: Doyle D, Hanks GWC, MacDonald N, eds. *Oxford Textbook of Palliative Medicine.* Oxford: Oxford University Press; 1993:577–605.
5. Portenoy RK. Issues in the management of neuropathic pain. In: Basbaum A, Besson J-M, eds. *Towards a New Pharmacotherapy of Pain.* New York: John Wiley & Sons; 1991:393–414.
6. Roberts WJ. A hypothesis on the physiologic basis for causalgia and related pains. *Pain* 1986; 24:297–311.
7. Asbury AK, Fields HL. Pain due to peripheral nerve damage: an hypothesis. *Neurology* 1984; 34:1587–1590.
8. Devor M. Neuropathic pain and injured nerve: peripheral mechanisms. *Br Med Bull* 1991; 47:3:619–630.
9. Wall PD, Gutnick M. Ongoing activity in peripheral nerves: the physiology and pharmacology of impulses originating from a neuroma. *Exp Neurol* 1974; 43:580–593.
10. Nordin M, Nystrom B, Wallin U, Hagbarth K-E. Ectopic sensory discharges and paresthesias in patients with disorders of peripheral nerves, dorsal roots, and dorsal columns. *Pain* 1984; 20:231–245.
11. Kajander KC, Wakisaka S, Bennett GJ. Early ectopic discharges are generated at the dorsal root ganglion in rats with a painful peripheral neuropathy. *Soc Neurosci Abstr* 1989; 15:816.
12. Devor M. The pathophysiology of damaged peripheral nerves. In: Wall PD, Melzack R, eds. *Textbook of Pain.* 2nd ed. London: Churchill-Livingstone; 1989:63–81.

13. Devor M, Rappaport ZH. Pain and the pathophysiology of damaged nerve. In: Fields H, ed. *Pain Syndromes in Neurology*. London: Butterworths; 1990:47–81.

14. Devor M, Janig W. Activation of myelinated afferents ending in a neuroma by stimulation of the sympathetic supply in the rat. *Neurosci Lett* 1981; 24:43–47.

15. Habler HJ, Janig W, Koltzenburg M. Activation of unmyelinated afferents in chronically lesioned nerves by adrenaline and excitation of sympathetic afferents in the cat. *Neurosci Lett* 1987; 82:35–40.

16. Scadding JW. Development of ongoing activity, mechanosensitivity, and adrenaline sensitivity in severed peripheral nerve axons. *Exp Neurol* 1981; 73:345–364.

17. Arnold JM, Teasell RW, MacLeod A, Brown JE, Carruthers SG. Increased venous alpha-adrenoceptor responsiveness in patients with reflex dystrophy. *Ann Intern Med* 1993; 118:619–621.

18. Bonica JJ. Causalgia and other reflex sympathetic dystrophies. In: Bonica JJ, Liebeskind JC, Albe-Fessard DG, eds. *Advances in Pain Research and Therapy*. Vol 3. New York: Raven Press; 1979:141–166.

19. Rasminsky M. Ephaptic transmission between single nerve fibers in the spinal nerve roots of dystrophic mice. *J Physiol* 1980; 305:151–169.

20. Devor M, Wall PD. Cross-excitation in dorsal root ganglia of nerve injured and intact rats. *J Neurophysiol* 1990; 64:1733–1746.

21. Nielsen WK. Pathophysiology of hemifacial spasm: I. Ephaptic transmission and ectopic excitation. *Neurology* 1984; 34:418–426.

22. Seltzer Z, Devor M. Ephaptic transmission in chronically damaged peripheral nerves. *Neurology* 1979; 29:1061–1064.

23. Yaari Y, Devor M. Phenytoin suppresses spontaneous ectopic discharge in rat sciatic nerve neuromas. *Neurosci Lett* 1985; 58:117–122.

24. Burchiel KJ. Carbemazepine inhibits spontaneous activity in experimental neuromas. *Exp Neurol* 1988; 102:249–253.

25. Swerdlow M. Anticonvulsant drugs and chronic pain. *Clin Neuropharmacol* 1984; 7:51–82.

26. Bowsher D. Neurogenic pain syndromes and their management. *Br Med Bull* 1991; 47:644–666.

27. Moulin DE, Foley KM, Ebers GC: Pain syndromes in multiple sclerosis. *Neurology* 1988; 38:12:1830–1834.

28. Tasker RR. Deafferentation. In: Wall PD, Melzack R, eds. *Textbook of Pain*. Edinburgh: Churchill Livingstone; 1984:119–132.

29. Wall PD. Neuropathic pain and injured nerve: central mechanisms. *Br Med Bull* 1991; 47:631–643.

30. Bennett GJ, Xie YK. A peripheral mononeuropathy in rat. *Pain* 1988; 33:87–108.

31. Loeser JD, Ward AA, White LE. Chronic deafferentation of human spinal cord neurons. *J Neurosurg* 1968; 29:48–50.

32. Lombard MC, Nashold BS, Pelissier T. Thalamic recordings in rats with hyperalgesia. In: Bonica JJ, Liebeskind JC, Albe-Fessard DG, eds. *Advances in Pain Research and Therapy*. Vol 3. New York: Raven Press; 1979:767–772.

33. Meyer RA, Campbell JN, Raja SN. Peripheral neural mechanisms of nociception. In: Wall PD, Melzack R, eds. *Textbook of Pain*. 3rd ed. Edinburgh: Churchill Livingstone; 1994:13–44.

34. Schott GD: Mechanisms of causalgia and related clinical conditions: the role of the central and of the sympathetic nervous system. *Brain* 1986; 109:717–738.

35. Elliott K, Foley KM. Neurologic pain syndromes in patients with cancer. In: Portenoy RK, ed. *Neurologic Clinics: Pain, Mechanisms and Syndromes.* Philadelphia: W.B. Saunders; 1989:333–360.

36. Bullit E, Tew JM, Boyd J, et al. Intracranial tumors in patients with facial pain. *J Neurosurg* 1986; 64:865–871.

37. Weinstein RE, Herec D, Friedman JH, et al. Hypotension due to glossopharyngeal neuralgia. *Arch Neurol* 1986; 43:90–92.

38. Wasserstrom WR, Glass JP, Posner JB. Diagnosis and treatment of leptomeningeal metastasis from solid tumors: experience with 90 patients. *Cancer* 1982; 49:759.

39. Byrne TN. Spinal cord compression from epidural metastases. *N Engl J Med* 1992; 327:614–619.

40. Graus F, Krol G, Foley KM. Early diagnosis of spinal epidural metastasis (SEM): correlation with clinical and radiological findings. *Proc Am Soc Clin Oncol* 1985; 4:269.

41. Cherny NI, Foley KM: Brachial plexopathy in patients with breast cancer. In: Harris JR, Lippman ME, Morrow M, Hellman S, et al., eds. *Diseases of the Breast.* Philadelphia: Lippincott-Raven, 1996: 796–808.

42. Jaeckle KA, Young DF, Foley KM. The natural history of lumbosacral plexopathy in cancer. *Neurology* 1985; 35:8–15.

43. Portenoy RK. Painful polyneuropathy. *Neurol Clin* 1989; 7:265–288.

44. Assa J. The intercostobrachial nerve in radical mastectomy. *J Surg Oncol* 1974; 6:123–126.

45. Watson CPN, Evans RJ, Watt VR. The postmastectomy pain syndrome and the effect of topical capsaicin. *Pain* 1989; 38:177–186.

46. Kanner R, Martini M, Foley KM. Nature and incidence of postthoracotomy pain. *Proc Am Soc Clin Oncol* 1982; 1:152.

47. Hollinshead WH. *Anatomy for Surgeons. Vol 1. The Head and Neck.* Philadelphia: Harper & Row; 1982:472–476.

48. Frederiks JAM. Phantom limb and phantom limb pain. In: Frederiks JAM, ed. *Handbook of Clinical Neurology. Vol 45. Clinical Neuropsychology.* New York: Elsevier Science Publishers; 1985: 395–404.

49. Kori SH, Foley KM, Posner JB. Brachial plexus lesions in patients with cancer: 100 cases. *Neurology* 1981; 31:45–50.

50. Lederman RJ, Wilbourne AJ. Brachial plexopathy: recurrent cancer or radiation? *Neurology* 1984; 34:1331–1335.

51. Harper CM, Thomas JE, Cascino TL, et al. Distinction between neoplastic and radiation-induced brachial plexopathy, with emphasis on the role of EMG. *Neurology* 1989; 39:502–506.

52. Thyagaran D, Cascino T, Harms G: Magnetic resonance imaging in brachial plexopathy of cancer. *Neurology* 1995; 45:421–427.

53. Thomas JE, Cascino TL, Earl JD, et al. Differential diagnosis between radiation and tumor plexopathy of the pelvis. *Neurology* 1985; 35:1–7.

54. Young DF, Posner JB. Nervous system toxicity of chemotherapeutic agents. In: Vinken PJ, Bruyn GW, eds. *Handbook of Clinical Neurology.* Amsterdam: North Holland Publishing Co; 1980:91–129.

55. Rusthoven JJ, Ahlgren P, Elhakim T, et al. Varicella-zoster infection in adult cancer patients: a population study. *Arch Intern Med* 1988; 148:1561–1566.

56. Watson CPN. Postherpetic neuralgia. *Neurol Clin* 1989; 7:231–248.

57. Demoragas JM, Kierland RR. The outcome of patients with herpes zoster. *Arch Dermatol* 1957; 75:193–196.

58. Ragozzino MW, Melton LJ, Kirland LT, et al. Population based study of herpes zoster and its sequelae. *Medicine* 1982; 21:310–316.

59. Gracely RH, Lynch SA, Bennett GJ. Painful neuropathy: altered central processing maintained dynamically by peripheral input. *Pain* 1992; 51:175–194.

60. Gilbert MR, Grossman SA. Incidence and nature of neurologic problems in patients with solid tumors. *Am J Med* 1986; 81:951–954.

61. Gonzales GR, Elliott KJ, Portenoy RK, Foley KM. The impact of a comprehensive evaluation in the management of cancer pain. *Pain* 1991; 47:141–144.

62. Bruera E, Ripamonti C, Brenneis C, Macmillan K, Hanson JA. A randomized double-blind crossover trial of intravenous lidocaine in the treatment of neuropathic cancer pain. *J Pain Symptom Manage* 1992; 7:138–140.

63. Elleman K, Sjogren P, Banning A, Jensen TS, Smith T, Geertson P. Trial of intravenous lidocaine on painful neuropathy in cancer patients. *Clin J Pain* 1989; 5:291–294.

64. Brose WG, Cousins MJ. Subcutaneous lidocaine for treatment of neuropathic cancer pain. *Pain* 1991; 45:145–148.

65. Eisenach JC, DuPen S, Dubois M, Miguel R, Allin D, the Epidural Clonidine Study Group. Epidural clonidine analgesia for intractable cancer pain. *Pain* 1995; 61:391–399.

66. Magni G, Arsie D, De Leo D. Antidepressants in the treatment of cancer pain: a survey in Italy. *Pain* 1987; 29:347–353.

67. Max MB, Culnane M, Schafer SC, et al. Amitriptyline relieves diabetic neuropathy pain in patients with normal or depressed mood. *Neurology* 1987; 37:589–596.

68. Max MB, Kishore-Kumar R, Schafer SC, et al. Efficacy of desipramine in painful diabetic neuropathy: a placebo controlled trial. *Pain* 1991; 45:3–9.

69. Kvinesdal B, Molin J, Froland A, Gram LF. Imipramine treatment of painful diabetic neuropathy. *JAMA* 1984; 251:1727–1730.

70. Watson CPN, Evans RJ, Reed K, Merskey H, Goldsmith I, Warsh J. Amitriptyline versus placebo in postherpetic neuralgia. *Neurology* 1982; 32:671–673.

71. Max MB, Schafer SC, Culnane M, Smoller B, Dubner R, Gracely RH. Amitriptyline but not lorazepam relieves postherpetic neuralgia. *Neurology* 1988; 38:1427–1432.

72. Watson CPN, Chipman M, Reed K, Evans RJ, Birkett N. Amitriptyline versus maprotiline in postherpetic neuralgia: a randomized, double-blind, crossover trial. *Pain* 1992; 48:29–36.

73. Kishore-Kumar R, Max MB, Schafer SC, et al. Desipramine relieves postherpetic neuralgia. *J Clin Pharm Ther* 1990; 47:305–312.

74. Max MB, Lynch SA, Muir J, et al. Effects of desipramine, amitriptyline and fluoxetine on pain in diabetic neuropathy. *N Engl J Med* 1992; 326:1250–1256.

75. Sindrup SH, Gram LF, Brøsen K, Eshøj O, Mogensen EF. The selective serotonin reuptake inhibitor paroxetine is effective in the treatment of diabetic neuropathy symptoms. *Pain* 1990; 42:135–144.

76. Rull JA, Quibrera R, Gonzalez-Millan H, et al. Symptomatic treatment of peripheral diabetic neuropathy with carbamazepine: double blind crossover trial. *Diabetologia* 1969; 5:215–220.

77. Wilton TD. Tegretol in the treatment of diabetic neuropathy. *S Afr Med J* 1974; 48:869–872.

78. Raftery H. The management of post herpetic pain using sodium valproate and amitriptyline. *J Irish Med Soc* 1979; 72:399–401.

79. Segal AZ, Rordorf G. Gabapentin as a novel treatment for postherpetic neuralgia *Neurology* 1996; 46:1175–1176

80. Fromm GH, Terence CF, Chatta AS. Baclofen in the treatment of trigeminal neuralgia. *Ann Neurol* 1984; 15:240–247.

81. Boas RA, Covino BG, Shahnarian A. Analgesic responses to IV lidocaine. *Br J Anaesth* 1982; 54:501–505.

82. Matzner O, Devor M. Sodium ion electrogenesis in nerve end neuroma. *Eur J Neurosci* 1988; (Suppl 1):173.

83. Rowbatham MC, Reisner-Keller LA, Fields HL. Both intravenous lidocaine and morphine reduce the pain of postherpetic neuralgia. *Neurology* 1991; 41:1024–1028.

84. Kastrup J, Petersen P, Dejgard A, Angelo HR, Hilsted J. Intravenous lidocaine infusion: a new treatment of chronic painful diabetic neuropathy. *Pain* 1987; 28:69–75.

85. Petersen P, Kastrup J, Zeeberg I, Boysen G. Chronic pain treatment with intravenous lidocaine. *Neurol Res* 1986; 8:189–190.

86. Backonja M, Gombar K. Response of central pain syndromes to intravenous lidocaine. *J Pain Symptom Manage* 1992; 7:172–178.

87. Galer BS, Miller KV, Rowbatham MC. Response to intravenous lidocaine infusion differs based on clinical diagnosis and site of nervous system injury. *Neurology* 1993; 43:1233–1235.

88. Dejgar A, Petersen P, Kastrup J. Mexiletine for treatment of chronic painful diabetic neuropathy. *Lancet* 1988; 1:9–11.

89. Lindstrom P, Lindblom U. Analgesic effect of tocainide in trigeminal neuralgia. *Pain* 1987; 28:45–50.

90. Max MB, Schafer SC, Culnane M, et al. Association of pain relief with drug side effects in postherpetic neuralgia: a single dose study of clonidine, codeine, ibuprofen, and placebo. *Clin Pharmacol Ther* 1988; 43:363–371.

91. Byas-Smith MG, Max MB, Muir J, Kingman A. Transdermal clonidine compared to placebo in painful diabetic neuropathy using a two-stage 'enriched enrollment' design. *Pain* 1995; 60:267–274.

92. Ghostine SY, Comair YG, Turner DM, Kassell NF, Azar CG. Phenoxybenzamine in the treatment of causalgia. *J Neurosurg* 1984; 60:1263–1268.

93. Watson CPN, Evans RJ, Watt VR. Postherpetic pain and topical capsaicin. *Pain* 1988; 33:333–340.

94. Capsaicin Study Group. Treatment of painful diabetic neuropathy with topical capsaicin. A multicenter, double-blind, vehicle-controlled study. *Arch Intern Med* 1991; 151:2225–2229.

95. Low PA, Opfer-Gehrking TL, Dyck PJ, Litchy WJ, O'Brien PC. Double-blind, placebo-controlled study of the application of capsaicin cream in chronic distal painful polyneuropathy. *Pain* 1995; 62:163–168.

96. Stow PJ, Glynn CJ, Minor B. EMLA cream in the treatment of postherpetic neuralgia. Efficacy and pharmacokinetic profile. *Pain* 1989; 39:301–306.

97. Rowbotham MC, Davies PS, Fields HL. Topical lidocaine gel relieves postherpetic neuralgia. *Ann Neurol* 1995; 37:246–253.

98. Arner S, Meyerson BA. Lack of analgesic effect of opioids on neuropathic and idiopathic forms of pain. *Pain* 1988; 33:11–23.

99. Kupers RC, Konings H, Adriaensen H, Gybels JM. Morphine differentially affects the sensory and affective pain rating in neurogenic and idiopathic forms of pain. *Pain* 1991; 47:5–12.

100. Bruera E, MacMillan D, Hanson J, MacDonald RN. The Edmonton staging system for cancer pain: preliminary report. *Pain* 1989; 37:203–210.

101. Porteney RK, Foley KM. Chronic use of opioid analgesics in nonmalignant pain: report of 38 cases. *Pain* 1986; 25:171–186.

102. Mercadante S, Maddaloni S, Roccella S, Salveggio L. Predictive factors in advanced cancer pain treated only by analgesics. *Pain* 1992; 50:151–155.

103. Galer BS, Coyle N, Pasternak GW, Portenoy RK. Individual variability in the response to different opioids: report of five cases. *Pain* 1992; 49:87–91.

104. Dellemijn PLI, Vanneste JAL. Randomised double-blind active-placebo-controlled crossover trial of intravenous fentanyl in neuropathic pain. *Lancet* 1997; 349:753–758.

105. Cherny NI, Thaler HT, Friedlander-Klar H, et al. Opioid responsiveness of cancer pain syndromes caused by neuropathic or nociceptive mechanisms: a combined analysis of controlled single-dose studies. *Neurology* 1994; 44:857–861.

105a. Gannon C. The use of methadone in the care of the dying. *Eur J Palliative Care* 1997; 4(5):152–158.

106. Jadad AR, Carroll D, Glynn CJ, Moore RA, McQuay HJ. Morphine responsiveness of chronic pain: double blind randomized crossover study with patient-controlled analgesia. *Lancet* 1992; 339:1367–1371.

107. McQuay HJ, Bullingham RES, Moore RA. Acute opiate tolerance in man. *Life Sci* 1981; 28:2513–2517.

108. Portenoy RK, Foley KM, Inturrisi CE. The nature of opioid responsiveness and its implications for neuropathic pain: new hypotheses derived from studies of opioid infusions. *Pain* 1990; 43:273–286.

109. Yamamoto T, Yaksh TL. Spinal pharmacology of thermal hyperesthesia induced by constriction injury of sciatic nerve. Excitatory amino acid antagonists. *Pain* 1992; 49:121–128.

110. Church J, Lodge D. N-Methyl-D-aspartate (NMDA) antagonism is central to the actions of ketamine and other phencyclidine receptor ligands. In: Domino EF, ed. *Status of Ketamine in Anesthesiology.* Ann Arbor, MI: NPP Books; 1990:501–519.

111. Stannard CF, Porter GE. Ketamine hydrochloride in the treatment of phantom limb pain. *Pain* 1993; 54:227–230.

112. Eide PK, Stubhaug A, Øye I, Breivik H. Continuous subcutaneous administration of the N-methyl-D-aspartate acid (NMDA) receptor antagonist ketamine in the treatment of postherpetic neuralgia. *Pain* 1995; 61:221–228.

113. Eide PK, Stubhaug A, Øye I, Breivik H. Relief of postherpetic neuralgia with the N-methyl-D-aspartate acid (NMDA) receptor antagonist ketamine: a double-blind, cross-over comparison with morphine and placebo. *Pain* 1994; 58:347–354.

114. Backonja M, Arndt G, Gombar KA, Check B, Zimmermann M. Response of chronic neuropathic pain syndromes to ketamine: a preliminary study. *Pain* 1994; 56:51–57.

115. Price DD, Mao J, Frenk H, Mayer DJ. The N-methyl-D-aspartate acid receptor antagonist dextromethorphan selectively reduces temporal summation of second pain in man. *Pain* 1994; 59:165–174.

116. McQuay HJ, Carroll D, Jadad AR, et al. Dextromethorphan for the treatment of neuropathic pain: a double-blind randomized controlled crossover trial with integral n-of-1 design. *Pain* 1994; 59:127–133.

117. Cousins MJ. Chronic pain and neurolytic neural blockade. In: Cousins MJ, Bridenbaugh PO, eds. *Neural Blockade in Clinical Anesthesia and Management of Pain.* 2nd ed. Philadelphia: J.B. Lippincott; 1988:1053–1084.

118. Swerdlow M. Subarachnoid and extradural neurolytic blocks. In: Bonica JJ, Ventafridda V, eds. *Advances in Pain Research and Therapy.* Vol 2. New York: Raven Press; 1979:325–337.

119. Raja SN, Treede R-D, David KD, Campbell JN. Systemic alpha-adrenergic blockade with phentolamine: a diagnostic test for sympathetically maintained pain. *Anesthesiology* 1991; 74:691–698.

120. Verdugo RJ, Ochoa JL. 'Sympathetically maintained pain'. I. Phentolamine block questions the concept. *Neurology* 1994; 44:1003–1010.

121. Verdugo RJ, Campero M, Ochoa JL. Phentolamine sympathetic block in painful polyneuropathies. II. Further questioning of the concept of 'sympathetically maintained pain'. *Neurology* 1994; 44:1010–1014.

122. White JC, Sweet WH. *Pain and the Neurosurgeon.* Springfield, IL: Charles C. Thomas, 1969.

123. Sanders M, Zuurmond W. Safety of unilateral and bilateral percutaneous cervical cordotomy in 80 terminally ill cancer patients. *J Clin Oncol* 1995; 13:1509–1512.

124. Ischia S, Ischia A, Luzani A, Toscano D, Steele A. Results up to death in the treatment of persistent cervico-thoracic (Pancoast) and thoracic malignant pain by unilateral percutaneous cervical cordotomy. *Pain* 1985; 21:339–355.

2

Opioids in the Treatment of Neuropathic Pain: A Systematic Review of Controlled Clinical Trials

ALEJANDRO R. JADAD

Neuropathic pain is a frequent problem and a great challenge for patients, clinicians, researchers, and policy makers. It is perhaps second only to low back pain as a cause for chronic nonmalignant pain.[1] In a recent, large case series, neuropathic pain was present in 34% of cancer patients attending a pain clinic.[2]

Despite increasing evidence that neuropathic pain involves multiple pathophysiological mechanisms,[3–5] adequate experimental methods to study, discriminate, and manipulate the putative abnormalities are lacking.[5,6] Such limitations in the understanding of the mechanisms responsible for neuropathic pain hinder any effort to classify patients in the clinical setting. In addition, clinical trials have consistently failed to identify patient characteristics that could predict the response of neuropathic pains to particular treatments.[6]

The treatment of patients with neuropathic pain can be very frustrating for both patients and clinicians. The number of treatments with proven effectiveness is so small that treatment has been described as "largely hit or miss, mostly miss."[7] Clinicians are usually forced to administer the same group of treatments regardless of the origin of the pain, hoping to find at least one that could give their patients adequate relief.[6] Nonetheless, extensive clinical experience and increasing numbers of clinical trials, suggest that some interventions can relieve neuropathic pain. Examples of the effective interventions are tricyclic antidepressants (amitriptyline in particular) and anticonvulsant drugs.[8,9]

The use of opioids for the treatment of neuropathic pain remains one of the most controversial issues in pain management.[10] During the past 10 years, clinicians and researchers have positioned themselves closer to one of two extreme positions. One position is that opioid responsiveness is a relative phenomenon and that most pains can be controlled satisfactorily by opioids, provided that adequate doses are given and adverse effects are controlled.[11] The other is that neuropathic pain is intrinsically unresponsive to opioids and that the lack of response can be predicted from the clinical characteristics of the pain; if a neuropathic pain responds to opioids, the response is attributed either to a placebo effect or to changes in the affective dimension of the pain sensation.[12,13] If the former is correct, then no patient with neuropathic pain should be denied opioid treatment on the grounds of presumptive inefficacy, especially if the pain is associated with a progressive and irreversible condition. If the latter is correct, the time and effort that would be spent on opioid therapy should be diverted to finding more effective interventions for the treatment of neuropathic pain.

This has been the background for the present systematic review of the literature, which has been designed to evaluate the evidence available on the effectiveness of opioids for the treatment of neuropathic pain. The remainder of this chapter includes information that has been created through the systematic assembly, critical appraisal, and synthesis of relevant controlled trials on opioids in neuropathic pain, prepared using strategies that limit bias and random error.[14,15]

Methods

Definition of neuropathic pain

For this review, neuropathic pain was defined as pain occurring in an area of somatosensory dysfunction which can be attributed to a discrete neurological lesion.[12,16] Trials in patients with diagnosis of reflex sympathetic dystrophy or sympathetically maintained pain were also included.

Inclusion criteria

The eligibility of a trial was determined by looking only at the methods section of the report. Each of the following criteria had to be met: (1) inclusion of patients of any age and gender with chronic neuropathic pain; (2) random and or double-blind allocation of treatments; (3) administration of an opioid agonist by any route to at least one of the treatment groups; and (4) availability of information on pain assessments.

Reports were excluded if any of the above inclusion criteria was not met or if the outcomes of patients with neuropathic pain could not be separated from those of patients with other types of pain (i.e., nociceptive or idiopathic).

Trial identification

The studies were identified using the following methods.

A systematic search of PARED 1950–1990 was conducted. PARED 1950–1990 is a database that contains references for more than 8000 analgesic trials in pain research, identified through a high-yield MEDLINE strategy and an extensive manual search of more than 40 biomedical journals.[8] The original search strategy in PARED was developed to identify any published randomized or double-blind trials in pain relief. For this review, the search of PARED from 1950 to 1990 was restricted to identify trials meeting the above inclusion criteria by using the additional medical subject heading and text words described in Table 2.1.

The search of PARED was complemented by a systematic search of MEDLINE (Ovid for UNIX, version 3.0, release 5.1) from January 1991 to September 1997 using the same strategies. The reference lists of the relevant

Table 2.1. Additional terms used to identify eligible trials in bibliographic databases

Terms	Type
Neuropathic pain	T
Neuropathy	T
Neuralgia	T, M
Nerve compression	T
Nerve compression syndrome	M
Nerve infiltration	T
Deafferentation	T
Denerv:	T
Plexus avulsion	T
Neoplasms	M
Cancer	T
Malign:	T
Paraplegia	T, M
Phantom limb	T, M
Diabetic neuropathy	T
Trigeminal neuralgia	T
Postherpetic neuralgia	T
Causalg:	T
Algodystrophy	T
Reflex sympathetic dystrophy	T, M

T = text word; M = medical subheading. The colon indicates that the term has been truncated to identify any text words with common characters (Malign, for instance, would identify articles in which malignant or malignancy appear as text words)

articles obtained were also searched for additional references, and selected publications were searched manually.

Assessment of trial validity

Once a trial was identified and included in the review, hard copies were obtained. Information on the identity and affiliation of the authors, the journal and date of publication, acknowledgements, and sources of funding was deleted from each of the copies. The masked copies were given to two observers who assessed the quality of each of the trial reports independently using a validated scale.[17] Both observers were health workers and had experience in health research methodology but were not familiar with the pain relief research literature. Any disagreement in the scores between them was solved by consensus. The scores produced on the validated scale range from 0 to 5 points and reflect the completeness of reporting of trial methodology and its likelihood of bias. Reports with scores of 2 points or less were regarded as having low quality and likely to yield biased estimates of treatment effects.[17] In addition, the observers assessed whether or not the trial reports described efforts to ensure that randomization codes had been concealed at least until treatment allocation occurred.[18]

Data extraction

The following information was extracted from each of the eligible reports: name of first author, publication year, study design, treatment arms, total number of patients with neuropathic pain, and the number of patients whose neuropathic pains responded to opioid treatment. For a response to opiods to be present, patients had to report at least moderate analgesia during the administration of the opioid. Analgesia was regarded arbitrarily as moderate or better when the magnitude of pain relief had been measured with any method and patients had reported it to be either moderate, adequate, satisfactory, acceptable, good, or complete, or if pain relief had been given more than 30% of the maximum possible score in a visual analogue scale (VAS). Alternatively, if only pain intensity measurements were available, analgesia was regarded as moderate or better when patients had reported pain intensity as none, slight, or mild, or had scored a reduction of more than 30% using a VAS or a numerical scale.

Results

Trials included and excluded

Eleven trials were identified as potentially eligible. Two trials were excluded; one because it was not double-blind or randomized[19] and the other because it included patients with neuropathic and nociceptive pains, but did not provide separate data from patients with neuropathic pain.[20]

Nine trials fulfilled all the eligibility criteria.[12,13,21–27] Morphine was the opioid used in seven trials, codeine was used in one, and fentanyl was used in one (Table 2.2). The total number of patients with neuropathic pain ranged from 6 to 53 in the individual trials; the total number of patients with neuropathic pain in the nine trials was 176. Three of the trials included a total of 29 patients with cancer,[21–23] two trials included 59 patients with postherpetic neuralgia,[24–25] one included mostly patients with reflex sympathetic dystrophy,[26] and one included patients with mixed neuropathic and deafferentation pain.[27] The route of administration was intravenous in seven trials, oral in three, epidural in one, and injection near the stellate ganglion in one (Table 2.2).

In three trials, the dose of opioid was titrated to an endpoint of adequate analgesia or unacceptable adverse effects, and in the remaining six trials the dose of opioid was fixed. The results of the three trials in which the dose of opioid was titrated suggest that neuropathic pain can respond to opioids.[21,23,27] Two of these studies used opioids as control and one used placebo and diazepam (Table 2.2). In one of the studies[23] a refined operational definition of opioid responsiveness was used and patients were allowed to self-administer morphine via a patient-controlled analgesia device. Three of six patients in that trial reported good analgesic response (more than 70% pain relief) with morphine.[23] In another trial, 13 of 18 patients reported more than 30% reduction in pain intensity following the administration of morphine orally or epidurally.[21] In this trial, patients with and without neuropathic pain achieved similar levels of analgesia, but patients with neuropathic pain required twice as much oral morphine as those without neuropathic pain (the epidural doses required by patients with and without neuropathic pain were similar). The incidence of adverse events in that trial was lower in patients receiving opioids epidurally than in those receiving opioids orally (10 events vs. 16 events, respectively. No statistical analysis was provided). In the remaining trial,[27] patients received two consecutive double-blind crossover infusions to evaluate the analgesic effects of fentanyl, diazepam, and placebo (saline solution) on neuropathic pain. Pain in 50%–65% of the patients who received fentanyl was reduced by at least 50% compared with 8% of those who received placebo and 15% of the patients who received diazepam.

Of the trials with fixed doses, four concluded that neuropathic pains are unresponsive to opioids[12,13,24,26] and two concluded that neuropathic pains can be responsive.[22,25] Two of the three studies with the highest methodological quality showed that neuropathic pains can respond to opioid treatment[22,25] (Table 2.3).

It was not appropriate to combine these results mathematically because the routes of administration of the opioid were so varied, the regimens and the indications were so different, the sample sizes were so small, and the analgesic outcomes were measured in such a heterogeneous fashion. One of the studies provided a detailed account of withdrawals and dropouts,[27] and two reports

Table 2.2. Randomized controlled trials of opioids in neuropathic pain

Trial	Patients[a]	Condition	Design	Experimental groups[b]	Control groups	Analgesic outcome[c]
Dellemijn, 1997	53	Mixed	C, R, DB	Fentanyl 5 μg/kg/h	Placebo and diazepam 0.2 mg/kg/h	PNS for pain intensity and unpleasantness
Jadad	6 (3)	Mixed	C, R, DB	Morphine high-dose IV PCA[d]	Morphine low-dose IV PCA[d]	PR (VAS)
Vainio	18	Cancer	P, R, O	Morphine 2–12 mg epidurally	Morphine 46–150 mg PO solution or slow release tablet	PID (VAS) at 24 hr and 2 weeks
Dellemijn, 1994	8	Cancer	C, R, DB	Morphine SR 60 mg/day PO	Naproxen 1500 mg/day PO	PNS
Rowbotham	19	PHN	C, R, DB	Morphine up to 0.3 mg/Kg IV	Placebo IV	PR and PI (VAS)
Max	40	PHN	C, R, DB	Codeine 120 mg single-dose PO	Placebo PO	PR, PI (CAT), MPQ
Arnér	12 (0)	Mixed	C, R, DB	Morphine 15 mg IV infusion	Placebo IV infusion	PI (VAS) and PR (CAT)
Kupers	14 (0)	Mixed	C, DB	Morphine 0.3 mg/Kg IV	Placebo IV	PNS for affective and sensory pain
Glynn	6	RSD	C, R, DB	Morphine 5 mg around the stellate ganglion	Bupivacaine 50 mg around the stellate ganglion	PR (binary scale)

[a]Total number of evaluable patients with neuropathic pain in all study arms. Numbers in parentheses indicate number of patients with diagnosis of cancer.
[b]Only includes arms in which opioids were used.
[c]Only one outcome is included in the table when the authors had chosen a primary outcome.
[d]High-dose morphine included a solution with 30 mg/ml and low-dose morphine included 10 mg/ml.

P = parallel design; C = cross-over design; R = randomized; O = open; DB = double-blind; PCA = patient-controlled analgesia; PID = pain intensity difference; PNS = pain numerical scale; CAT = categorical; MPQ = McGill Pain Questionnaire; PR = pain relief; PHN = Postherpetic neuralgia; RSD = Reflex sympathetic dystrophy.

Table 2.3. Opioids in neuropathic pain: dose titration, responsiveness and quality of evidence

Trial	Quality	Titration	Titration endpoint Analgesia	Titration endpoint Adverse effects	Results	Conclusion[a]
Dellemijn, 1997	5	Yes	Yes	Yes	S (compared with placebo and diazepam). See text.	Responsive
Jadad	4	Yes	Yes	Yes	NR $3/6$ achieved good response.[a]	Responsive
Vainio	1	Yes	Yes	Yes	NR (between groups or compared with baseline). $13/18$ PID > 30%	Responsive
Dellemijn, 1994	3	No	NA	NA	S (compared with baseline). $4/8$ had at least moderate relief.	Responsive
Rowbotham	3	No	NA	NA	S (compared with placebo). No individual data.	Responsive
Max	3	No	NA	NA	NS (compared with placebo). $8/40$ had at least moderate relief.	Unresponsive
Arnér	2	No	NA	NA	NR (compared with placebo). $1/8$ had at least moderate relief.[b]	Unresponsive
Kupers	1	No	NA	NA	S (for affective); NS (for sensory pain). No individual data.	Unresponsive
Glynn	2	No	NA	NA	NR No pain relief was reported by any of the 6 patients.	Unresponsive

NA = nonapplicable; NR = statistical significance not reported in the trial; S = statistically significant results; NS = nonsignificant.

[a] Good response was defined as pain relief more than 70 mm in a 100 mm VAS on more than one assessment time.

[b] Only 8 of 12 patients had pain assessed with a categorical scale. No individual data were available for the other 4 patients.

[c] Refers to the author's conclusions as to whether neuropathic pain can respond to the opioid treatment administered in the study.

(contributing 59 patients) described adequate concealment of the randomization codes until allocation of treatment occurred.[23,27]

Discussion

Despite an intense controversy spanning more than 10 years, only nine controlled trials appear to have been reported evaluating the responsiveness of neuropathic pain to opioids. The trials have not only had very small sample sizes, but also very heterogenous patient populations and designs.

It has been proposed that during the study of opioid responsiveness, meaningful results would be obtained if the trials are rigorously designed and conducted, if they include both pain relief and adverse effects as endpoints, and if patients are given increasing doses of opioids until either unacceptable analgesia or analgesia are achieved.[11] Most of the trials available do not fulfill those requirements. The lack of information on the strategies to allocate patients and the incomplete reporting of withdrawals and dropouts raise concerns about bias in most of the studies.[18]

The best evidence available, however, seems to support the contention that neuropathic pain can respond to opioids. This evidence derives both from trials in which the dose of opioids was titrated[21,23,27] and most of the trials with the highest methodological quality among those with titrated[23,27] or fixed doses.[22,25] The information they offer is very fragile, however, as it represents the evaluation of only 104 patients.

Given the magnitude of the problem and the weakness of the evidence available, the main challenge is to ensure that trials of sufficient size and rigorous design are conducted to establish whether or not neuropathic pain responds to opioids. In addition, research is urgently required to address some other fundamental questions that still remain unanswered. The answers to those questions would not only improve the understanding of neuropathic pain and its treatment but also contribute to improving the management of any type of pain amenable to opioid treatment.

One of the trials included in this review is perhaps the first randomized clinical trial to show that opioids given by different routes (in this case, oral and epidural) may have different adverse effects profiles. The validity of the results of this study, however, is limited by its sample size (18 patients), by the lack of information on the method of randomization used, by inadequate description of withdrawals and dropouts, and by the fact that the observations were not carried out under blind conditions.[21] If the results of this trial are confirmed by randomized, double-blind studies of adequate size, patients may obtain additional relief at a lower adverse effect penalty by a simple change in the route of administration of the opioid. Another small randomized clinical trial has shown that the adverse effect profile of opioids may be different, even when they are given by the same route.[20] If this is also confirmed, patients may get additional benefit not only by changes in the route of administration but also by changing the opioid.

Another remaining challenge is the study of patients in whom opioids fail to provide adequate analgesia, despite careful dose titration and aggressive adverse effect management. Research is needed to assess the effects of a combination of opioids with other analgesics, the use of more selective opioids, and on the measurement, and the management of adverse effects.

Given the limitations on large, randomized, clinical trials in pain research, and in palliative medicine in particular, it is unlikely that a single research group would be able to conduct studies of the size required to address reliably the fundamental research issues that remain unanswered. Meeting the challenge will depend largely on effective collaboration and communication among multiple research groups. If the magnitude of the challenge and the need for collaboration are ignored, isolated efforts are likely to continue, producing incomplete answers to complex questions and preventing us from offering our patients the strong, evidence-based care that we desire and they deserve.

References

1. McQuay HJ, Machin L, Moore RA. Chronic non-malignant pain: a population prevalence study. *Practitioner* 1985; 229:1109–1111.
2. Zech DFJ, Grond S, Lynch J, Hertel D, Lehmann KA. Validation of World Health Organization Guidelines for cancer pain relief: a 10-year prospective study. *Pain* 1995; 63:77–84.
3. Dubner R. A call for more science, not more rhetoric, regarding opioids and neuropathic pain. *Pain* 1991; 47:1–2.
4. Fields HL, Rowbotham MC. Multiple mechanisms of neuropathic pain: a clinical perspective. In: Gerbhart GF, Hammond DL, Jensen TS, eds. *Proceedings of the 7th World Congress on Pain. Progr Pain Res Manage* 1994; 2:437–454.
5. Bennett GJ. Neuropathic pain. In: Wall PD, Melzack R, eds. *Textbook of Pain.* New York: Churchill-Livingstone; 1994:201–224.
6. Max MB. Towards physiologically based treatment of patients with neuropathic pain. *Pain* 1990; 42:131–133.
7. Fields HL. Peripheral neuropathic pain: an approach to management. In: Wall PD, Melzack R, eds. *Textbook of Pain.* New York: Churchill-Livingstone; 1994;991–996.
8. Jadad AR. Meta-analysis of randomised clinical trials in pain relief. D Phil thesis. University of Oxford, 1994.
9. McQuay HJ, Carroll D, Jadad AR, Wiffen P, Moore A. Anticonvulsant drugs for the management of pain: a systematic review. *BMJ* 1995; 311:1047–1052.
10. Jadad AR. Neuropathic pain. In: *Proceedings of the Refresher Course on Cancer Pain. 7th World Congress on Pain.* Seattle: International Association of the Study of Pain, 1993: 245–249.
11. Portenoy RK, Foley KM, Inturrisi CE. The nature of opioid responsiveness and its implications for neuropathic pain: new hypotheses derived from studies of opioid infusions. *Pain* 1990; 43:273–286.

12. Arné S, Meyerson BA. Lack of analgesic effect of ipioids on neuropathic and idiopathic forms of pain. *Pain* 1988; 33:11–23.

13. Kupers RC, Konings H, Adriaensen H, Gybels JM. Morphine differentially affects the sensory and affective pain ratings in neurogenic and idiopathic forms of pain. *Pain* 1991; 47:5–12.

14. Chalmers I, Altman DG, eds. *Systematic Reviews*. London: BMJ Publishing Group, 1995.

15. Cook DJ, Sackett DL, Spitzer WO. Methodologic guidelines for systematic reviews of randomized control trials in health care from the Postdam consultation on meta-analysis. *J Clin Epidemiol* 1995; 48:167–171.

16. Portenoy RK. Issues in the management of neuropathic pain. In: Basbaum AI, Besson J-M, eds. *Towards a New Pharmacology of Pain*. New York: Wiley; 1991:393–414.

17. Jadad AR, Moore RA, Carroll D, Jenkinson C, Reynolds DJM, Gavaghan DJ, McQuay HJ. Assessing the quality of randomized clinical trials: is blinding necessary? *Controlled Clin Trials* 1996;17:1–12.

18. Schulz KF, Chalmers I, Hayes RJ, Altman DG. Empirical evidence of bias: dimensions of methodological quality associated with estimates of treatment effects in controlled trials. *JAMA* 1995;273:408–412.

19. Tasker RR, Tsuda T, Hawrylsyshyn P. Clinical neurophysiological investigation of deafferentation pain. In: Bonica JJ, Lindblom U, Iggo A, eds. *Proceedings of the 3rd World Congress on Pain. Advances Pain Research and Therapy*. Vol 5. New York: Raven Press; 1983:713–718.

20. Kalso E, Vainio A. Morphine and oxycodone hydrochloride in the management of cancer pain. *Clin Pharmacol Ther* 1990;47:639–646.

21. Vainio A, Tigerstedt I. Opioid treatment for radiating cancer pain: oral administration vs. epidural techniques. *Acta Anaesthesiol Scand* 1988; 32:179–185.

22. Dellemijn PLI, Verbiest HBC, van Vliet JJ, Roos PJ, Vecht CJ. Medical therapy of malignant nerve pain: a randomised double-blind explanatory trial with naproxen versus slow-release morphine. *Eur J Cancer* 1994; 30A:1244–1250.

23. Jadad AR, Carroll D, Glynn CJ, Moore RA, McQuay HJ. Morphine responsiveness of chronic pain: double-blind randomised crossover study with patient-controlled analgesia. *Lancet* 1992; 339:1367–1371.

24. Max MB, Schafer SC, Culnane M, Dubner R, Gracely RH. Association of pain relief with drug side effects in postherpetic neuralgia: a single-dose study of clonidine, codeine, ibuprofen, and placebo. *Clin Pharmacol Ther* 1988; 43:363–371.

25. Rowbotham MC, Reisner-Keller LA, Fields HL. Both intravenous lidocaine and morphine reduce the pain of postherpetic neuralgia. *Neurology* 1991; 41:1024–1028.

26. Glynn CJ, Casale R. Morphine injected around the stellate ganglion does not modulate the sympathetic nervous system nor does it provide pain relief. *Pain* 1993; 53:33–37.

27. Dellemijn PLI, Vanneste JAL. Randomised double-blind active-placebo-controlled crossover trial of intravenous fentanyl in neuropathic pain. *Lancet* 1997; 349:753–58.

3

Adjuvant Drugs for
Neuropathic Cancer Pain

DAVID J. HEWITT AND RUSSELL K. PORTENOY

Neuropathic pain refers to any syndrome in which pain is imputed to have a pathophysiology related to aberrant somatosensory processing in the peripheral or central nervous systems. Neuropathic pain can result from injury to nervous tissue at any point along afferent pathways, including peripheral nerves, nerve plexus, nerve root, spinal cord, brainstem, thalamus, or cortex. Cancer can produce neuropathic pain through direct compression or invasion of neural structures by tumor or by injury caused by antineoplastic therapies. These therapies include neurotoxic drugs (e.g., vinca alkaloids, cis-platinum, and paclitaxel), radiation, and surgery.

Adjuvant analgesics are drugs that have primary indications other than pain, but are analgesic in some painful conditions (Table 3.1). Some of these drugs are used in populations with nonmalignant pain syndromes as multipurpose, nonspecific analgesics; others are used for more specific indications. In patients with cancer pain, these drugs are typically combined with an opioid to enhance pain relief or reduce the analgesic dose of an opioid to limit side effects. Their largest role in this population is in the treatment of neuropathic pain that has been poorly responsive to opioids. Adjuvant analgesics should also be considered when a comorbid condition may respond to the nonanalgesic effect of the drug. For example, antidepressants are used when pain is accompanied by depression and tricyclic antidepressants might be particularly useful when pain and depression are accompanied by insomnia.

General Principles

Several principles guide the appropriate use of all analgesic medications, including the adjuvant analgesics. Effective therapy requires a comprehensive assess-

Table 3.1. Major classes of adjuvant analgesics for neuropathic pain

Antidepressants
Anticonvulsants
GABA agonists
Benzodiazepines
Local anesthetics
Alpha-2 adrenergic agonists
Sympatholytics
Corticosteroids
N-methyl-D-aspartate receptor blockers
Neuroleptics

ment, which includes a careful history and physical examination, review of medical records, pertinent laboratory work, and imaging studies. This assessment should yield information about important characteristics of the pain, such as temporal features, location, severity, and quality; etiology and its relationship to the underlying disease process; and impact of pain and other physical and psychosocial concerns on the patient's quality of life and functional ability. The stage of disease and the goals of therapy must be clearly understood.

In the palliative care setting, adjuvant analgesics should be administered after the opioid regimen has been optimized. This guideline reflects the observation that adjuvant analgesics are generally less reliable analgesics than the opioids. For example, in contrast to survey data that demonstrate adequate analgesia within days for 70%–90% of cancer patients treated with opioids, treatment with tricyclic antidepressants (TCAs) may require weeks to obtain >50% relief for 50%–75% of patients with neuropathic pain.[1,2]

The addition of an adjuvant analgesic may alter the metabolism of other drugs or produce pharmacodynamic interactions among coadministered drugs. Common interactions should be anticipated. TCAs, for example, can directly increase the plasma morphine concentration[3] or produce additive sedative effects independent of changes in drug concentration.

Adjuvant Analgesic Classes and Drugs

The proper selection and use of an adjuvant analgesic requires a familiarity with the drug's approved indications, unapproved indications accepted in medical practice, likely side effects and potential serious adverse effects, specific dosing guidelines for pain, important drug interactions, usual time–action relationship, and pharmacokinetics. The heterogeneity of symptoms described by patients with neuropathic pain suggests the existence of mechanisms that could respond differently to drugs with varying modes of action.

Antidepressant drugs

Compelling evidence has shown that tricyclic antidepressants are analgesic in a variety of chronic pain syndromes.[3-7] In the treatment of neuropathic pains, anecdotal observation suggests that antidepressants are more useful for pains characterized by continuous dysesthesias (Table 3.2) than pains described as lancinating, notwithstanding data from controlled clinical trials that suggest the efficacy of amitriptyline and desipramine for both types.[1,2]

The analgesic effects of tertiary amine tricyclic antidepressants have been well characterized in both controlled and uncontrolled studies. Amitriptyline has been shown to be effective in diverse types of chronic pain, including many neuropathic pains such as postherpetic neuralgia,[8,9] painful polyneuropathies (e.g., diabetic polyneuropathy),[1,10,11] central pain,[12] and neuropathic pain associated with cancer or its treatment.[13] Other TCAs have similar actions.[2,10,11,14–19]

Some of the "newer" antidepressants have also been studied, with more equivocal results. Maprotiline[9,20] and trazodone[13] may be analgesic, but the evidence is less certain than that acquired in studies of the tricyclic compounds.

The selective serotonin reuptake inhibitors (SSRIs) paroxetine[21] and citalopram[22] have demonstrated some efficacy in the treatment of painful diabetic neuropathy. Although SSRIs in general appear to be weaker analgesics than the

Table 3.2. Selective adjuvant analgesics for neuropathic pain

Continuous dysesthesias	
First-line	
Tricyclic antidepressants	Amitriptyline, doxepin, imipramine, clomipramine, desipramine, nortriptyline
"Newer" antidepressants	Paroxetine, trazodone, maprotiline
Oral local anesthetics	Mexiletine, tocainide, flecainide
Gabapentin	
Second-line	
Alpha-2 adrenergic agonists	Clonidine
Anticonvulsants	Carbamazepine, phenytoin, valproate, clonazepam, lamotrigine
Topical agents	Capsaicin, local anesthetics
Neuroleptics	Methotrimeprazine, prochlorperazine, haloperidol
NMDA receptor antagonists	Ketamine, dextromethorphan
Calcitonin	
Baclofen	

tricyclics,[21] they might be considered for the treatment of neuropathic pain because of a relatively good side effect profile.[23,24]

Monamine oxidase inhibitors, including phenelzine and tranylcypromine, have demonstrated efficacy in a number of pain syndromes.[25] Although these drugs could be used to treat neuropathic pain, they are rarely used because of the risk of serious toxic reactions induced by sympathomimetic compounds in the diet or coadministered drugs. Alprazolam, a benzodiazepine with antidepressant effects, may have some efficacy in the treatment of neuropathic pain due to cancer.[26]

Mechanism of action

The mechanisms responsible for antidepressant analgesia are not dependent on a primary antidepressant effect. The effective analgesic dose is often lower than the antidepressant dose and the onset of action typically occurs much sooner.[8,12,14–21] The findings that nondepressed patients can experience analgesia and depressed patients can report pain relief without a change in mood[1,11,21] further support the dissociation between these analgesic and antidepressant effects.

Antidepressants block the reuptake of monoamines and presumably increase activity in endogenous monoamine-mediated pain-modulating pathways. Well-characterized pathways descend from the brainstem and use serotonin or norepinephrine as neurotransmitters.[27,28] Clinical studies support the concept that an increase in neurotransmitter availability in either the serotonergic or norepinephrine pathways can produce analgesia. The TCAs are not highly selective and also interact with other types of receptors that may be important in the development of analgesia, including acetylcholine and histamine receptors.[29–32]

Adverse effects

Although serious adverse side effects are uncommon at the TCA doses usually administered for pain, pharmocokinetic variability may lead to relatively high plasma concentrations in some patients, despite low doses. Less serious side effects are frequent and may limit the usefulness of some of these drugs. Patients on multiple other drugs or those with major organ dysfunction are at particular risk. To minimize the risk of adverse side effects, initial doses should be low and dose escalation gradual.

The most serious complication of TCAs, cardiotoxicity, is very uncommon. Patients with serious heart disease, including conduction disorders, arrhythmia or failure, should not be selected for treatment. A monoamine oxidase inhibitor or an SSRI with demonstrated efficacy for analgesia should be considered instead.

Orthostatic hypotension is a more common side effect of the tricyclic antidepressants.[33] Nortriptyline is the least hypotensive TCA, and should be considered in patients who develop this symptom.[34]

Somnolence and mental clouding are common side effects of TCAs, but acute delirium is rare. The risk of these side effects is increased in persons who have pre-existing encephalopathy. Desipramine is the TCA least likely to cause somnolence and confusion.

The anticholinergic effects of the tricyclic antidepressants can produce gastrointestinal disturbances, dry mouth, blurred vision, urinary retention, and other problems. These effects are more likely to occur with the tertiary amine than the secondary amine compounds. Among the TCAs, they are least likely to occur with desipramine. Serious anticholinergic side effects (precipitation of acute angle closure glaucoma, obstipation, and urinary retention) necessitate discontinuation of the drug. Men should be asked about the symptoms of prostatism prior to therapy and a compound with less anticholinergic effect should be used in those who are symptomatic.

The SSRIs are much better tolerated than the TCAs. They lack anticholinergic effects and are less sedating. Instead, SSRIs may produce a sense of activation, with distressing anxiety, tremulousness, akithesia, or insomnia.[23,35]

Clinical guidelines

Unless relatively contraindicated, a trial of amitriptyline is usually considered first when an antidepressant is selected for the treatment of neuropathic pain. Amitriptyline may be preferred because of the numerous trials that support its efficacy as an analgesic. If treatment with amitriptyline has failed or is contraindicated because of possible side effects, an alternative TCA should be considered (Table 3.3). Desipramine has a more favorable side effect profile, as well as evidence for analgesic efficacy,[2,11] and it is a reasonable choice. Intraindividual variability in the analgesic response to different antidepressants suggests the utility of sequential trials if needed.

Table 3.3. Selective adjuvant analgesics for neuropathic pain

Lancinating or paroxysmal dysesthesias	
First-line	
Anticonvulsants	Carbamazepine, phenytoin, valproate, clonazepam, gabapentin, lamotrigine
Baclofen	
Second-line	
Oral local anesthetics	Mexiletine, tocainide, flecainide
Tricyclic antidepressants	Amitriptyline, doxepin, imipramine, clomipramine, desipramine, nortriptyline
"Newer" antidepressants	Paroxetine, trazodone, maprotiline
Neuroleptics	Pimozide
Alpha-2 adrenergic agonists	Clonidine
Topical agents	Capsaicin, local anesthetics
NMDA receptor antagonists	Dextromethorphan, ketamine
Calcitonin	

The starting dose for TCAs is 10 mg in the elderly or medically ill and 25 mg in younger patients. The dose should be increased every few days by increments equal to the starting dose. The effective dose for both desipramine and amitriptyline is usually between 50 and 150 mg per day, although some patients may benefit from doses above or below this range. Based on clinical experience, dose escalation should continue until analgesia ensues, side effects preclude higher doses, or the dose (and plasma concentration) are in the antidepressant range. Analgesia is usually obtained within 1 week after achieving an effective dosing level. The patient must be informed about this potentially long trial period, during which the dose is escalated and side effects may occur in the absence of analgesia.

Anticonvulsant drugs

Anticonvulsant drugs are now widely accepted for the management of lancinating (stabbing) neuropathic pain and paroxysmal neuropathic pains (acute in onset, peak very rapidly, and remit after a brief period).[36] Anecdotally, continuous dysesthesias appear to respond occasionally, but there is little evidence of benefit comparable to that attained in lancinating dysesthesias. The exception to this observation is gabapentin, a newer anticonvulsant that has rapidly gained acceptance as an analgesic for all types of neuropathic pain because of very favorable anecdotal experience.

Numerous controlled and uncontrolled trials support the use of carbamazepine and phenytoin in the treatment of lancinating pain, regardless of the specific pathology. These drugs have been studied in trigeminal neuralgia, postherpetic neuralgia, painful diabetic neuropathy, paroxysmal pain in multiple sclerosis, postsympathectomy pain, stabbing pain following laminectomy, lancinating pain due to cancer, and post-traumatic mononeuropathy.[37–44]

Case reports and uncontrolled surveys have suggested that clonazepam and valproic acid may also be useful in lancinating pain. Clonazepam was reported to be effective in patients with trigeminal neuralgia[43] and paroxysmal postlaminectomy pain;[44] valproate was beneficial for patients with trigeminal neuralgia and postherpetic neuralgia.[45,46]

"Newer" anticonvulsants may also be effective for neuropathic pain. As noted, gabapentin is now widely used for all types of neuropathic pain; this acceptance is based on favorable clinical experience[47] and a relatively good safety profile. Lamotrigine has been effective in reducing hyperalgesia in an animal model of neuropathic pain[48] and, on this basis, has also been used anecdotally in humans. Felbamate demonstrated some promise as an analgesic for neuropathic pain,[49] but the potential for lethal aplastic anemia limits its utility.

Mechanism of action
Although the specific mechanisms by which analgesia is produced by anticonvulsant drugs are not known, they likely relate to their anticonvulsant mechanisms.

Most of these drugs reduce neuronal hyperexcitability and suppress paroxysmal discharges and their spread from their site of origin,[50] an effect that could suppress aberrant electrical activity linked to neuropathic pain.[51-56] The mechanism of gabapentin is not known.

Adverse effects

The common side effects of carbamazepine (sedation, dizziness, nausea, and unsteadiness) can be minimized by low initial doses and gradual dose titration. More serious side effects include leukopenia and/or thrombocytopenia (2% of patients); aplastic anemia is even more rare. A complete blood count should be obtained prior to the start of therapy, after several weeks, then every 3–4 months thereafter. A leukocyte count below 4000 is a contraindication to treatment and a decline to less than 3000 (or an absolute neutrophil count of less than 1500) should lead to the discontinuation of the drug. Hepatic damage, hyponatremia due to inappropriate secretion of antidiuretic hormone, and congestive heart failure are rare adverse effects of carbamazepine. Monitoring requires baseline measurement of liver and renal function and electrolytes prior to the initiation of therapy.

The common side effects of phenytoin—sedation, mental clouding, unsteadiness, and diplopia—are dose dependent and usually occur at plasma concentrations above the therapeutic range for seizure control. Some patients experience toxicity at lower concentrations. Ataxia, progressive encephalopathy, and even seizures may occur at toxic levels. The most serious adverse effects, hepatotoxicity and exfoliative dermatitis, are idiosyncratic. The appearance of a maculopapular rash mandates discontinuation of the drug. A rare permanent cerebellar degeneration has been reported in patients with chronic phenytoin intoxication.

The side effects of valproate include sedation, nausea, tremor, and sometimes increased appetite. Dose-dependent side effects are reduced by the use of low initial doses and gradual dose titration. Gastrointestinal disturbances are minimized with use of an enteric-coated tablet. Rare idiosyncratic reactions include hepatotoxicity, encephalopathy, dermatitis, alopecia, and a hyperammonemia syndrome that can occur without abnormalities in other liver function tests.

Drowsiness is the most common and troubling side effect of clonazepam. Tachyphylaxis to this effect often develops within weeks after dosing has begun. At higher doses, patients may develop ataxia. Very rare idiosyncratic reactions include dermatitis, hepatotoxicity and hematologic effects. Like other benzodiazepines, a withdrawal syndrome may occur with abrupt discontinuation of relatively high doses.

Gabapentin and lamotrigine are associated with favorable side effect profiles.[57-59] Experience with these drugs is still limited and the spectrum of toxicities may still expand.

Clinical guidelines

Gabapentin is now commonly administered as an early trial for any type of neuropathic pain. The other anticonvulsants are considered first-line adjuvant analgesics for episodic paroxysmal and lancinating neuropathic pain (Table 3.3). Studies comparing the relative efficacy of the anticonvulsants have not been performed and variability in the response to these drugs is great. Clinical experience supports the use of sequential trials in patients with refractory pain.

After gabapentin, carbamazepine is usually the first anticonvulsant considered for the management of neuropathic pain, but it may have limited value in the cancer population because of the potential for leukopenia and thrombocytopenia. When chronic pain is associated with anxiety or insomnia, an early trial of clonazepam may be warranted.

The dosing guidelines used in the management of pain are extrapolated from the treatment of seizures. Most of these drugs are started at low initial doses followed by a gradual escalation to favorable effects, or side effects or plasma concentrations at the upper limit of the therapeutic range for the treatment of seizures. Phenytoin can be initiated at the expected therapeutic dose (e.g., 300 mg per day), or a loading dose can be given first (500 mg twice, separated by hours).

GABA$_B$ agonists

Baclofen is another important drug for the treatment of lancinating pain. An agonist at the GABA$_B$ receptor, it is primarily used for the treatment of spasticity. Controlled trials have conclusively demonstrated efficacy in trigeminal neuralgia[60] and, on this basis, it has been used in other neuropathic pains characterized by an episodic lancinating or paroxysmal phenomenology.

The starting dose of baclofen is 5 mg two to three times per day. The dose is gradually escalated to the range of 30–90 mg per day and sometimes higher. Dose escalation should continue until pain is relieved or limiting side effects occur. Dizziness, somnolence, and gastrointestinal distress are the common side effects and are minimized by low starting doses and gradual dose escalation. Doses should always be tapered before discontinuation of this drug because there is the potential for a serious withdrawal syndrome (delirium and seizures) with abrupt discontinuation following prolonged use.[61]

Corticosteroids

Corticosteroids have been used to treat reflex sympathetic dystrophy[62] and diverse types of neuropathic cancer pain resulting from infiltration or compression of neural structures (e.g., nerve, plexus, root, or spinal cord). Patients administered high doses of dexamethasone (96 mg per day for 2 weeks) for malignant spinal cord compression observed pain relief within hours of the initial dose.[63] Another study confirmed the analgesic effect of dexamethasone in spinal cord compression but did not identify a difference between high (100 mg) and low (10 mg) initial dose.[64] Analgesic differences among the corticosteroids have not been discerned, and there are no data by which to judge dose–response relationships, relative potency, and long-term efficacy.

Mechanism of action

The mechanism of action of corticosteroids in producing analgesia is unknown. Reduction of peritumoral edema, direct cytolytic effect on neoplasm, and a reduction in tissue concentrations of inflammatory mediators resulting in a decrease in the activation of nociceptors may all play some role.

Adverse effects

Although generally well tolerated in the palliative care setting, chronic administration of corticosteroids can lead to cushingoid habitus, changes in integument, weight gain, hypertension, osteoporosis, myopathy, increased risk of infection, and gastrointestinal perforation. Withdrawal of steroids can cause a flare in symptoms, or malaise, headache, mood disturbances, disturbances associated with hypocortisolism, or steroid "pseudorheumatism."[65]

Clinical guidelines

Dexamethasone has relatively low mineralocorticoid effects, and it may be preferred on this basis. Prednisone and methylprednisolone are also frequently used. A high-dose regimen with dexamethasone starts with a single dose of 100 mg followed by 96 mg per day in divided doses and can be used in episodes of severe acute pain, e.g., malignant plexopathy[66] or pain associated with epidural cord compression.[63] A lower-dose regimen uses 1–2 mg of dexamethasone once or twice daily and may be helpful for a variety of less severe chronic pain syndromes, especially when pain is associated with other target symptoms such as anorexia or malaise.

Alpha-2 adrenergic agonists

Clonidine, tizanidine, medetomidine, and dexmedetomidine have all demonstrated antinociceptive effects in a variety of experimental and clinical models, including neuropathic pain.[67,68] Systemic administration of clonidine via the oral or transdermal route or via intraspinal infusions can be effective in pain syndromes that are relatively less opioid-responsive, including neuropathic cancer-related pain.[67–70]

Mechanism of action

The mechanism of action of the alpha-adrenergic agonists is probably complex.[71] Interactions with alpha-2 receptors in the spinal cord[72,73] or brainstem[74] activate endogenous systems that reduce nociceptive input to the central nervous system thought to be involved in the processing of noxious stimuli.[71] Through a reduction in sympathetic tone, these drugs may also interfere with mechanisms that perpetuate sympathetically maintained pain.

Adverse effects
Important side effects of clonidine include somnolence, orthostatic hypotension, and dry mouth. A controlled trial of epidural clonidine in cancer patients demonstrated that the drug produced sustained hypotensive effects in almost one-half of patients.[67] Consequently, clonidine should be limited to patients with opioid-refractory pain of neuropathic origin who are hemodynamically stable and not predisposed to serious hypotension. Given the limited experience in patients with cancer pain, it is generally used after other adjuvants, (e.g., antidepressants, oral local anesthetics, and anticonvulsants) have failed.

Clinical guidelines
Oral and transdermal clonidine administration begin with low doses to avoid adverse side effects (0.1 mg orally per day). If lower doses are desired, the transdermal system can be cut into pieces without change in the delivery properties. Doses should be escalated slowly with careful attention to possible side effects. Anecdotal experience suggests that patients can benefit from relatively high doses and it is reasonable to continue dose escalation until dose-limiting toxicity is encountered.

Neuroleptics

Some neuroleptic drugs have shown antinociceptive effects in animal models[75] and analgesia in diverse pain syndromes.[76–80] The phenothiazine methotrimeprazine is analgesic in cancer pain, including neuropathic pain.[77] Pimozide has been shown to be effective in trigeminal neuralgia.[80] Unfortunately, side effects, including physical and mental slowing, tremor, and Parkinsonism, limit the value of the latter drug. Other studies suggest that neuroleptics may be coanalgesic when used in combination with other psychotropic or opioid analgesics.[81–83] An opioid-sparing effect has been described in several,[81,84] but not all,[85] surveys of patients with cancer pain.

Mechanism of action
The mechanism of action of neuroleptics may involve dopaminergic blockade within endogenous pain-modulating systems. The D_2 receptor subtype may mediate this action. Metoclopramide (a D_2 and $5HT_3$ receptor agonist) is also analgesic in humans.[86,87]

Adverse effects
Sedation, orthostatic dizziness, and anticholinergic effects are common side effects of neuroleptics. Phenothiazines are more likely to produce these effects than the butyrophenones (e.g., haloperidol). These effects can be minimized with low initial doses and continuous dose escalation.

Extrapyramidal side effects are perhaps the greatest concern in the clinical use of neuroleptic drugs. These effects vary with the drug, duration of therapy, and dose. Fluphenazine and haloperidol are relatively more likely to produce these side effects. Acute dystonic reactions (e.g., trismus, torticollis, and even opisthotonus), akithisia, and Parkinsonism may occur early in treatment. Management involves discontinuation of the neuroleptic and administration of an anticholinergic drug such as benztropine if the reaction is severe. A rare and serious condition, neuroleptic malignant syndrome, is characterized by fever, rigidity, autonomic instability, and encephalopathy. Successful management requires prompt diagnosis, discontinuation of the neuroleptic, supportive measures, and in some cases, treatment with a dopamine agonist and muscle relaxant. Tardive syndromes, including dyskinesias and dystonias, occur more commonly in the elderly and women. Treatment requires tapering and discontinuation of the drug.

Clinical guidelines

Although not specific for neuropathic pain, methotrimeprazine has been useful in the treatment of pain in patients with advanced cancer, particularly bedridden patients who are experiencing pain associated with anxiety, restlessness, or nausea. Methotrimeprazine may be given by continuous subcutaneous administration,[88] subcutaneous bolus injection, or brief intravenous infusion (20–30 min). Dosing begins with 5 mg every 6 hours, or a comparable dose delivered by infusion, which is gradually increased as needed. Trials of other neuroleptics are usually considered only after numerous other adjuvant analgesics have failed.

Local anesthetics

The oral and parenteral local anesthetics are an important class of adjuvant analgesics for the treatment of neuropathic pain. A brief intravenous infusion of lidocaine or procaine can relieve a variety of chronic pains, including neuropathic pain. Well-controlled studies have established the efficacy of this technique in postherpetic neuralgia[89] and painful diabetic neuropathy[90] but have not confirmed benefit in neuropathic cancer pain.[91,92] Anecdotal experience, however, includes the long-term use of subcutaneous lidocaine for the relief of refractory neuropathic pain in cancer patients.[93] There have been no controlled comparisons of the analgesic effects produced by brief intravenous infusion of the various parenteral local anesthetics.

The advent of oral local anesthetic formulations has facilitated long-term use. Controlled trials have demonstrated that tocainide is effective for trigeminal neuralgia[94] and mexiletine lessens the pain of diabetic neuropathy.[95] A survey of cancer patients with pain due to infiltration of nerve[96] suggested that flecainide might be an effective drug.

Mechanism of action

When applied to peripheral nerves, local anesthetics block sodium channels and create a nondepolarizing conduction block of the action potential.[97] This effect does not explain the analgesia produced by systemic administration.[98] Experimental models suggest that local anesthetics suppress the activity of dorsal horn neurons that are activated by C fiber input,[99] as well as the spontaneous firing of neurons and dorsal root ganglion cells.[100,101] Hence, systemic administration probably produces analgesic effects by suppression of aberrant electrical activity or hypersensitivity in neural structures involved in the pathogenesis of neuropathic pain, such as sensitized central neurons and neuroma.

Adverse effects

Local anesthetics produce dose-dependent adverse effects that involve the central nervous system and the cardiovascular system. The former include dizziness, tremor, perioral numbness, and other paresthesias at lower dosages, followed by progressive encephalopathy and seizures at higher plasma concentrations.[97] Cardiac disorders include cardiac conduction disturbances, with prolongation of the PR interval and QRS duration, followed by bradycardia and other arrythmias at higher plasma levels. Myocardial depression[97] may also occur and can be severe enough to cause pump failure. Both the central nervous system and cardiovascular side effects are correlated with the potency of the local anesthetic at the sodium channel.

Systemically administered local anesthetic drugs must be used cautiously in patients with pre-existing heart disease. Typically, they are not administered to patients with cardiac rhythm disturbances, those receiving antiarrhythmic drugs, and those who have cardiac insufficiency. Although mexiletine, tocainide, and flecainide have all been used for long-term systemic treatment, flecainide may be less preferred because of an association with sudden death during a trial of therapy for patients immediately post-myocardial infarction.[102] The generalizability of the latter finding is uncertain, but the potential for increased risk with flecainide is also supported by its relatively greater potency and negative inotropic effects.

Side effects associated with tocainide include nausea, dizziness, lightheadedness, tremors, palpitations, vomiting, and paresthesias. Rare serious side effects include interstitial pneumonitis, severe encephalopathy, blood dyscrasia, hepatitis, and dermatologic reactions. Mexiletine may produce nausea and vomiting, tremor, dizziness, unsteadiness, and paresthesias, which are frequently intolerable and lead to the discontinuation of the drug.[103,104] Liver damage and blood dyscrasias may occur but are very rare.

Clinical guidelines

Systemic local anesthetic therapy has been used in the long-term management of opioid-refractory neuropathic pain of both peripheral and central origin.[105] Both continuous dysesthesias and lancinating pains can respond favorably.[94,95] Based on clinical experience, these drugs are usually considered after several of the more commonly used drugs (e.g., antidepressants and anticonvulsants) have failed.

Some patients experience immediate analgesia with brief intravenous local anesthetic infusions, which may continue for some period. The use of an intravenous infusion to predict the response to oral local anesthetic treatment has not been adequately studied for pain and cannot be advocated for this purpose. A trial of a brief local anesthetic infusion may be useful in patients with severe neuropathic pain that has not responded promptly to an opioid and requires immediate relief.

Mexiletine has been the preferred oral local anesthetic in the United States. Low initial doses and slow dose titration may reduce the likelihood of adverse effects. Mexiletine dosing should start at 150 mg once or twice a day with food. The dose is increased slowly every few days, to a usual maximum dose of 300 mg three times a day. Plasma drug concentration can be monitored to guide further dose escalation. Lidocaine infusions have been administered at varying doses, typically within a range of 2–5 mg/kg infused over 20–30 minutes, with the lower range indicated for medically frail patients. Sequential infusions allow exploration of varied doses and may be the safest method of parenteral local anesthetic administration in the medically ill.

N-Methyl-D-Aspartate (NMDA) receptor antagonists

N-methyl-D-aspartate antagonists are undergoing investigation as potential multipurpose analgesics. There is great interest in their use for the treatment of neuropathic pain.

Excitatory amino acids are now recognized as integral to the central processing of pain-related information. Primary afferent neurons release glutamate and aspartate in response to noxious stimuli. These transmitters bind to the NMDA receptor and produce changes in the central nervous system that may, in pathologic conditions, underlie chronic pain. For example, the NMDA receptor is involved in the sensitization of central neurons following injury and in the development of the "wind-up" phenomenon, a change in the response of central neurons that has been associated with neuropathic pain.[106,107] Changes mediated by the NMDA receptor also modulate opioid mechanisms, including tolerance.

Two NMDA receptor antagonists are currently available in the United States. Both the antitussive dextromethorphan and the general anesthetic ketamine have been shown to produce analgesic effects in experimental and clinical pain.[108–113]

Clinical guidelines

Current data are sufficient to justify a trial of dextromethorphan or ketamine in patients with neuropathic pain that has been refractory to other analgesics. Dextromethorphan has a good safety profile, but ketamine is associated with psychotomimetic effects and should only be used by experienced practitioners. Delirium, severe nightmares, hallucinosis, and dysphoria can be daunting side effects especially in the medically ill and frail. The risk of serious toxicity at the subanesthetic ketamine doses used for neuropathic pain is low, however, and a trial may be justified when pain has been intractable to many routine approaches.

Based on clinical experience, a trial of dextromethorphan may be initiated using a proprietary cough suppressant lacking alcohol and other active drugs. A starting dose of 45–60 mg daily can be gradually increased until favorable effects occur, side effects supervene, or a maximal dose of 1 gm is achieved.

A ketamine trial can be initiated at low doses (0.1–0.15 mg/kg) in a brief infusion or 0.1–0.15 mg/kg/hour continuous infusion. The dose is gradually escalated with close monitoring of pain and side effects. Patients have been maintained on long-term therapy using continuous subcutaneous infusion or repeated subcutaneous injections of ketamine.

Calcitonin

Calcitonin may have several pain-related indications in the cancer population. Controlled trials that have demonstrated efficacy for this drug in populations with sympathetically maintained pain[114] and acute phantom limb pain[115] justify an empirical trial in refractory neuropathic pain of diverse types. The mechanisms that underlie the analgesic effects are unknown.

Clinical experience suggests that a low initial dose (e.g., 25 IU per day) reduces the incidence of nausea, the major side effect. This side effect is also less likely if an intranasal formulation is used. If parenterally administered, skin testing with 1 IU prior to the start of therapy is recommended because of a small risk of serious hypersensitivity reactions. Doses can be increased gradually to 100–200 IU/day; dose escalation may identify a lower effective dose. Initially, doses are given daily, but the frequency can be decreased to every other day or less in some cases.

Drugs for sympathetically maintained pain

Sympathetically maintained pain may occur in patients with cancer and is characterized by dysesthesias presumed to be sustained through efferent activity in the sympathetic nervous system. The syndromes of reflex sympathetic dystrophy and causalgia are believed to have a high likelihood of being sympathetically maintained pain states. Focal autonomic dysregulation, focal motor disturbances, or trophic changes are characteristic of these pain syndromes. Sympathetic block serves as both an important diagnostic test and as a first line of treatment.

Any of the aforementioned drugs may be used in the treatment of sympathetically maintained pain. Therapy also may focus on trials of drugs that influence sympathetic function or have been specifically studied in this condition, such as clonidine, phenoxybenzamine, prazosin, calcium channel blockers, or phentolamine infusion.[116–119] Phentolamine infusion has also been used as a diagnostic tool for sympathetically maintained pain.[116]

Topical analgesics

Topical analgesics, such as capsaicin, formulations containing aspirin or a nonsteroidal anti-inflammatory drug, local anesthetic preparations,[120] and prostaglandin E1 ointment,[121] have been used for continuous neuropathic pain with a predominating peripheral mechanism. Topical therapy may be useful in medically ill patients who are often predisposed to side effects from systemically administered drugs.

Topical capsaicin has been used to treat neuropathic pain, such as postherpetic neuralgia, postmastectomy pain, painful diabetic neuropathy, and pain due to osteoarthritis. Capsaicin presumably lessens pain by reducing the concentration of small peptides (including substance P) in primary afferent neurons, which activate nociceptive systems in the dorsal horn of the spinal cord.[122] Capsaicin may cause a local burning that can create enough discomfort to discontinue therapy. This burning may disappear with repeated administrations over days to weeks. Prior administration of a local anesthetic or ingestion of an analgesic increases the ability of some patients to tolerate a trial of this drug.

Topical use of anti-inflammatory drugs has been investigated for neuropathic pain with mixed results. Although topical aspirin, indomethacin, and diclofenac have been effective in patients with acute herpetic neuralgia or postherpetic neuralgia,[123] other data are less convincing and suggest that the efficacy of topical anti-inflammatory drugs for neuropathic pain remains unproven.

The eutectic mixture of local anesthetics (EMLA), which contains a 1:1 mixture of prilocaine and lidocaine, is capable of penetrating the skin to produce a dense local cutaneous anesthesia. This preparation is widely used to prevent the pain of needle puncture and incision and has demonstrated efficacy in postherpetic neuralgia.[124] High concentrations of topical lidocaine and a 5% lidocaine gel can also be effective in patients with postherpetic neuralgia. Commercially available lower concentrations have been less effective.

The risk of toxicity from systemic absorption of a topical local anesthetic is remote.[124,125] There is a small risk of methemoglobinemia from the prilocaine contained in EMLA. Consequently, this preparation should be used cautiously in infants, patients with histories of methemoglobinemia, and those who are taking coadministered drugs that may also cause this complication, such as sulfonamides.

To create an area of dense sensory loss, the eutectic mixture of lidocaine and prilocaine must be applied thickly under an occlusive dressing (e.g., plastic wrap) for at least 1 hour. Cutaneous anesthesia may not be necessary to gain benefit from a topical local anesthetic, however, and some patients seem to respond favorably to a thin application applied without a dressing.

Conclusion

The number of adjuvant analgesic drugs for the treatment of neuropathic cancer pain is large and continues to expand. Successful use requires an understanding of pharmacokinetics and pharmacodynamics, including potential adverse effects. Pain management can be optimized only if an initial assessment is followed by ongoing reassessment and adjustment of therapy. The ultimate success in the use of adjuvant analgesics relies on a strong therapeutic alliance between the health care provider and the patient. Given the empirical nature of therapeutic trials, patients must be educated about the process. Expectations must be appropriate lest patients become frustrated and lose hope of obtaining benefit.

References

1. Max MB, Culnane M, Schafer SC, et al. Amitriptyline relieves diabetic neuropathy pain in patients with normal or depressed mood. *Neurology* 1987; 37:589–596.

2. Kishore-Kumar R, Max MB, Schafer SC, et al. Desipramine relieves postherpetic neuralgia. *Clin Pharmacol Ther* 1990; 47:305–312.

3. Ventafridda V, et al. Studies on the effects of antidepressant drugs on the antinociceptive action of morphine and on plasma morphine in rat and man. *Pain* 1990; 43:155–162.

4. Monks R. Psychotropic drugs. In: Wall PD, Melzack R, eds. *Textbook of Pain*. 3rd ed. New York: Churchill Livingstone; 1994:963–990.

5. France RD, Krishnan KRR. Psychotropic drugs in chronic pain. In: France RD, Krishnan KRR, eds. *Chronic Pain*. Washington, DC: American Psychiatric Press; 1988:322–374.

6. Onghena P, Van houdenhove B. Antidepressant-induced analgesia in chronic non-malignant pain: a meta-analysis of 39 placebo-controlled studies. *Pain* 1992; 49:205–219.

7. Magni G. The use of antidepressants in the treatment of chronic pain: a review of the current evidence. *Drugs* 1991; 42:730–748.

8. Watson CPN, Evans RJ, Reed K, Merskey H, Goldsmith L, Warsh J. Amitriptyline versus placebo in postherpetic neuralgia. *Neurology* 1982; 32:671–673

9. Watson CPN, Chipman M, Reed K, Evans RJ, Birkett N. Amitriptyline versus maprotiline in postherpetic neuralgia: a randomized double-blind, crossover trial. *Pain* 1992; 48:29–36.

10. Turkington RW. Depression masquerading as diabetic neuropathy. *JAMA* 1980; 243:1147–1150.

11. Max MB, Lynch SA, Muir J, Shoaf SE, Smoller B, Dubner R. Effects of desipramine, amitriptyline, and fluoxetine on pain in diabetic neuropathy. *Engl J Med* 1992; 326:1250–1256.

12. Leijon G, Boivie J. Central post-stroke pain: a controlled trial of amitriptyline and carbamazepine. *Pain* 1989; 36:27–36.

13. Ventafridda V, Bonezzi C, Caraceni A, et al. Antidepressants for cancer pain and other painful syndromes with deafferentation component: comparison of amitriptyline and trazadone. *Ital J Neurol Sci* 1987; 8:579–587.

14. Kvinesdal B, Molin J, Froland A, Gram LF. Imipramine treatment of painful diabetic neuropathy. *JAMA* 1984; 251:1727–1730.

15. Sindrup SH, Ejlertsen B, Froland A, Sindrup EH, Brosen K, Gram LF. Imipramine treatment in diabetic neuropathy: relief of subjective symptoms without changes in peripheral and autonomic nerve function. *Eur J Clin Pharmacol* 1989; 37:151–153.

16. Sindrup SH, Gram LF, Skjold T, Froland A, Beck-Nielsen H. Concentration-response relationship in imipramine treatment of diabetic neuropathy symptoms. *Clin Pharmacol Ther* 1990; 47:509–515.

17. Panerai AE, Monza G, Movillia P, Bianchi M, Francucci BM, Tiengo M. A randomized, within-patient crossover, placebo-controlled trial on the efficacy and tolerability of the tricyclic antidepressants chlorimipramine and nortriptyline in central pain. *Acta Neurol Scand* 1990; 82:34–38.

18. Langohr HD, Stohr M, Petruch F. An open and double-blind crossover study on the efficacy of clomipramine (Anafranil) in patients with painful mono- and poly-neuropathies. *Eur Neurol* 1982; 21:309–317.

19. Sindrup SH, Gram LF, Skjold T, Grodum E, Brosen K, Beck-Nielsen H. Clomipramine vs. desipramine vs. placebo in the treatment of diabetic neuropathy symptoms. A double-blind cross-over study. *Br J Clin Pharmacol* 1990; 30:683–691.

20. Eberhard G, Von Knorring L, Nilsson HL, et al. A double-blind randomized study of clomipramine versus maprotiline in patients with idiopathic pain syndromes. *Neuropsychobiology* 1988; 19:25–34.

21. Sindrup SH, Gram LF, Brosen K, Eshoj O, Mogensen EF. The selective serotonin reuptake inhibitor paroxetine is effective in the treatment of diabetic neuropathy symptoms. *Pain* 1990; 42:135–144.

22. Sindrup SH, Bjerre U, Dejgaard A, et al. The selective serotonin reuptake inhibitor citalopram relieves the symptoms of diabetic neuropathy. *Clin Pharmacol Thera* 1992; 52:547–552.

23. Cooper GL. The safety of fluoxetine: an update. *Br J Psychiatry* 1988: 153 (Suppl 3):77–86.

24. Kerr JS, Fairweather DB, Mahendran R, Hindmarch I. The effects of paroxetine, alone and in combination with alcohol on psychomotor performance and cognitive function in the elderly. *Int Clin Psychopharmacol* 1992; 7:101–108.

25. Anthony M, Lance JW. Monoamine oxidase inhibitors in the treatment of migraine. *Arch Neurol* 1969; 21:263–268.

26. Fernandez F, Adams F, Holmes VF. Analgesic effect of alprazolam in patients with chronic, organic pain of malignant origin. *J Clin Psychopharmacol* 1987; 3:167–169.

27. Basbaum AI, Fields HL. Endogenous pain control systems: brainstem spinal pathways and endorphin circuitry. *Annu Rev Neurosci* 1984; 7:309–338.

28. Yaksh TL. Direct evidence that spinal serotonin and noradrenaline terminals mediate the spinal antinociceptive effects of morphine in the periaqueductal gray. *Brain Res* 1979; 160:180–185.

29. Richelson E. Tricyclic antidepressants and neurotransmitter receptors. *Psychiatric Ann* 1979; 9:186–194.

30. Charney DS, Menkes DB, Heninger FR. Receptor sensitivity and the mechanism of action of antidepressant treatment. *Arch Gen Psychiatry*, 1981; 38:1160–1180.

31. Potter WZ, Scheinin M, Golden RN, et al. Selective antidepressants and cerebrospinal fluid: lack of specificity in norepinephrine and serotonin metabolites. *Arch Gen Psychiatry* 1985; 42:1171–1177.

32. Cross JA, Horton RW. Effects of chronic oral administration of the antidepressants, desmethylimipramine and zimelidine on rat cortical GABA-B binding sites: a comparison with 5HT2 binding site changes. *Br J Pharmacol* 1988; 93:331–336.

33. Glassman AH, Bigger JT. Cardiovascular effects of therapeutic doses of tricyclic antidepressants. *Arch Gen Psychiatry* 1981; 38:815–820.

34. Roose SP, Glassman AH, Giardina EG. Nortriptyline in depressed patients with left ventricular impairment. *JAMA* 1986; 256:3253–3257.

35. Boyer WF, Blumhardt CL. The safety profile of paroxetine. *J Clin Psychiatry* 1992; 53 (Suppl 2):61–66.

36. Swerdlow M. Anticonvulsant drugs and chronic pain. *Clin Neuropharmacol* 1984; 7:51–82.

37. Hatangdi VS, Boas RA, Richards EG. Postherpetic neuralgia: management with antiepileptic and tricyclic drugs. In: Bonica JJ, Albe-Fessard D, eds. *Advances in Pain Research and Therapy.* Vol 1. New York: Raven Press; 1976:583–587.

38. Gerson GR, Jones RB, Luscombe DK. Studies on the concomitant use of carbamazepine and clomipramine for the relief of postherpetic neuralgia. *Postgrad Med J* 1977; 53:104–109.

39. Raskin NH, Levinson SA, Hoffman PM, Pickett JBE, Fields HL. Postsympathectomy neuralgia: amelioration with diphenylhydantoin and carbamazepine. *Am J Surg* 1974; 128:75–78.

40. Swerdlow M, Cundill JG. Anticonvulsant drugs used in the treatment of lancinating pains. A comparison. *Anesthesia* 1981; 36:1129–1132.

41. Espir MLE, Millac P. Treatment of paroxysmal disorders in multiple sclerosis with carbamazepine (Tegretol). *J Neurol Neurosurg Psychiatry* 1970; 33:528–531.

42. Chadda VS, Mathur MS. Double-blind study of the effects of diphenylhydantoin sodium in diabetic neuropathy. *J Assoc Physicians India* 1978; 26:403–406.

43. Caccia MR. Clonazepam in facial neuralgia and cluster headache: clinical and electrophysiological study. *Eur Neurol* 1975; 13:560–563.

44. Martin G. The management of pain following laminectomy for lumbar disc lesions. *Ann R Coll Surg Engl* 1981; 63:244–252.

45. Peiris JB, Perera GLS, Devendra SV, Lionel NDW. Sodium valproate in trigeminal neuralgia. *Med J Aust* 1980; 2:278.

46. Raftery H. The management of postherpetic pain using sodium valproate and amitriptyline. *J Irish Med Assoc* 1979; 72:399–401.

47. Rosenberg JM, Harrell C, Ristic H, Werner RA, de Rosayro AM. The effect of gabapentin on neuropathic pain. *Clin J Pain* 1997; 13:251–255.

48. Nakamura-Craig M, Follenfant RL. Lamotrigine and analogs: a new treatment for chronic pain? In: Gebhardt GF, Hammond DL, Jensen TS, eds. *Progress in Pain Research and Management.* Vol 2. Seattle: IASP Press; 1994:725–730.

49. Mellick GA. Hemifacial spasm: successful treatment with felbamate. *J Pain Symptom Manage* 1995; 10:392–395.

50. Weinberger J, Nicklas WJ, Berl, S. Mechanism of action of anticonvulsants. *Neurology* 1976; 26:162–173.

51. Devor M. The pathophysiology of damaged peripheral nerves. In: Wall PD, Melzack R, eds. *Textbook of Pain.* Churchill Livingstone: Edinburgh; 1994:79–100.

52. Albe-Fessard D, Lombard MC. Use of an animal model to evaluate the origin of deafferentation pain and protection against it. In: Bonica JJ, Lindblom U, Iggo A, eds. *Advances in Pain Research and Therapy.* Vol 5. New York: Raven Press; 1982:691–700.

53. Lenz FA, Kwan HC, Dostrovsky JO, Tasker RR. Characteristics of the bursting pattern of action potentials that occurs in the thalamus of patients with central pain. *Brain Res* 1989; 496:357–360.

54. Nystrom B, Hagbarth KE. Microelectrode recordings from transected nerves in amputees in phantom limb pain. *Neurosci Lett* 1981; 27:211–216.
55. Loeser JD, Ward AA, White LE. Chronic deafferentation of human spinal cord neurons. *J Neurosurg* 1968; 29:48–50.
56. Devor M, Govrin-Lippman R, Raber P. Corticosteroids reduce neuroma hyperexcitability. In: Fields HL, Dubner R, Cervero F, eds. *Advances in Pain Research and Therapy. Vol 9. Proceedings of the Fourth World Congress on Pain.* New York: Raven Press; 1985:451–455.
57. Goa KL, Sorkin EM. Gabapentin: a review of its pharmacological properties and clinical potential in epilepsy. *Drugs* 1993; 46:409–427.
58. Matsuo F, Bergen D, Faught E, et al. Placebo-controlled study of the efficacy and safety of lamotrigine in patients with partial seizures. *Neurology* 1993; 43:2284–2291.
59. Messenheimer J, Ramsay RE, Willmore LJ, et al. Lamotrigine therapy for partial seizures: a multicenter, placebo-controlled, double-blind, cross-over trial. *Epilepsia* 1994; 35:113–121.
60. Fromm GH, Terrence CF, Chattha AS. Baclofen in the treatment of trigeminal neuralgia: double-blind study and long-term follow-up. *Ann Neurol* 1984; 15:240–244.
61. Kofler M, Leis AA. Prolonged seizure activity after baclofen withdrawal. *Neurology* 1992; 42:697.
62. Kozin F, Ryan LM, Carerra GF, Soin LS, Wortmann RL. The reflex sympathetic dystrophy syndrome (RSDS). III. Scintigraphic studies, further evidence for the therapeutic efficacy of systemic corticosteroids, and proposed diagnostic criteria. *Am J Med* 1981; 70:23–29.
63. Greenberg HS, Kim J, Posner JB. Epidural spinal cord compression from metastatic tumor: results with a new treatment protocol. *Ann Neurol* 1980; 8:361–366.
64. Vecht Ch.J, Haaxma-Reiche H, van Putten WLJ, de Visser M, Vries EP, Twijnstra A. Initial bolus of conventional versus high-dose dexamethasone in metastatic spinal cord compression. *Neurology* 1989; 39:1255–1257.
65. Dixon RA, Christy NP. On the various forms of corticosteroid withdrawal syndrome. *Am J Med* 1980; 68:224–230.
66. Ettinger AB, Portenoy RK. The use of corticosteroids in the treatment of symptoms associated with cancer, *J Pain Symptom Manage* 1988; 3:99–103.
67. Eisenach JC, Du Pen S, Dubois M, Miguel R, Allin D, the Epidural Clonidine Study Group. Epidural clonidine analgesia for intractable cancer pain. *Pain* 1995; 61:391–400.
68. Coombs DW, Saunders R, Gaylor M, LaChance B, Jensen L. Clinical trial of intrathecal clonidine for cancer pain. *Reg Anesth* 1984; 9:34–35.
69. Coombs DW, Saunders RL, LaChance D, Savage S, Ragnarsson TS, Jensen LE. Intrathecal morphine tolerance: use of intrathecal clonidine, DADLE and intraventricular morphine. *Anesthesiology* 1985; 62:357–363.
70. Coombs DW, Saunders RL, Fratkin JD, Jensen LE, Murphy CA. Continuous intrathecal hydromorphone and clonidine for intractable cancer pain. *J Neurosurg* 1986; 64:890–894.
71. Kayser V, Desmeules J, Guilbaud G. Systemic clonidine differentially modulates the abnormal reactions to mechanical and thermal stimuli in rats with peripheral mononeuropathy. *Pain* 1995; 60:275–285.

72. Puke MJC, Wiesenfeld-Hallin Z. The differential effects of morphine and the alpha 2 adrenoceptor agonists clonidine and dexmedetomidine on the prevention and treatment of experimental neuropathic pain. *Anesth Analg* 1993; 77:105–109.

73. Yaksh TL. Pharmacology of spinal adrenergic systems which modulate spinal nociceptive processing. *Pharmacol Biochem Behav* 1985; 22:845–858.

74. Sagen J, Proudfit H. Evidence for pain modulation by pre-and postsynaptic noradrenergic receptors in the medulla oblongata. *Brain Res* 1985; 331:285–293.

75. Yjritsy-Roy JA, Standish SM, Terry LC. Dopamine D-1 and D-2 receptor antagonists potentiate analgesic and motor effects of morphine. *Pharmacol Biochem Behav* 1989; 32:717–721.

76. Bloomfield S, Simard-Savoie S, Bernier J, Tetreault L. Comparative analgesic activity of levomepromazine and morphine in patients with chronic pain. *Can Med Assoc J* 1964; 90:1156–1159.

77. Beaver WT, Wallenstein S, Houde RW, Rogers A. A comparison of the analgesic effects of methotrimeprazine and morphine in patients with cancer. *Clin Pharmacol Ther* 1966; 7:436–446.

78. Lasagna L, DeKornfeld TJ. Methotrimeprazine, a new phenothiazine derivative with analgesic properties. *JAMA* 1961; 178:887–890.

79. Hakkarainen H. Fluphenazine for tension headache: double-blind study. *Headache* 1977; 17:216–218.

80. Lechin F, van der Dijs B, Lechin ME, et al. Pimozide therapy for trigeminal neuralgia. *Arch Neurol* 1989; 9:960–962.

81. Breivik H, Rennemo F. Clinical evaluation of combined treatment with methadone and psychotropic drugs in cancer patients. *Acta Anaesthesiol Scandi* 1982; 74:135–140.

82. Cavenar JO, Maltbie AA. Another indication for haloperidol. *Psychosomatics* 1976; 17:128–130.

83. Weis O, Sriwatanakul K, Weintraub M. Treatment of postherpetic neuralgia and acute herpetic pain with amitriptyline and perphenazine. *S African Med J* 1982; 62:274–275.

84. Taub A. Relief of postherpetic neuralgia with psychotropic drugs. *J Neurosurg* 1973; 39:235–239.

85. Hanks GW, Thomas PJ, Trueman T, Weeks E. The myth of haloperidol potention. *Lancet* 1983; 2:523–524.

86. Rosenblatt WH, Cioffi AM, Sinatra R, Saberski LR, Silverman DG. Metoclopramide: an analgesic adjunct to patient-controlled analgesia. *Anesth Analg* 1991; 73:553–555.

87. Kandler D, Lisander B. Analgesic action of metoclopramide in prosthetic hip surgery. *Acta Anaesthesiol Scandi* 1993; 37:49–53.

88. Storey P, Hill HH, St. Louis R, Tarver EE. Subcutaneous infusions for control of cancer symptoms. *J Pain Symptom Manage* 1990; 5:33–41.

89. Rowbotham MC, Reisner-Keller LA, Fields HL. Both intravenous lidocaine and morphine reduce the pain of postherpetic neuralgia. *Neurology* 1991; 41:1024–1028.

90. Kastrup J, Petersen P, Dejgard A, Angelo HR, Hilsted J. Intravenous lidocaine infusion—a new treatmen· for chronic painful diabetic neuropathy. *Pain* 1987; 28:69–75.

91. Bruera E, Ripamonti C, Brenneis C, MacMillan K, Hanson J. A randomized double-blind crossover trial of intravenous lidocaine in the treatment of neuropathic cancer pain. *J Pain Symptom Manage* 1992; 7:138–140.

92. Elleman K, Sjogren P, Banning A, Jensen TS, Smith T, Geertsen P. Trial of intravenous lidocaine on painful neuropathy in cancer patients. *Clin J Pain* 1989; 5:291–294.

93. Brose WG, Cousins MJ. Subcutaneous lidocaine for treatment of neuropathic cancer pain. *Pain* 1991; 45:145–148.

94. Lindstrom P, Lindblom U. The analgesic effect of tocainide in trigeminal neuralgia. *Pain* 1987; 28:45–50.

95. Dejgard A, Petersen P, Kastrup J. Mexiletine for treatment of chronic painful diabetic neuropathy. *Lancet* 1988; 1:9–11.

96. Dunlop R, Davies RJ, Hockley J, Turner P. Letter to the Editor. *Lancet* 1989; 1;420–421.

97. Covino BG. Local anesthetics. In: Ferrante FM, VadeBoncouer TR, eds. *Postoperative Pain Management*. New York: Churchill Livingstone; 1993:211–253.

98. deJong RH, Nace R. Nerve impulse conduction during intravenous lidocaine injection. *Anesthesiology* 1968; 29:22–28.

99. Woolf CJ, Wiesenfeld-Halli Z. The systemic administration of local anesthetic produces a selective depression of C-afferent evoked activity in the spinal cord. *Pain* 1985; 23:361–374.

100. Chabal C, Russell LC, Burchiel KJ. The effect of intravenous lidocaine, tocainide and mexiletine on spontaneously active fibers originating in rat sciatic neuromas. *Pain* 1989; 38:333–338.

101. Devor M, Wall PD, Catalan N. Systemic lidocaine silences ectopic neuroma and DRG discharge without blocking nerve conduction. *Pain* 1992; 48:261–268.

102. CAST (Cardiac Arrhythmia Suppression Trial) Investigators. Preliminary report: effect of encainide and flecainide on mortality in a randomized trial of arrhythmia suppression after acute myocardial infarction. *N Engl J Med* 1989; 321:406–412.

103. Kreeger W, Hammill SC. New antiarrhythmic drugs: tocainide, mexiletine, flecainide, encainide and amiodarone. *Mayo Clin Proc* 1987; 62:1033–1050.

104. Campbell RWF. Mexiletine. *N Engl J Med* 1987; 316:29–34.

105. Galer BS, Miller KV, Rowbotham MC. Response to intravenous lidocaine infusion differs based on clinical diagnosis and site of nervous system injury. *Neurology* 1993; 43:1233–1235.

106. Woolf CJ, Thompson SWN. The induction and maintenance of central sensitization is dependent on N-methyl-D-aspartic acid receptor activation: implications for the treatment of post-injury pain hypersensitivity states. *Pain* 1991; 44:293–299.

107. Dickenson AH, Sullivan AF. Evidence for a role of the NMDA receptor in the frequency dependent potentiation of deep dorsal horn nociceptive neurons following C fibre stimulation. *Neuropharmacology* 1987; 26:1235–1238.

108. Price DD, Mao J, Frenk H, Mayer DJ. The N-methyl-d-aspartate antagonist dextromethorphan selectively reduces temporal summation of second pain in man. *Pain* 1994; 59:165–174.

109. Park KM, Max MB, Robinovitz E, Gracely RH, Bennett GJ. Effects of intravenous ketamine and alfentanil on hyperalgesia induced by intradermal capsaicin. In: Gebhardt GF, Hammond DL, Jensen TS, eds. *Proceedings of the 7th World Congress on Pain*. Seattle: IASP Press; 1994:647–655.

110. Persson J, Axelsson G, Hallin RG, Gustafsson LL. Beneficial effects of ketamine in a chronic pain state with allodynia, possibly due to central sensitization. *Pain* 1995; 60:217–222.

111. Stannard CF, Porter GE. Ketamine hydrochloride in the treatment of phantom limb pain. *Pain* 1993; 54:227–230.

112. Backonja M, Arndt G, Gombar KA, Check B, Zimmerman M. Response of chronic neuropathic pain syndromes to ketamine: a preliminary study. *Pain* 1994; 56:51–57.

113. Eide PK, Jorum E, Stubhaug A, Bremnes J, Breivik H. Relief of post-herpetic neuralgia with the N-methyl-D-aspartic receptor antagonist ketamine: a double-blind, crossover comparison with morphine and placebo. *Pain* 1994; 58:347–354.

114. Gobelet C, Waldburger M, Meier JL. The effect of adding calcitonin to physical treatment on reflex sympathetic dystrophy. *Pain* 1992; 48:171–175.

115. Jaeger H, Maier C. Calcitonin in phantom limb pain: a double blind study. *Pain* 1992; 48:21–27.

116. Raja SN, Treede RD, Davis KD, Campbell JN. Systemic alpha-adrenergic blockade with phentolamine: a diagnostic test for sympathetically-maintained pain. *Anesthesiology* 1991; 74:691–698.

117. Ghostine SY, Comair YG, Turner DM, Kassell NF, Azar CG. Phenoxybenzamine in the treatment of causalgia. *J Neurosurg* 1984; 60:1263–1268.

118. Abram SE, Lightfoot RW. Treatment of longstanding causalgia with prazosin. *Reg Anesth* 1981; 6:79–81.

119. Tabira T, Shibasaki H, Kuroiwa Y. Reflex sympathetic dystrophy (causalgia) treatment with guanethidine. *Arch Neurol* 1983; 40:430–432.

120. Rowbotham MC. Topical analgesic agents. In: Fields HL, Liebeskind JC, eds. *Pharmacological Approaches to the Treatment of Chronic Pain: New Concepts and Critical Issues.* Seattle: IASP Press; 1994:211–229.

121. Mashimo T, Tomi K, Pak M, Demizu A, Yyoshiya I. Relief of causalgia with prostaglandin E_1 ointment. *Anest Analg* 1991; 72:700–701.

122. Dubner R. Topical capsaicin therapy for neuropathic pain. *Pain* 1991; 47:247–248.

123. DeBenedittis G, Besana F, Lorenzettit A. A new topical treatment for acute herpetic neuralgia and postherpetic neuralgia: the aspirin/diethyl ether mixture. An open-label study plus a double-blind controlled clinical trial. *Pain* 1992; 48:383–390.

124. Stow PJ, Glynn CJ, Minor B. EMLA cream in the treatment of postherpetic neuralgia: efficacy and pharmacokinetic profile. *Pain* 1989; 39:301–305.

125. Rowbotham MC, Davies PS, Fields HL. Topical lidocaine gel relieves postherpetic neuralgia. *Ann Neurol* 1995; 37:246–253.

4

Invasive Techniques for Neuropathic Pain in Cancer

TESS CRAMOND

The conventional management of patients with cancer pain involves anticancer therapy; oral analgesics; support for the patient and family, and psychological techniques, including modification of lifestyle; and the control of other distressing symptoms. It is generally agreed that effective pain control is achieved in 85%–90% of patients by these standard means.[1]

When pain persists and definitive treatment of the lesion is not possible, invasive techniques must be considered (Fig. 4.1). The proper use of these techniques for the treatment of neuropathic pain is challenging and demands an understanding of the underlying pathophysiology.

Neuropathic pain may be defined as pain due to dysfunction of the peripheral or central nervous system in the absence of nociceptor (nerve terminal) stimulation by trauma or disease.[2] It is associated with abnormal somatosensory processes resulting from physical (e.g., injury, infection, or stroke) or functional (e.g., diabetic neuropathy and trigeminal neuralgia) disturbance of some part of the nervous system.

Neuropathic pain may appear immediately after nerve injury or may have delayed onset. It may be constant and independently maintained, or include superimposed intermittent exacerbations that are described as lancinating, shooting, stabbing, or like electric shocks. The pain is usually dysesthetic, i.e., altered sensations described as burning, tingling, itching, or even numbness, and it may or may not be associated with abnormal evoked sensation (e.g., allodynia, hyperesthesia, or hyperpathia).

Portenoy's[3] classification (Fig. 4.2) demonstrates that neuropathic pain can be sustained by central nervous system processes, peripheral nervous system processes, or both central and peripheral components in some circumstances. Peripherally, nerve lesions may result from section (partial or complete), traction, com-

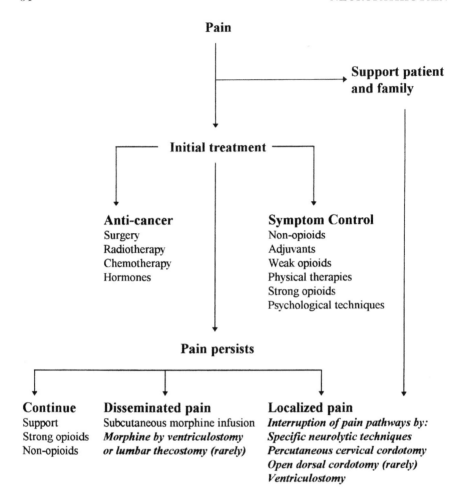

Figure 4.1. Management plan for patients with cancer pain.

pression, or ischemia. This may be associated with infiltration or compression by tumor, viral infection, or treatment with surgery, radiotherapy or chemotherapy.

Although it is said that neuropathic pain does not respond to opioids (which is true for conventional routes of administration), this is controversial and there may be a component of nociceptive pain that will respond to opioids. This combination of pain types resembles that seen characteristically in patients with partial thickness burns who need opioids for relief of the nociceptive pain but also suffer burning dysesthesia, which emanates especially from donor sites and requires adjuvant medication, such as an infusion of lidocaine or oral mexiletine.

An element of sympathetically maintained pain may be present in both central and peripheral pain but is more commonly associated with peripheral le-

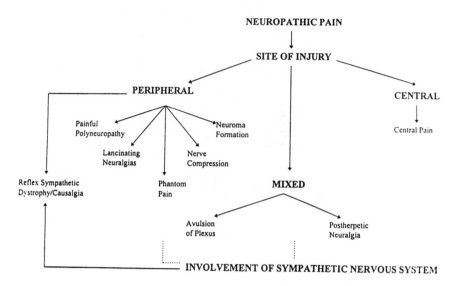

Figure 4.2. Pathways of neuropathic pain. (Reprinted with permission from Portenoy RK: Issues in the management of neuropathic pain. In: Basbaum AI, Besson JM (eds.) *Towards a New Pharmacology of Pain*, p. 393. Chichester, England: John Wiley and Sons, 1991.[3])

sions[3,4] (Fig. 4.2 and 4.3). The presence of pain that is sustained by sympathetic efferent activity will influence treatment.

Treatment of Neuropathic Pain

The treatment of neuropathic pain must begin with a careful history, including a pain history and assessment of any precipitating incident or accident. This history should be followed by a thorough physical examination and appropriate investigations. These, together with an understanding of any psychosocial problems, will enable the development of a reliable management plan.

The aim must be to treat any reversible conditions and relieve the pain so that an exercise and activity program will enable rehabilitation within the limits of the patient's clinical status. Apart from interventional anesthetic and surgical techniques, treatment may involve anticancer treatment, pharmacological means, stimulation techniques, physical therapies, and always psychosocial support.

The common interventional procedures that are available for the treatment of cancer-related neuropathic pain include: *(1)* local anesthetic blocks of the neuraxis and the sympathetic chain; *(2)* neurolytic blocks; *(3)* percutaneous cervical cordotomy; *(4)* spinal opioids; and *(5)* ventriculostomy for administration of morphine by direct injection into the lateral ventricle.

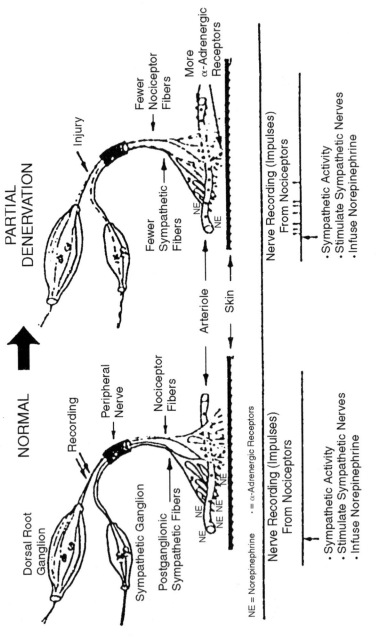

Figure 4.3. Pain responses to sympathetic activity after injury. (Reprinted with permission from Perl E: *Pain: Clinical Updates*. International Association for the Study of Pain. 1993; 1:1–4.[4])

This review of invasive techniques for neuropathic pain represents a personal view based on over 30 years' experience in the Royal Brisbane Hospital Multidisciplinary Pain Center, a tertiary referral center now serving a population of 3.5 million people.

Anesthetic Techniques

Neural blockade may fulfill diagnostic, prognostic, or therapeutic roles in the management of pain. It can be used to identify the anatomical origin of the pain, differentiate somatic and visceral components of thoracoabdominal pain, and determine whether peripheral pain is sympathetically maintained.

However, it is unwise to rely on the prognostic value of local anesthetic blocks before decisions for surgery or neurolytic blockade are made. Successful blockade does not necessarily guarantee long-term pain relief. Therapeutically, local anesthetic blocks can provide effective short-term pain relief while diagnosis is established or definitive treatment determined.

Local anesthetic blocks

Management of acute herpes zoster and prevention of postherpetic pain
Acute herpes zoster is common in patients with cancer. Patients frequently present with severe pain before the appearance of the characteristic vesicles that confirm the diagnosis. Severe constant background pain is often associated with distressing hyperesthesia, present with stimulation; light touch and temperature can both increase the severity of the pain. There may also be episodes of severe neuralgic pain. Neither the lancinating pain nor the burning dysesthesia are reliably relieved by opioid drugs.

Those most at risk of developing postherpetic neuralgia are the elderly (aged 55 or more) and those with cancer and HIV/AIDS. Active treatment of the acute pain is indicated in an attempt to prevent this unpleasant sequela,[5] which is usually associated with physical and emotional distress, sometimes extreme. Antiviral treatment with aciclovir or one of the newer antiviral drugs (e.g., famciclovir or valaciclovir) should be commenced within 48 hours of the appearance of the rash.[6] Anticonvulsant drugs may modify the neuralgic pain.[7] This is well accepted in the management of postherpetic neuralgia and may be considered as well for some patients with acute zoster. Although carbamazepine has been used traditionally, caution is needed in the elderly because of the risk of inducing confusion and ataxia. The risk of leukopenia may also relatively contraindicate this drug in patients who are receiving cytotoxic therapy or have limited bone marrow reserve. Sodium valproate is our preferred drug, starting with 400 mg a day and adjusting the dose to control the pain. It is not necessary to achieve the therapeutic levels essential for the control of epilepsy, but liver function must be monitored.

Bowsher[2] has suggested the value of pre-emptive treatment with amitriptyline, 25 mg at the time of diagnosis of acute shingles. This drug is known to be effective for postherpetic neuralgia and this pre-emptive role awaits confirmation. Although therapy is not always completely effective in controlling pain, amitriptyline will also assist sleep. Provided there are no cardiac contraindications, the oral analogues of lidocaine, such as mexiletine, may also be useful in controlling burning dysesthesia.[7] Again, the approach is well accepted for chronic pain and can be considered in some cases of severe acute pain.

Although not always successful, there is evidence that sympathetic blockade commenced within the first 48 hours and continued for 7 days can modify the course of the disease. Reports of the efficacy of sympathetic blockade in the management of the pain of acute herpes zoster have appeared in the literature since the work of Rosenak.[8] The literature contains the considerable experience of Colding[9] and, more recently, of Winnie.[10] Unfortunately, the value of this technique is not recognized by many of those who see the patient when acute herpes zoster is first diagnosed, i.e., primary care physicians, dermatologists, ophthalmologists, and oncologists. Interdisciplinary education must be the objective if patients are to benefit from this treatment.

Winnie[10] has recommended that the earlier the treatment, the more successful the blockade will be in aborting the acute episode and, perhaps, in preventing the development of postherpetic neuralgia. He set 8 weeks as the upper time limit. The form of the sympathetic blockade will depend on the site of the lesion. For lesions involving thoracic, lumbosacral, or low cervical nerves (C6–C7), an epidural infusion will provide excellent pain relief while maintaining motor function. Although Winnie used repeated epidural injections, it is our practice to use an infusion to prevent the return of pain. Lesions involving the trigeminal nerve or cervical nerves above C6–C7 will require stellate ganglion blocks, which will have to be repeated while pain persists.

In performing sympathetic blockade, it is necessary first to use a concentration of bupivacaine that will achieve a sensory blockade to confirm that the level of the blockade is appropriate for the level of the lesion. The concentration can then be reduced to maintain sympathetic blockade. If dural puncture or other complications are to be avoided, these epidurals should be undertaken only by experienced anesthesiologists, especially for thoracic blocks.

Our own experience reinforces the extensive experience of Colding[9] and Winnie,[10] who found that sympathetic blockade is effective in relieving the pain of acute herpes zoster and in modifying the severity of the disease. Sympathetic blockade may also prevent the development of postherpetic neuralgia if undertaken within 8 weeks. Finally, amitriptyline can improve the quality of pain relief, even if this is not complete, and it will assist sleep.

Diagnosis and treatment of sympathetically maintained pain
In 1872, Weir Mitchell[11] first used the term "causalgia" to describe the intractable pain that followed nerve injuries sustained by casualties in the American Civil

War. It took another 75 years before the association of the sympathetic nervous system to causalgia was described by the French surgeon Rene Leriche.[12] It is now generally accepted that pain associated with sympathetic efferent function in peripheral nerves is classified as sympathetically maintained pain.[13] The patient may exhibit disturbances of sensation and motor function, and autonomic regulation, and there may be evidence of psychological distress. Sympathetically maintained pain is exemplified in cancer patients by invasion or irritation of the sympathetic chain, as in Pancoast's syndrome and in lumbosacral plexopathy.

Patients with possible sympathetically maintained pain may present with burning dysesthesia exacerbated by warmth, cold, or stress; hyperesthesia; allodynia; hyperpathia; and sympathetic effector activity. The spontaneous or evoked pain may occur any time from just days to weeks after the injury. The pain varies from "irritating but tolerable to totally immobilising and preoccupying."[4]

Sympathetically maintained pain must be distinguished from pain associated with abnormal impressions of sympathetic activity in a painful area.[13] The presence of pain in response to mild cooling is a sensitive, but not a specific, marker for sympathetically maintained pain. Only about 50% of patients with sympathetically independent pain show cooling hyperalgesia.

While local anesthetic sympathetic ganglion blocks are useful as screening tests for sympathetically maintained pain, Charlton[14] has warned that they should be interpreted with caution because of the problems of diffusion of the local anesthetic drugs, the systemic effects of these drugs, and the placebo effect. In 1991, Arner[15] advocated a more conclusive test in which phentolamine, an adrenergic blocking agent, is infused intravenously (with appropriate resuscitation and monitoring facilities available). Because the pathology is peripheral rather than central in the early stages, it is also appropriate to use peripheral blocking techniques to facilitate restoration of function. Of particular interest is whether continuous epidural blockade with bupivacaine is better than repeated regional sympathetic blockade, e.g., with guanethidine, bretylium, or phentolamine with bupivacaine.

If the blocks facilitate active physiotherapy, they should be continued. The objective should be to decrease the number of blocks and increase the patient's role in active physiotherapy. If there is no progress after one month, ongoing sympathetic blockade is unlikely to be successful. If the patient has advanced cancer, cordotomy or ventriculostomy could then be considered (see below). Although some clinicians support the use of spinal opioids, their justification has yet to be established.

The concept of causalgia as a tissue receptor disorder has been advanced by Perl[4] and implies development of new therapeutic regimens. Future approaches may use selective adrenergic blocking agents parenterally, or locally as a cream, patch, or ointment.[16,17]

Stellate ganglion block

The indications for cervicodorsal sympathetic block using local anesthetic include regional circulatory insufficiency, presumed sympathetically maintained pain (e.g., associated with herpes zoster), and burning dysesthetic pain associated with brachial plexopathy (possibly sympathetically maintained). All authors question the advisability of neurolytic stellate ganglion block.[18]

Blockade of the stellate ganglion is achieved by injection at the transverse process of C6 or C7 to lessen the risk of pneumothorax. Lateral traction of the sterno-mastoid muscle and the carotid artery facilitates safe injection. It is much easier to have an assistant inject 15–20 ml of local anaesthetic solution through sterile extension tubing while the anesthetist stabilizes the needle. Immediately after the injection, the patient may experience temporary hoarseness or dysphagia. Horner's syndrome is a recognized sign of a successful block but does not necessarily imply blockade of the sympathetic supply to the arm. To obtain a therapeutic effect, a series of blocks is usually required, commonly daily for 5 days then every other day.

Phantom pain and stump pain
Phantom sensations occur very commonly after amputation, when a major nerve has been severed. The patient may complain of a shrunken, deformed part, or feel intense shooting pain into an amputated foot when a stump neuroma is palpated or when there is any clearly defined trigger point and a positive Tinel's sign. Phantom pain is usually described as burning, lancinating, or shooting pain, and there may be complaint of "vice-like" pain.

Sherman[19] has reviewed the therapies for phantom pain, most of which are unreliable in achieving sustained relief. It is essential to ensure that the prosthetic device fits properly; in this regard, the advice of an interdisciplinary amputee clinic is invaluable. Regular intravenous injections of lidocaine (3 mg/kg), given slowly over 30 minutes daily for 5 days, can reduce the size of the phantom and ablate the burning sensitivity.[20] While the duration of relief may be short lived—4 to 6 weeks—it may last for months and can be repeated without burden. Although peripheral nerve stimulation has some advocates, it may be necessary to use dorsal column stimulation to influence the Aβ primary afferents that are stimulated when transcutaneous electrical nerve stimulation is used.[2]

Psychiatric support and counseling assume major importance, especially in the young patient facing amputation. Such support may not be possible in emergency amputation, but it should be provided as soon as possible. It should always be part of the preoperative preparation for elective amputations for cancer or peripheral vascular disease, and it should continue postoperatively.

Pre-emptive analgesia using 5 days of sensory blockade with epidural analgesia for lower limb amputations or appropriate upper limb blockade may lessen the incidence of severe phantom pain.[21] In below-knee amputations, another useful technique is placement of an epidural catheter close to the lateral popliteal nerve at the time of surgery to permit instillation of 10 ml of bupivacaine 0.25% three times a day. Again, interdisciplinary cooperation among surgeons, anesthesiologists, and psychiatrists will ensure the best results in preventing phantom limb pain. Once pain is established, the treatment is not satisfactory.

Neurolytic blockade of the neuraxis

Neurolytic blockade has been used for many years in management of intractable cancer pain. Benefits must be weighed against the known side effects and potential complications. The aim is to produce a chemical posterior rhizotomy. Neurolytic blockade is usually reserved for patients with pain of cancer origin and short expectation of life, in whom somatic pain is limited to two or three dermatomes and is not responsive to accepted doses of opioid drugs.[22]

There is always the risk of motor as well as sensory loss when mixed nerves are involved. Because of abnormal anatomy, there is the potential for damage to other than the targeted nerves. This is very significant if there is a risk of alteration in sphincter function or impairment of mobility because neurolysis may exacerbate an incipient neurological problem.

While it is inappropriate to subject patients to unnecessary investigations, appropriate imaging will be essential to exclude tumor within the spinal canal. Patt[23] has warned that neurolytic blocks may precipitate dysesthesias when used peripherally, although the time span for onset makes this less significant in cancer patients.

Neurolytic blocks have a limited place in the management of neuropathic pain. If they are used, there must be a clear understanding by the patient and the caregivers of the aims of the treatment, the expected duration of effect, and the potential for side effects. There must always be full documentation of the neurological state and other significant physical findings prior to and following neurolytic blockade.

Spinal subarachnoid blocks

Precise unilateral segmental sensory blocks can be performed at any level from the cervical region to the perineum, but they are most useful for patients with neuropathic pain localized to two or three dermatomes who are not suitable for percutaneous cervical cordotomy.[24] These blocks might be very useful, for example, in the treatment of a patient who has a paralyzed diaphragm or has had a pneumonectomy with recurrent tumor causing neuralgic pain and dysesthesia in the chest wall. The risk of motor paresis or interruption of bladder or bowel function is unlikely with thoracic injections, so this technique has a useful, if limited, role.

Provided the patient can lie on the painful side, phenol 6.67% in glycerine is an appropriate neurolytic agent. If the patient cannot lie on the painful side, alcohol is used instead. After the needle is placed correctly, the patient is postured appropriately, depending on the neurolytic agent used.

Lumbosacral block

Intrathecal neurolysis of the sacral nerves is a very useful technique for the relief of deep, central perineal pain associated with pelvic malignancy. Because neurolysis of the second and third sacral nerve roots will compromise bladder and bowel sphincters, these blocks are done only if the patient already has a colostomy and has or will accept an indwelling urinary catheter.

Lumbar puncture is performed between L5 and S1 with the patient seated. Once the needle is correctly placed, the table is tilted backwards to 45°. Increments of 0.25 ml phenol 6.67% in glycerine are injected with a maximum at one time of 1.0 ml. Pain relief is usually immediate but the full effect may not be apparent for 2–3 days. Some patients receive long-lasting benefit—up to 6 months—but in others it may be short-lived. The block may be repeated. Injections of alcohol are painful and the maximum benefit may not appear for 3–5 days.

Peripheral neurolysis and neurectomy

Cranial nerves. The intractable pain associated with head and neck cancer is often complicated by an inability to open the mouth, gross ulceration of the floor of the mouth, lytic lesions of the cervical spine, fixation of the neck muscles due to tumor, and fungating lesions of the mouth, face, and neck. The pain is frequently exacerbated by speaking, swallowing saliva, or eating, or by movements of the head and coughing. Dwyer[25] has shown the efficacy of neurolytic blockade in the management of malignant pain associated with carcinoma of the tongue and floor of the mouth. Apart from trigeminal thermocoagulation or neurolysis, however, the indications for peripheral neurolysis/neurectomy for craniocervical pain are few. The availability of intraventricular opioid therapy may provide a greater likelihood of pain relief with few side effects.[26]

Management of the pain may be complicated by distortion of the normal anatomy by tumor, previous surgery, or radiation therapy, and by the overlapping contributions of the cranial nerves, particularly V, IX, and X, and the upper cervical nerves. While all of these nerves may be sectioned through the posterior fossa, this is a major procedure in a patient with advanced malignancy.

Blockade of the glossopharyngeal nerve may be useful when the pain involves the base of the tongue, the external auditory canal, and the tonsillar fossa. Although the glossopharyngeal supplies the nasopharynx, the uvula, and the Eustachian tube, pain from these areas is difficult to localize.

The vagus contributes to the nerve supply to the ear, the external auditory canal, and the larynx. Laryngeal pain is often bilateral, but bilateral blockade of the glossopharyngeal and the vagus is contraindicated because of the risk of airway difficulties and interference with swallowing.

Peripheral sensory neurolysis. Blockade of the peripheral sensory nerves is associated with a relatively high incidence of neuritis and tissue necrosis. Nonetheless, Doyle[27] has reported successful pain relief following neurolytic block of intercostal nerves.

Neurolytic blocks of the sympathetic axis

As discussed, sympathetically maintained pain, a subtype of neuropathic pain, may be associated with tumor involvement of nerve plexuses, as in lumbosacral plexopathy and Pancoast's syndrome. Such involvement is accompanied by dysesthetic pain and, at times, vasomotor changes. Sympathetic blocks may be effective in this type of pain. A sympathetic block may also be helpful if afferent nerves that traverse sympathetic structures carry nociceptive messages from injured viscera. The most useful sympathetic blocks in the latter case are celiac plexus block, hypogastric plexus block, and block of the ganglion impar.

Sympathetic blockade has the advantage of providing effective pain relief without a decrease in muscle power and without sensory loss. Alcohol 50% is the drug of choice for celiac plexus block and phenol with contrast is the preferred drug for block of the hypogastric plexus and the ganglion impar. The availability of screening techniques has rendered more accurate placement of needles and identification of the spread of contrast solution. Moore[28] has advocated CT for this purpose.

Celiac plexus and splanchnic block. Celiac plexus block is used to ablate the constant gnawing upper abdominal pain moving through to the back, which is a feature of the pain of carcinoma of the pancreas and other upper abdominal organs. If somatic nerves are also involved, other forms of pain relief will be necessary. The most widely used technique is the classical retro-crural approach dating from 1918 when it was described by Kappis.[29] Later it was modified by Moore in 1965.[30] The anatomical landmarks for these blocks are the twelfth ribs and the spine of T12 (which is at the level of the body of L1). Both Singer[31] and Boas[32] have recommended the transcrural approach, with appropriate radiographic guidance. For celiac plexus block, the use of 50 ml of alcohol 50% is recommended.

When splanchnic block is performed, the needles are placed more cephalad near the anterolateral margin of the body of T12. Lesser volumes of the neurolytic agent are needed (e.g., 15 ml of phenol 10%). The risk of pneumothorax is greater with splanchnic than with celiac plexus block and the value of radiographic control is undisputed. The incidence of postural hypotension is lessened by proper attention to hydration, the use of support stockings, and care when posture is changed.

Sympathetic blocks for pelvic pain

Neuropathic pelvic pain is particularly difficult to manage because it is often poorly localized and tends to spread to both sides.

Superior hypogastric plexus block. Block of the superior hypogastric plexus provides very effective pain relief for visceral pain associated with pelvic malignancy. It is especially useful for the burning tenesmus that may follow radiotherapy. A 15- to 20-cm short bevelled needle is inserted through skin wheals 5–7 cm from the midline at the level of the L4–L5 interspace. The needles are directed towards the antero-lateral aspect of the body of L5 and 6–8 ml of aqueous phenol 10% is injected through each needle after injection of contrast to determine that placement is accurate.[33]

Block of the ganglion impar. This block has been introduced recently to alleviate perineal pain, which is characterized by burning and urgency.[34] The ganglion impar is located at the sacrococcygeal junction and identifies the termination of the paired paravertebral sympathetic chains. The block is performed with the patient in the lateral position. The 22-gauge, 10-cm spinal needle is inserted through the anococcygeal ligament after being bent about 2.5 cm from the hub to form a 30° angle. The concavity is directed posteriorly and the needle is placed anterior to the coccyx and advanced until its tip reaches the sacrococcygeal junction. Care that the needle remains against the coccyx will lessen the risk of rectal penetration. An injection of contrast will confirm correct placement, reducing the risk of caudal epidural injection. Six milliliters of phenol 6.67% is used for the neurolytic block.

Surgical Therapies

Percutaneous cervical cordotomy

Percutaneous cervical cordotomy has been performed in our unit since 1979. A detailed analysis of the results of the first 253 patients was reported in 1993.[24] Our experience, now based on the care of 400 patients managed by one neurosurgeon, has shown that this procedure provides a satisfactory surgical method of interrupting the pain pathways to achieve effective pain relief in properly selected patients with unilateral cancer pain below the neck. It obviates the need for opioid medication with its attendant disadvantages, especially nausea, constipation, drowsiness, and decreased concentration.

Being able to withdraw opioid medication is particularly advantageous in the aged, many of whom have slowly growing tumors and are particularly susceptible to the undesirable side effects of opioids. Although open cordotomy would be effective for some of these patients, there is no justification for submitting these often frail and elderly patients to further major surgery under general anesthesia, unless degenerative disease of the cervical spine precludes an effective percutaneous cervical cordotomy. Patients who have open cordotomy involving hemilaminectomy can expect painful movements of at least one arm for 2 or 3 weeks.

Percutaneous cervical cordotomy relieves visceral, somatic, and neuropathic pain. It provides very effective relief of pain associated with weight-bearing and other incident pain. Some patients with neuropathic pain have a specific, sometimes urgent, need for percutaneous cordotomy. For example, it can be a highly effective method for the arm pain associated with Pancoast's tumor or other brachial plexopathy, which cannot be relieved by open dorsal cordotomy and is poorly responsive to opioids. The technique also has a particular role in the relief of unilateral chest wall pain, especially that associated with mesothelioma or intercostal nerve involvement from other tumors. These patients together form a group with a critical need for percutaneous cordotomy which is too often ignored.

The decision to recommend percutaneous cervical cordotomy will depend on the severity and nature of the pain, the age and general condition of the patient, and the expectation of life. Further, the patient must be able to lie flat for the duration of the procedure (about 1 hour) and be able to indicate the effects of the passage of the electrical stimuli. Thus, they must be both rational and cooperative. Frequently, prior adjustment of medication is necessary as the patient may be confused because of unrelieved pain or inappropriate doses of opioid drugs.

An 82-year-old woman presented in 1987 with intractable neuropathic buttock and leg pain associated with a large pararectal recurrence of bowel cancer. She could neither sit nor stand without pain and ate her meals lying down, but she was still incapacitated by lancinating pain and burning dysesthesia. Following percutaneous cervical cordotomy she has been pain-free for 8 years and continues to play golf and travel overseas.

Information for patients. The procedure, and its benefits, potential complications, and side effects, are explained in detail to the patient and the spouse. Patients are advised that the procedure is for the relief of pain only and will not influence weakness or general lethargy and discomfort. It will not alter the progression of the cancer. It also will not prevent the onset of neuromuscular deficit when there is already nerve plexus involvement on the painful side, and there is a 1% chance of weakness on the ipsilateral side (of the cordotomy).

Patients are also told that they will be withdrawn gradually from opioid drugs and can expect less nausea and constipation and improved concentration as the opioid dose is reduced. They are assured of access to physical therapies that ensure rehabilitation to maximum independence that is compatible with the physical condition.

The patient must want the cordotomy and must not be persuaded to have it. The decision becomes a mutual decision of the patient, the referring doctor, the neurosurgeon, and the director of the pain relief service.

Preoperative preparation. Preoperative preparation includes general medical care, psychosocial support, and treatment of hematological and biochemical abnormalities, if possible, with particular emphasis given to hemoglobin, platelet levels, serum creatinine, and calcium. Chest radiographs and respiratory function tests are routine and arterial blood gas tensions are measured.

As a general rule, we exclude those patients with an arterial oxygen tension of less than 8.66 kPa. We have been more conservative about this requirement than Ischia et al.,[35] some of whose patients had an arterial oxygen tension of 6.67 kPa. We also exclude patients whose respiratory function shows compromise of respiratory reserve. A previous pneumonectomy or a paralyzed diaphragm is an absolute contraindication irrespective of arterial oxygen tension.

The operation. The usual dose of opioid medication is given on the morning of cordotomy. It may be necessary to give an additional dose intravenously prior to moving the patient to the radiography table. The procedure is performed with minimal awake sedation. Oxygen is administered by intranasal cannula at 4 L/min with oxygen saturation monitored by pulse oximetry.

The technique follows that of Lipton[36] and Ischia et al.[37] For a detailed consideration of anatomical factors and a meticulous description of the technique, interested readers are referred to Lipton's excellent textbook account.[38] A lateral cervical spinal puncture is made at C1–C2 under radiographic control and image intensification. Myelography with water-soluble dye outlines the anterior surface of the spinal cord, the dentate ligament, and the posterior margin of the theca. The cord is punctured with the electrode anterior to the dentate ligament. Once the spinothalamic tract has been located by electrical stimulation, the lesion is made progressively by radiofrequency current from a Radionic's lesion generator (Radionics, Burlington, MA) until the desired hypalgesia is obtained. Hypalgesia is considered satisfactory when there is loss of appreciation of deep pinprick. This is usually accompanied by loss of temperature sensation on the side of the pain, and Horner's syndrome on the side of the lesion. Failure to achieve a Horner's syndrome is a sign of an incomplete cordotomy and the risk of inadequate pain relief is high.

After surgery, patients have specialized nursing supervision for the first night to monitor respiratory function and oxygen saturation. Under the supervision of physiotherapists, mobilization begins on the day after the procedure. Progressive withdrawal of opioid drugs begins in the immediate postoperative period. The time taken to achieve complete withdrawal depends on the preoperative dose, but discharge from hospital is usually within 7 days.

Percutaneous cordotomy is not a procedure for the "occasional" operator. It requires attention to detail in the preoperative assessment and postoperative care of the patient, gentleness and dexterity in placing the electrode, and a willingness to desist should the patient be distressed or show any evidence of weakness on the side of the lesion.

Because analgesia is achieved some two or three segments below the lesion, which is made at C1–C2, analgesia above C5 will not necessarily be attained. Relief of shoulder pain is therefore unpredictable. Lower segmental pains of unilateral origin will benefit from the procedure.

When the patient has lumbar or sacral segment pain, the cause of the pain must be identified carefully. Many of these patients will already have spread of tumor to the opposite side, even though they report pain on one side only at initial presentation. Relief of really severe pain on one side may "unmask" pain on the other side, but it may be possible to control this with open cordotomy or a lower dose of opioid.

For all of these patients, thorough assessment and appropriate imaging (CT or MRI) will identify those with spread of tumor to the other side or into the spinal epidural space. A myelogram is not necessary and causes unnecessary discomfort for patients already in severe pain. The reticulospinal tract that controls unconscious automatic breathing, as opposed to conscious controlled voluntary breathing, is between the spinothalamic homunculus and the ventral horn and is strictly ipsilateral (Fig. 4.4). Many patients are dependent on the lung on the side of the cordotomy and the neurosurgeon cannot control the spillover of the thermocoagulation current to the reticulospinal tract.[39,40] Such patients are also usually excluded from consideration of cordotomy. Rosomoff et al.[41] and Ischia et al.[42] have emphasized the risks of the bilateral operation. Bilateral percutaneous cervical cordotomies are no longer performed in our unit because of the risk of sleep apnea.

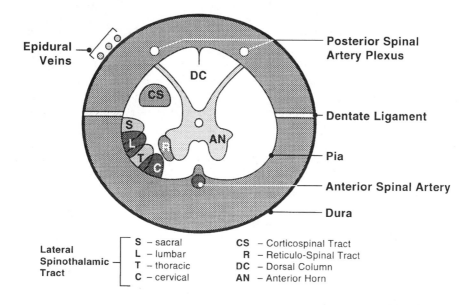

Figure 4.4. The proximity of the reticulospinal tract in cordotomy.

The importance of early referral. Freedom from pain without the need for opioid drugs will mean for the patient maximum improvement in quality of life; this is best enjoyed if the patient is referred early before the disease is far advanced or opioid tolerance has developed. Although effective analgesia can be achieved even when patients are referred late, the limitation of respiratory reserve will make the procedure more hazardous. The stress of an hour-long procedure must be weighed against the benefit for these patients, many of whom can at this stage achieve satisfactory pain relief from intraventricular morphine.

Patients who are referred early and have their pain relieved by percutaneous cervical cordotomy may experience spread to the other side or rostral spread to the axial skeleton. An effort is made to exclude this by appropriate imaging. In the case of spread to the other side, if it is low enough, an open dorsal cordotomy would be done. Patients with secondary deposits in the axial skeleton would be referred for radiation therapy if suitable, or for appropriate hormone therapy or chemotherapy. For diffuse pain, ventriculostomy would be considered for the administration of intraventricular morphine.

It is impossible to predict the long-term prognosis of patients with severe pain associated with cancer. Fading in the density of the block produced by percutaneous cordotomy has not been a problem in those of our patients who have survived for 8, 6, and 5 years. We believe that meticulous attention to detail in the production of the lesion contributes to this.

In patients whose unilateral pain is below the waist, ideally, the induction of hemianalgesia should be restricted to below the innervation of the arm, avoiding the reticulospinal tracts, especially in younger patients. This is attempted in the production of the lesion in the spinal cord and is achieved in about half the suitable patients; but if pain relief can be obtained only by inclusion of the arm and trunk in the area of analgesia, this is accepted. One patient in whom analgesia below T10 was induced for hip and leg pain required a repeat cordotomy 6 years later on the same side for pain developing above the limit of analgesia.

Particular reference needs to be made to patients (148 in our series) suffering from primary lung malignancy, including mesothelioma (an increasing problem). Our experience has paralleled that of Ischia et al.,[35] who state that unilateral percutaneous cordotomy is the only method of controlling, in a stable manner until death, refractory cervicothoracic pain from Pancoast's tumor and from mesothelioma, as well as other unilateral pain of malignancy of lower cervical or upper thoracic origin, or brachial neuropathy caused by radiotherapy (fortunately, rarely seen now). We also agree with Ischia et al.[35] that many of these patients are, regrettably, referred very late, but there is no reason that late diagnosis and referral should preclude satisfactory pain relief by percutaneous cervical cordotomy, provided patients meet the other selection criteria.

Open cordotomy

Open cordotomy produces equally effective pain relief in suitable patients and is practiced in most neurosurgical units. However, if performed at the standard level of T2–T3, pain relief will be only below T5–T6, and this will not control upper trunk or limb pain, which was present in over 50% of our patients. The open operation is a major procedure necessitating general anesthesia and laminectomy. It carries a higher mortality (10%) and morbidity rate in cancer patients.[43] Nonetheless, it still has a place in the relief of neuropathic pain.

Cordotomy: personal experience

In our series of 347 patients who underwent percutaneous cervical cordotomy up to the end of 1995, 186 (53.5%) had neuropathic pain in the arm, shoulder and arm, and arm and chest wall. Of these, 148 (42.7%) suffered from primary lung malignancy (carcinoma 117 or mesothelioma 31). In all of these patients, the pain was too high for open dorsal cordotomy. The other major group was comprised of patients with "malignant psoas syndrome" and lumbosacral plexopathy; but some of these patients had nociceptive pain as well.

Patients' ages ranged from 19 to 90 years, including 14 in the 80- to 90-years group. The greatest number were in the 60- to 70-years group.

Effective pain relief was achieved in 316 patients (91.1%), 30 of them at the second attempt. Eleven patients (3.2%) died in the first postoperative week. One of these was a patient who had undergone the second stage of a bilateral procedure and experienced respiratory arrest on the fifth day. None of the other first-week deaths was considered to be directly related to the procedure. Two patients who developed sleep apnea after the bilateral procedure lived for 2 and 4 months, respectively. No patients suffered persistent hemiplegia. Five had persistent significant hemiparesis, but none was rendered unable to walk. Other complications included persistent urinary retention (4), pathological fracture in analgesic limb (1), burn in analgesic hand (1), and ulcer on analgesic heel (1). Only two patients developed anesthesia dolorosa. This low incidence may be due to the thoroughness of the lesion.

Spinal Opioids

Spinal opioids are never used as the primary method of pain control. Patients are stabilized on oral or subcutaneous medication first. Combined with local anesthesia, spinal opioids offer excellent relief for movement-related pain that is not responsive to reasonable doses of parenteral or oral morphine.

Intrathecal opioid therapy provides very effective relief of pain that is midline, bilateral, or diffuse, particularly when present in the trunk or pelvis.[44] On the other hand, Samuelson and colleagues[45] have shown poor response to epidural morphine in patients with neuropathic pain, certain types of visceral pain, and incident pain.

Intraventricular Morphine

Among the most difficult pain management problems are those associated with advanced head and neck cancer, either primary or metastatic, and those associated with midline, bilateral, or diffuse pain.[46] Some of these patients can have pain relieved by opioids but experience unacceptable side effects, especially drowsiness and confusion. Others, especially those with neuropathic pain, experience only partial relief, if any. If the dose of morphine is increased in the latter patients in an attempt to relieve pain, they will exhibit myoclonic jerks, hyperesthesia, allodynia, and cognitive impairment. Some patients may have these unpleasant side effects lessened by changing from morphine to methadone, although this is not always successful;[47,48] by conversion from the oral to the subcutaneous route or to a combination of morphine and bupivacaine by the epidural route; or simply by reduction in the dose of subcutaneous morphine. In our experience, methadone is not an easy drug to use because of its long and unpredictable half-life, a difficulty compounded in the elderly, who may experience respiratory depression and confusion.

In 1986, we first used ventriculostomy for the percutaneous injection of small doses of morphine into the lateral cerebral ventricle and reported our first 52 cases in 1993.[26] Our experience up to the end of 1995 extended to 136 patients, of whom 107 were suffering from major, unrelieved neurophatic pain. Many had nociceptive or bone pain as well. Table 4.1 lists the principal conditions causing the neuropathic pain, which, under ordinary circumstances, would have been described as "morphine resistant" or "morphine nonresponsive."

The Ommaya reservoir can be inserted under local analgesia—a distinct advantage in patients with head and neck cancer and those in whom respiratory function is already compromised. Only a small incision is required. The technique is suitable for persons of all age groups. The youngest patient was almost 10 years old and the oldest was 82 years. In all patients, pain relief has been greatly improved. Weight-bearing pain in disease of the axial skeleton, while considerably relieved, has required some form of spinal orthosis.

Morphine tolerance has not been a problem. For initial stabilization of pain relief, most patients required 5 mg or less daily, the lowest dose being 0.15 mg. One patient required 15 mg daily (7.5 mg twice daily). In the majority of patients,

Table 4.1. Principal groups of conditions causing neuropathic pain in 107 ventriculostomy patients

Condition	No. of patients
Malignancies of the oropharynx and larynx	15
Advanced primary and secondary squamous cell carcinoma of the neck	7
Cervical plexopathy or nerve root compression from lytic lesions of the cervical spine due to metastases from breast carcinoma (8), miscellaneous (4)	12
Primary lung carcinoma (18) or mesothelioma (9) with cervical plexopathy or chest wall infiltration	27
Lung secondaries infiltrating chest wall from breast carcinoma (3), renal cell carcinoma (3), miscellaneous (5)	11
Lumbar plexopathy ("malignant psoas syndrome") from colonic carcinoma (3), miscellaneous (4)	7
Infiltration of abdominal plexuses (coeliac and hypogastric) from carcinoma of esophagus and gastrointestinal tract	2
Infiltration of pelvic and sacral plexuses from carcinoma of cervix (4), rectum (3), prostate (3), bladder (2), Ewing's sarcoma	13
Lumbar nerve root compression from vertebral secondaries from carcinoma of prostate (2), miscellaneous (3)	5
Canal stenosis with cord compression from vertebral body secondaries from carcinoma of breast, prostate, and kidney	3
Neuralgic pain from skeletal secondaries from carcinoma of prostate	2
Meningeal secondaries from squamous cell carcinoma of lung	1
Neurofibrosarcoma of sacral plexus	1
Recurrence of malignant melanoma of arm with perineural spread	1

the dose remained unchanged from stabilization to death. In some, the dose decreased and in some it increased; the highest dose was 20 mg daily (10 mg twice daily). For most patients, freedom from the unpleasant side effects usually experienced with morphine given by other routes, especially constipation, has been a feature.

Considering that most patients were debilitated, often very ill and immuno-compromised, complications have been minimal. Colonization or infection of the reservoir has occurred in five patients. These can be treated successfully with intraventricular and intravenous vancomycin. In every case, the organism has been staphylococcus epidermidis. Removal of the reservoir is unnecessary. One patient developed postoperative meningitis due to staphylococcus epidermidis when a reservoir was reinserted after the previous one had become blocked and had been removed. Again, the infection was successfully treated with vancomy-cin.

Rigid asepsis is necessary for performing the intraventricular injections. When the patient returns home, injections are given by domiciliary nurses trained in the Pain Center. Family members are not instructed. The domiciliary nurses are already trained in asepsis and when they visit the patient they are able to assess the efficacy of pain relief and other symptoms and provide support to the caregiver. The procedure has now been performed on 170 of our patients.

In a patient suffering from beta-cell lymphoma of the pharynx, who is still alive, the daily dose of intraventricular morphine remained stable at 3 mg for 24 months in spite of the fact that he had in the past been an intravenous diamor-phine user. His disease went into unexpected remission and he was able to be withdrawn from intraventricular morphine and converted to oral methadone without any adverse effects or relapse into addictive behavior during a further 22 months. Among the deceased patients are some who survived 75, 65, 51, and 49 weeks. One patient received over 900 injections into the reservoir.

The use of the intraventricular route for the administration of morphine has provided our research group with the opportunity to study the relative concentrations of morphine and its metabolites, morphine-3-glucuronide and morphine-6-glucuronide, in plasma and cerebrospinal fluid (CSF).[49] This may lead to an explanation for the effectiveness of intraventricular morphine in neuropathic pain. Results so far reveal that after chronic oral or subcutaneous administration of morphine, the CSF concentration of M3G is in the range of 2 to 10 times that of morphine and 1 to 5 times that of M6G. Occasionally, no M6G is found in the CSF. The CSF concentration of morphine is highly variable in the range of 0.05 to 1 times plasma concentration.

With the administration of a small intraventricular dose of morphine, the CSF concentration of morphine, when measured 24 hours later (i.e., before the next dose), increases 100-fold compared with the concentration found immediately pre-ventriculostomy. There is a simultaneous 10- to 15-fold decrease in the M3G concentration, and at this stage there is no M6G detectable in the CSF, despite its presence in the plasma. Subsequent CSF concentrations of M3G remain relatively constant for the duration of treatment. Once the intraventricular dose of morphine is stabilized, the CSF concentration of morphine is also stable.

These data suggest that no pain is nonresponsive to morphine if the morphine is delivered in a sufficiently high concentration to the supraspinal receptors adjacent to the lateral ventricle, in the absence of very high CSF levels of M3G. A simple case history illustrates the complications of high-dose subcutaneous morphine in a patient with mesothelioma, and the efficacy of intraventricular morphine.

F.D., a 69-year-old male, was referred to the Pain Center by a respiratory physician in a relatively large peripheral city. Mesothelioma of the left chest had been diagnosed 8 months previously when he presented with severe chest wall pain. His pain had been made much worse by pleurectomy 6 months before presentation to the Pain Center and had assumed a neuropathic character.

At that time, he was eminently suitable for right percutaneous cervical cordotomy, but he decided to "consider and let us know." Twelve months later he was referred to the Royal Brisbane Hospital as an urgent admission. He was confused and restless with myoclonic jerks and clutching at the bed clothes. Allodynia of the left chest wall necessitated the use of a bed cradle as he could not tolerate contact with the bed clothes. He was receiving 4600 mg of morphine daily by subcutaneous infusion.

Imaging showed gross extension of the mesothelioma with encasement of the left chest wall and hemidiaphragm and encroachment on the mediastinum. His esophagus was encased and dilated above the obstruction. His poor respiratory function was indicated by an arterial oxygen tension of 6.65 kPa and an arterial carbon dioxide tension of 7.45 kPa. He was by this time unsuitable for percutaneous cervical cordotomy.

The dose of morphine was reduced gradually and his mental state cleared. After 10 days, the morphine had been reduced to 1100 mg and he was competent to agree to ventriculostomy. Ventriculostomy was performed and his pain was controlled completely for 8 weeks with 3 mg morphine daily by intraventricular injection. During his last 48 hours, he complained of shortness of breath and showed signs of superior vena caval obstruction. He was kept comfortable on 10 mg morphine and 2 mg midazolam administered by subcutaneous infusion over 24 hours.

F.D. had neuropathic pain at the time of the original referral. This had been made worse by pleurectomy. The excitatory side effects and allodynia were exacerbated by the ever-increasing doses of morphine administered by continuous subcutaneous infusion. Laboratory studies confirmed the very high ratio of M3G to morphine in his CSF before ventriculostomy and the subsequent dramatic reversal (Table 4.2). This patient was one of those in whom no M6G was found in the CSF.

Experience with the use of intraventricular morphine suggests the following:

1. Effective pain relief can be provided for patients with neuropathic cancer pain that has not been controlled adequately with standard pharmacological techniques and is unsuitable for percutaneous cordotomy.

Table 4.2. CSF concentrations in nM

Day	M3G	Morphine	M6G
0	1752	1353	0
1	512	6109	0
2	156	18933	0
3	199	20274	0
5	140	18902	0
6	50	18439	0
10	?	20893	0

2. Other patients with advanced cancer whose pain is difficult to relieve may also benefit from this technique.
3. The approach is suitable for patients of all ages.
4. The reservoir can be inserted under local analgesia with minimum operative risk.
5. A short prognosis is not a contraindication.
6. Tolerance has not been a problem, but some patients may request supplemental oral analgesics, and one drug-dependent patient has proved difficult to manage.
7. Rigid asepsis is essential to prevent infection.
8. The very small dose of morphine needed to provide effective pain relief lessens the incidence and severity of side effects, especially drowsiness and constipation.
9. Laboratory studies have provided useful new information about morphine and its metabolites in the CSF. Further collaborative work is needed.

Acknowledgments

The research on morphine and its metabolites in plasma and CSF would not be possible without the input from the scientists in our research group from the Department of Pharmacy, University of Queensland, led by Dr. Maree Smith, Ph.D.

References

1. Foley KM. The treatment of cancer pain. *N Engl J Med* 1985; 313:84–95.
2. Bowsher D. Neurogenic pain syndromes and their management. *Br Med Bull* 1991; 47:644–666.

3. Portenoy RK. Issues in the management of neuropathic pain. In: Basbaum AI, Besson JM, eds. *Towards a New Pharmacotherapy of Pain.* Chichester: John Wiley and Sons, 1991:393.

4. Perl E. Causalgia: sympathetically aggravated chronic pain from damaged nerves. *Pain Clin Updates.* International Association for the Study of Pain. 1993; 1:1–4.

5. Colding A. The effect of regional sympathetic blocks in the treatment of herpes zoster. *Acta Anaesthesiol Scand* 1969; 13:133–141.

6. Crooks RJ, Bell AR, Fiddian AP. Treatment of shingles and postherpetic neuralgia. *Br Med J* 1989; 299:392–393.

7. Dejgard A, Petersen P, Kastrup J. Mexiletine for treatment of chronic painful diabetic neuropathy. *Lancet* 1988; 1:9–11.

8. Rosenak S. Paravertebral blocks for the treatment of herpes zoster. *NY State J Med* 1956; 56:2684.

9. Colding A. Treatment of pain: organisation of a pain clinic. Treatment of acute herpes zoster. *Proc R Soc Med* 1973; 66:541–543.

10. Winnie AP. Acute herpes zoster and postherpetic neuralgia. Pathophysiology and treatment. In: Winnie AP, Waldman SD, eds. *Interventional Pain Management— Principles and Current Management.* San Antonio: Dannemiller Memorial Educational Foundation; 1993; 106:1–13.

11. Mitchell SW. *Injuries of Nerves and Their Consequence.* Philadelphia: J.B. Lippincott, 1872.

12. Le Riche R. *La Chirurgie de la Douleur.* Paris: Masson et Cie, 1949.

13. Campbell JN, Raja SN, Selig DF, Selzberg AJ, Meyer RA. Diagnosis and management of sympathetically maintained pain. In: Fields HJ, Lieberkind JC, eds. *Pharmacological Approaches to the Treatment of Pain: New Concepts and Critical Issues.* Seattle: IASP Press; 1994:85–97.

14. Charlton JE. The management of sympathetic pain. *Br Med Bull* 1991; 47:601–618.

15. Arner S. Intravenous phentolamine test. Diagnostic and prognostic use in reflex sympathetic dystrophy. *Pain* 1991; 46:17–22.

16. Davis KD, Treede RD, Raja SN, Meyer RA, Campbell JN. Topical application of clonidine relieves hyperalgesia in patients with sympathetically maintained pain. *Pain* 1991; 47:309–371.

17. Kirkpatrick AF, Derasari M. Transdermal clonidine: treating reflex sympathetic dystrophy (Letter). *Reg Anaesth* 1993; 18:140–141.

18. Plancarte R, Velazquez R, Patt RB. Neurolytic block of the sympathetic axis. In: Patt RB, ed. *Cancer Pain.* Philadelphia: J.B. Lippincott; 1993:377–425.

19. Sherman RA, Sherma CJ, Parker L. Chronic phantom and stump pain among American veterans. Results of a survey. *Pain* 1984; 18:83.

20. Bach F, Jensen TS, Kastrup T, Stigsby B, Dejgard A. The effect of intravenous lignocaine on nociceptive processing in diabetic neuropathy. *Pain* 1990; 40:29–34.

21. Bach S, Noreng MF, Tjellden NU. Phantom limb pain in amputees during first twelve months following limb amputation after lumbar epidural blockade. *Pain* 1988; 33:297–302.

22. Dwyer B, Gibb D. Chronic pain and neurolytic neural blockade. In: Cousins MJ, Bridenbaugh PO, eds. *Neural Blockade in Clinical Anaesthesia and Management of Pain.* 1st ed. Philadelphia: J.B. Lippincott; 1988:637–650.

23. Patt RB. Peripheral neurolysis and the management of cancer pain. In: Patt RB, ed. *Cancer Pain.* Philadelphia: J.B. Lippincott; 1993:359–376.

24. Stuart G, Cramond T. Role of percutaneous cervical cordotomy for pain of malignant origin. *Med J Aust* 1993; 158:667–670.

25. Dwyer B. Treatment of pain of carcinoma of the tongue and floor of mouth. *Anaesth Intensive Care* 1972; 1:59–61.

26. Cramond T, Stuart G. Intraventricular morphine for intractable pain of advanced cancer. *J Pain Symptom Manage* 1993; 8:465–473.

27. Doyle D. Nerve blocks in advanced cancer. *Practitioner* 1982; 226:539–544.

28. Moore DC, Bush WH, Burnett LL. Celiac plexus block: a roentgenographic anatomic study of technique and spread of solution in patients and corpses. *Anesth Analg* 1981; 60:369–379.

29. Kappis M. Die Antshesierung der Nervus splanchnicus. *Zenralbl Chir* 1918; 45:709.

30. Moore DC. Regional Block. *A Handbook of Use in Clinical Practice of Medicine and Surgery.* 1st ed. Springfield IL: Charles C Thomas, 1965.

31. Singer RC. An improved technique for alcohol neurolysis of the coeliac plexus. *Anesthesiology* 1982; 56:137–141.

32. Boas RA. Sympathetic blocks in clinical practice. *Int Anesthesiol Clin* 1978; 16:149–182.

33. Plancarte R, Amescua C, Patt RB, Aldrete JA. Superior hypogastric plexus block for pelvic cancer pain. *Anesthesiology* 1990; 73:236–239.

34. Plancarte R, Amescua C, Patt RB, Allenby S. Presacral blockade of the ganglion of Walther (ganglion impar). *Anesthesiology* 1990; 73 (Supplement):Abstract A 751.

35. Ischia S, Ischia A, Luzzani A, Toscano D, Steele A. Results up to death in the treatment of persistent cervico-thoracic (Pancoast) and thoracic malignant pain by unilateral percutaneous cervical cordotomy. *Pain* 1985; 21:339–355.

36. Lipton S. Percutaneous electrical cordotomy in the relief of intractable pain. *BMJ* 1968; 2:210–212.

37. Ischia S, Luzzani A, Maffezzolli GF, Pacini L, Nicolini F. Percutaneous cordotomy: technical considerations and results in 400 treated cases. In: Rezzi R, Vissentin M, eds. *Pain Therapy.* Amsterdam: Elsevier Biomedical Press; 1983:367–379.

38. Lipton S. Percutaneous cervical cordotomy and pituitary injection of alcohol. In: Swerdlow M, ed. *Relief of Intractable Pain.* 3rd ed. Amsterdam: Elsevier Science Publishers; 1983:267–304.

39. Nathan PW. The descending respiratory pathway in man. *J Neurol Neurosurg Psychiatry* 1963;26:487–499.

40. Hitchcock E, Leece B. Somatotropic representation of the respiratory pathways in the spinal cord of man. *J Neurosurg* 1967; 27:320–329.

41. Rosomoff HL. Bilateral percutaneous cervical radio-frequency cordotomy. *J Neurosurg* 1969; 31:41–46.

42. Ischia S, Luzzani A, Ischia A, Maffezzoli G. Bilateral percutaneous cervical cordotomy: immediate and long term results in 36 patients with neoplastic disease. *J Neurol Neurosurg Psychiatry* 1984; 47:141–147.

43. Rosomoff HL, Carroll F, Brown J, Sheptak P. Percutaneous radiofrequency cervical cordotomy technique. *J Neurosurg* 1965; 23:639–644.

44. Wang JK. Intrathecal morphine for intractable pain secondary to cancer of the pelvic organs. *Pain* 1985; 21:99–102.

45. Samuellson H, Malmberg F, Eriksson M, Hedner T. Outcomes of epidural morphine treatment in cancer pain: nine years of clinical experience. *J Pain Symptom Manage* 1995; 10:(2):105–112.

46. Raj PP, Phero JC. Pain control in cancer of head and neck. In: Thawley SE, Pauje WR, eds. *Comprehensive Management of Head and Neck Tumors.* Philadelphia: W.B. Saunders; 1987:42–68.
47. Ettinger DS, Vitale PJ, Trump DL. Important clinical pharmacological considerations in the use of methadone in cancer patients. *Cancer Treat Rep* 1979; 63:457–459.
48. Foley KM. Current controversies in opioid therapy. In: Foley KM, Inturrissi CE, eds. *Advances in Pain Research and Therapy,* Vol 8. New York: Raven Press; 1986:3–11.
49. Cramond T, Wright AWE, Stuart GS, Smith M. Plasma and CSF concentrations of morphine, M3G and M6G in cancer patients receiving morphine by the intracerebroventricular route. In: *Abstracts of 7th World Congress on Pain.* Seattle: IASP Publications; 1993:531–532.

II

CACHEXIA/ANOREXIA

Introduction: Anorexia:
An Evolving Understanding

Anorexia is a frequent and devastating symptom in patients with advanced cancer.[1,2] It occurs more frequently in patients having solid participating tumors than in those having hematological malignancies and in patients with severe depression.[3]

During the early 1980s, anorexia was suspected to be one of the main mechanisms for cancer-induced malnutrition. Tumor by-products were considered responsible for anorexia and decreased food intake, which resulted in progressive weight loss.[2-4] This belief prompted a number of clinical trials of aggressive enteral and parental nutrition in cancer patients.[2,5] These studies were overwhelmingly disappointing. Aggressive nutrition treatment was found to have no significant impact on survival, response to antineoplastic therapy, or toxicity of antineoplastic treatments, and it had only minimal effects on the overall nutritional status of cancer patients.[2,5]

These studies led to the emerging view of cancer cachexia as resulting from major metabolic abnormalities. Tumor by-products and host cytokines were capable of causing massive lipolysis and major metabolic abnormalities that did not allow for the appropriate utilization of energy. Anorexia was considered one of the results of these metabolic abnormalities, rather than the cause of malnutrition. Therefore, anorexia remained a relatively uninteresting phenomenon for researchers on cancer cachexia. However, this symptom remained as one of the more frequent and distressing symptoms for cancer patients and their families.

During recent years, a number of researchers have focused on anorexia as a symptom similar to pain, nausea, or dyspnea. As a result, clinical trials have been designed that focus on anorexia and quality-of-life constructs as the main outcomes instead of the more traditional nutritional outcomes. A number of pharmacological interventions including corticosteroids and megestrol acetate have been found to be effective in the management of anorexia.[6,7] Other drugs, including cannabinoid derivatives or melatonin, are currently entering clinical trials.

These studies are important because safe and effective drugs for the management of anorexia are badly needed. However, perhaps the main contribution of these clinical trials has been the recognition that for terminally ill cancer patients, the traditional "objective" outcomes, such as response to antineoplastic therapies or nutritional status, are irrelevant. The indication for therapeutic interventions in these patients will be based on the ability of those interventions to significantly modify "subjective" outcomes such as the intensity of different symptoms, physical and psychosocial function, and overall quality of life.

References

1. Dunlop R. Clinical epidemiology of cancer cachexia. In: Bruera E, Higginson I, eds. *Cachexia–Anorexia in Cancer Patients.* Oxford: Oxford University Press; 1996:76–82.
2. Bruera E, MacDonald RN. Nutrition in cancer patients: an update and review of our experience. *J Pain Symptom Manage* 1988; 3:133–140.
3. Bruera E, Roca E, Carraro S. Association between malnutrition and caloric intake, emesis, psychological depression, glucose taste and tumor mass. *Cancer Treat Rep* 1984; 68:873–876.
4. Bruera E. Clinical management of cachexia and anorexia in patients with advanced cancer. *Oncology* 1992; 49(Suppl 2):35–42.
5. Vigano A, Bruera E. Enteral and parenteral nutrition in cancer patients. In: Bruera E, Higginson I, eds. *Cachexia–Anorexia in Cancer Patients.* Oxford: Oxford University Press; 1996:110–127.
6. Fainsinger R. Pharmacological approach to cancer anorexia and cachexia. In: Bruera E, Higginson I, eds. *Cachexia–Anorexia in Cancer Patients.* Oxford: Oxford University Press; 1996:128–140.
7. Bruera E, Roca E, Cedaro L, Carraro S, Chacon R. Action of oral methylprednisolone in terminal cancer patients: a prospective randomized double-blind study. *Cancer Treat Rep* 1985;69:751–754.

5

Prevalence and Pathophysiology of Cancer Cachexia

GRACE MA AND H. RICHARD ALEXANDER

The word "cachexia," descriptive of emaciative disease states, comes from the Greek words "kakos" meaning bad, and "hexis," meaning condition. Cancer cachexia is a complex metabolic syndrome characterized clinically by progressive, involuntary weight loss, which, if left unchecked, can ultimately lead to death of the host. The precise mechanism by which a cancer-bearing patient develops anorexia leading to body compositional changes associated with a severely malnourished state remains largely unknown. This syndrome represents an array of nutritional abnormalities found in a majority of cancer patients at some point in their illness, and includes the clinical features associated with the progressive growth of a cancer, including abnormalities of carbohydrate, fat, protein, and energy metabolism.

Cancer cachexia develops in a majority of patients with advanced malignancy, has a negative impact on the ability of patients to undergo cancer treatment,[1,2] and is a major contributing cause of death in up to 50% of these patients.[1] Patients who are malnourished on the basis of cachexia cannot tolerate effective therapy and may be more prone to the adverse effects of anticancer treatments such as surgery, chemotherapy, and radiation therapy. Attempts at replenishment of the cachectic patient with enteral or parenteral nutrition has been effective in interrupting or reversing some of the metabolic sequelae of advancing malignancy.[3-6] However, although total parenteral nutrition appears to decrease operative morbidity and mortality in some groups of patients[7] and to benefit patients undergoing high-dose chemotherapy and bone-marrow transplant,[8] it has not been shown to improve survival in other groups of cancer patients.[9-12] Treatment strategies utilizing insulin or progestational agents such as megestrol acetate have been shown to increase appetite and restore weight gain, and hydrazine sulphate, a drug which inhibits hepatic gluconeogenesis, has been used to ameliorate the accelerated gluconeogenesis that is well characterized in cancer cachexia. The clinical efficacy of these approaches has not been established conclusively, although preliminary results in experimental settings and in cancer patients appear promising.[13-17] Better understanding of the mechanisms of cachexia should improve the ability to support these patients during anticancer treatment.

For over half a century, the complex metabolic changes that occur in tumor-bearing laboratory animals and in patients with cancer have been the focus of extensive studies. The major host deficit is a negative energy balance, in which food intake is inappropriately less than energy output such that the net effect is loss of lean body mass.[2,18] Although some suggest that these changes associated with cancer cachexia merely represent the increased metabolic and nutritional demands of the tumor itself,[19-22] it has become increasingly clear that the host response to the tumor-bearing state is more complex. Recently, there has been much interest in the role of endogenously produced cytokines, specifically, tumor necrosis factor (TNF), interleukin-1 (IL-1), interleukin-6 (IL-6), leukemia inhibitory factor (LIF), and interferon gamma (IFN-γ), in the development of cancer cachexia.[23-27]

This chapter will briefly review the prevalence of cancer cachexia, the pathophysiology, and the predominant host changes associated with the tumor-bearing state; discuss prevailing theories of the causes and mechanisms of these changes; and examine the role of the endogenous cytokines involved.

Prevalence

Cachexia is so common in progressive and end-stage cancer that its true incidence is difficult to quantitate. Although the cachectic changes associated with progressive tumor growth can be carefully observed and quantified in laboratory models, parallel studies in humans are not possible. In rats bearing an experimental sarcoma, it was clear that weight loss was dependent on the presence of tumor, because following recovery from tumor resection, surviving animals began to eat normally and regained all the weight which they had lost.[28,29] In addition, similar to the finding that weight loss is associated with decreased survival following cancer therapy in humans[1] (Table 5.1), approximately 50% of these cachectic rats that had experienced tumor-induced weight loss failed to survive tumor resection[28] or had a poorer response to doxorubicin chemotherapy.[30] Therefore, studies in rats suggest that tumor-associated weight loss is dependent on the presence of tumor and that the animals with weight loss have a poorer response to antitumor therapy. Similarly, in 35 patients who underwent surgical resection, adjuvant chemotherapy, and radiation therapy for soft-tissue sarcomas of the head, neck, and trunk, anticancer treatment caused significant weight loss in all patients.[31] However, patients in whom sarcomas did not recur showed little long-term nutritional morbidity after completion of this aggressive regimen; but, patients whose sarcomas recurred showed severe nutritional morbidity and progressive

Table 5.1. Effect of weight loss on survival

	Median survival (weeks)		
Tumor type	*No weight loss*	*Weight loss*°	*P value*[†]
Favorable non-Hodgkin's lymphoma	‡	138	<0.01
Breast	70	45	<0.01
Acute nonlymphocytic leukemia	8	4	N.S.
Sarcoma	46	25	<0.01
Unfavorable non-Hodgkin's leukemia	107	55	<0.01
Colon	43	21	<0.01
Prostate	46	24	<0.05
Lung, small cell	34	27	<0.05
Lung, non-small cell	20	14	<0.01
Pancreas	14	12	N.S.
Nonmeasurable gastric	41	27	<0.05
Measurable gastric	18	16	N.S.

Source: Reproduced with permission from DeWys et al.[1]
°All categories of weight loss (0–5%, 5%–10%, and 10%) have been combined.
[†]The P values refer to a test of the hypothesis that the entire survival curves are identical, not merely a test of the medians. However, in all disease sites under study, the median is a representative indicator of the survival distribution, and consequently, its use as a summary statistic is acceptable.
[‡]Only 20 of 199 patients have died, so median survival cannot be estimated. However, the observed rate of failure predicts that the survival will be significantly longer than for the group with weight loss.

weight loss. Anorexia leading to profound weight loss and cachexia has been shown to be the common pathway to death during progressive malignancy in many experimental models. Some experimental tumors produce cachexia at very small tumor volumes, illustrating that tumors have varying abilities to cause cachexia. This phenomenon is also seen in cancer patients with different tumor histologies.

Older data on condition at death and mortality rates from various kinds of cancer estimated that approximately two-thirds of people who die of cancer are cachectic at the time of death,[32] with incidence varying with cancer type. Table 5.2 summarizes the prevalence of symptoms in 275 consecutive patients with advanced cancer.[33] Anorexia was present in 85% of these patients, this symptom being more prevalent than pain and second only to asthenia. When one considers the components of cachexia (relative hypophagia, weakness, and weight loss), the incidence in treated cancer patients approaches 100%. This is because one cannot clearly separate the cachectic component of treatment from disease; the two factors go hand in hand. For example, in a study by Kinsella et al., patients who underwent radiotherapy with or without surgery for pelvic tumors often developed weight loss during and following treatment.[34] In addition, many

Table 5.2. Prevalence of symptoms in 275 consecutive advanced cancer patients

Symptom	Prevalence %	95% Confidence interval
Asthenia	90	81–100
Anorexia	85	78–92
Pain	76	62–85
Nausea	68	61–75
Constipation	65	40–80
Sedation-confusion	60	40–75
Dyspnea	12	8–16

Source: Reproduced with permission from Bruera.[33]

chemotherapeutic agents cause severe nausea, vomiting, and anorexia. However, these side effects usually resolve after each cycle of chemotherapy and do not necessarily result in weight loss. Drugs that cause desquamative mucositis lead to a chronic reduction in food intake and more significant weight loss.

The frequency of weight loss in cancer patients derived from a study by the Eastern Cooperative Oncology Group is listed in Table 5.3. In over 3000 patients studied, the average percentage of cancer patients with no weight loss was 46%.[1] The remainder had lost weight, and 32% had lost greater than 5% of their preillness weight. Gastric and pancreatic cancer patients had lost the greatest amount of weight, probably because the organ in which the cancer originated was directly involved with alimentation. Non-small-cell and small-cell lung cancer patients also had a high percentage of weight loss despite their generally small tumor burdens which do not affect their ability to aliment themselves. In these cases, weight loss is probably secondary to a systemic effect of the tumor.[1] This same study carefully documented the effect of weight loss on subsequent survival with chemotherapy (Table 5.4). In all cancer patient groups studied except patients with leukemia and pancreatic and measurable gastric cancer, the median survival was significantly shorter in the patients with weight loss compared with the patients with no weight loss.[1] These findings suggested that weight loss, a measure of cachexia, affected the patients' ability to respond to anticancer treatment and ultimately affected their outcome from cancer treatment.

Other studies have documented the incidence of malnutrition in cancer patients undergoing major surgery. Buzby et al.[35,36] used a prognostic nutritional index (PNI) (a linear regression model relying on serum albumin measurements to predict malnutrition and operative risk) and showed that 58% (92 of 159) of cancer patients undergoing major surgical procedures had evidence of severe malnutrition. However, PNI may not accurately or specifically reflect nutritional status since it relies heavily on serum albumin measurements and delayed cutaneous hyposensitivity, both indicators of degree of illness. In other words, PNI

Table 5.3. Frequency of weight loss in cancer patients

Tumor type	Patients (no.)	Weight loss in the previous 6 months (%)[a]			
		0	0–5	5–10	>10
Favorable non-Hodgkin's lymphoma[b]	290	69	14	8	10
Breast	289	64	22	8	6
Acute nonlymphocytic leukemia	129	61	27	8	4
Sarcoma	189	60	21	11	
Unfavorable non-Hodgkin's lymphoma[c]	311	52	20	13	15
Colon	307	46	26	14	14
Prostate	78	44	28	18	10
Lung, small cell	436	43	23	20	14
Lung, non-small cell	590	39	25	21	15
Pancreas[d]	111	17	29	28	26
Nonmeasurable gastric	179	17	21	32	30
Measurable gastric	138	13	20	29	38

Reproduced with permission from Dewys et al.[1]

[a] Data shown are percentage of line total in each weight loss category.

[b] The favorable non-Hodgkin's lymphoma protocol includes nodular lymphocytic well differentiated, nodular lymphocytic poorly differentiated, nodular lymphocytic poorly differentiated, nodular mixed, nodular histioctic, and diffuse lymphocytic well differentiated.

[c] The unfavorable non-Hodgkin's lymphoma protocol includes diffuse lymphocytic poorly differentiated, diffuse mixed, diffuse histiocytic, diffuse undifferentiated, and mycosis fungoides.

[d] Data for pancreatic cancer are weight loss in previous 2 months.

may indicate surgical morbidity or mortality that is totally unrelated to patient nutrition.

Nixon et al.[37] surveyed 84 hospitalized cancer patients at Emory University and found a nearly universal prevalence of protein-calorie undernutrition in patients with advanced cancer. Malnutrition was demonstrated by loss of adipose tissue, visceral protein, and skeletal muscle, which varied from patient to patient. Anthropometric measurements were used to quantitate the composition of host weight loss. Of the patients, 88% had a creatinine-to-height ratio <80% of standard, and 42% had abnormal triceps skin fold measurements. In this study, the degree of malnutrition significantly correlated with survival, with the highest mortality rate found in patients who had a creatinine-to-height ratio <60% of standard, albumin ≤3.5 g/dl, or triceps skin fold thickness <60% of standard.[37]

Although the true prevalence of cancer cachexia is difficult to determine, these studies suggest that cancer cachexia, including asthenia, weight loss, and anorexia, is present in approximately 50% of cancer patients during treatment[1]

Table 5.4. Metabolic abnormalities in experimental and human cancer cachexi

Metabolic component	Parameter	Effect
Lipid	Body lipid mass	Decreased
	Lipoprotein lipase activity	Decreased
	Fat synthesis	Decreased
	Fat breakdown	Increased
	Serum lipid levels	Increased
	Serum triglyceride levels	Increased
Water	Total body water	Increased
Protein	Body muscle mass	Decreased
	Skeletal protein synthesis	Decreased
	Skeletal protein breakdown	Increased
	Liver protein synthesis	Increased
	Whole body protein synthesis	Increased
	Nitrogen balance	Decreased
Carbohydrate	Body glycogen mass	Decreased
	Body glucose consumption	Increased
	Glucose production	Increased
	Insulin effects	Blunted
	Cori's cycle	Increased
Energy	Energy expenditure	Increased/decreased
	Energy balance	Negative
	Energy stores	Decreased

Source: Reproduced with permission from Langstein and Norton.[45]

and increases to nearly 100% as the disease progresses.[31] If there are nutritional complications of cancer treatment, these complications cease with the cessation of treatment, but if the tumor progresses or recurs, the nutritional debility will progress similarly.[31] Cachexia appears to have a negative impact on the outcome of therapy and its severity is a biologic predictor of survival.

Manifestations of Cancer Cachexia

Anorexia and weight loss

Declining food intake and tumor–host interactions result in an imbalance in body homeostatic mechanisms such that energy intake falls short of energy expenditure. If the energy and substrate requirements of the organism are not met, the negative energy balance results in loss of adipose tissue and protein mass, which eventually leads to death of the patient. The precise etiology of this anorexia or relative hypophagia, although not completely understood, is probably multifactorial[38] (Fig. 5.1). There may be alterations in food perception, including taste and smell, that result in decreased food intake,[2,19] or a mechanical gastrointestinal obstruction, such as a large malignant tumor in the aerodigestive tract, that may make the ingestion of adequate nutrients impossible. Vigorous anticancer treatment in the form of chemotherapy, radiation therapy, immunotherapy, or surgery may be associated with varying degrees of nausea, vomiting, anorexia, and diminished food intake.[2,39,40] Psychologic causes including depression may also reduce feeding. Learned food aversions can develop if certain types of food are given just prior to anticancer treatment, and these will also contribute to anorexia.[41] DeWys et al. found that tumors of different histological types cause varying degrees of anorexia and/or cachexia.[1] Whereas patients with lung carcinoma may have marked anorexia and weight loss at a relatively early stage of disease, breast cancer patients do not reduce their food intake (unless as a result of therapy) until a very advanced stage. This suggests that different circulating factors produced either by the tumor (such as bombesin, secreted by oat cell carcinomas) or by the host (such as cytokines) in response to the tumor may cause the diminished

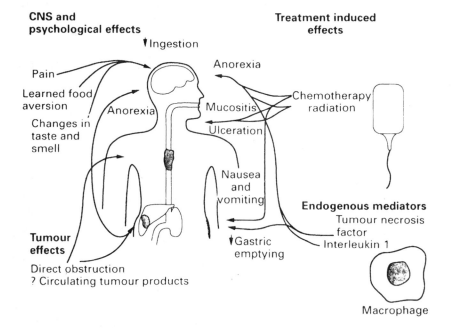

Figure 5.1. Multifactorial aetiology of cancer anorexia. The figure demonstrates four different factors that influence the food intake of cancer patients. (Reproduced with permission from Alexander, HR. *Oxford Textbook of Palliative Medicine,* 1993, p. 318.)

appetite/anorexia commonly observed with some types of malignancy. Therefore, reduced food intake is central to the condition of cancer cachexia and may be mediated by a direct effect of either tumor- or host-derived factors. In addition, the physical and psychologic consequences of either tumor or antitumor therapy may also exacerbate anorectic effects.[2,40,42]

Alterations in host metabolism

Patients with cancer cachexia often demonstrate accelerated mobilization and oxidation of energy substrates and loss of body proteins.[43] In the 1920s, Cori and Cori observed that the venous effluent from a chick wing bearing a sarcoma had decreased concentrations of glucose and elevated levels of lactate compared with the contralateral nontumor-bearing wing.[44] This suggested that the sarcoma was using glucose and producing large amounts of lactic acid. Since that sentinel observation, the metabolic abnormalities present in tumor-bearing laboratory animals and cancer patients have been studied in detail. Some of these metabolic abnormalities of cancer cachexia are listed in Table 5.4.[45] The failure of cachetic patients to gain lean body mass despite seemingly adequate nutritional support is related to these widespread metabolic abnormalities. In general, despite anorexia and declining food intake, the cancer-bearing host usually has evidence of accelerated catabolism, with either normal[46] or increased energy expenditure[47-50] and mobilization of peripheral protein and lipid stores with augmented liver gluconeogenesis.[51-56] This may provide substrate and nutrients for the host to combat the tumor or it may provide nutrients for a metabolically active tumor. Specific metabolic alterations can also be detected in the host at sites remote from the tumor and occur in the presence of a very small tumor burden,[57] suggesting that either the host or the tumor produces circulating substances that induce the metabolic alterations described. Further support that the metabolic sequelae of cancer cachexia may be mediated via the host production of humoral factors is given by the finding that patients with different types of cancer all suffer similar metabolic derangements.

The cachectic syndrome exhibited by cancer patients demonstrates numerous metabolic perturbations involving overall energy expenditure as well as alterations in glucose, protein, and lipid metabolism. These changes are unlike the metabolism of starvation and are more closely related to the metabolic picture of severe trauma and sepsis.[43] Forced feeding, paired feeding, and caloric restriction experiments in tumor-bearing animals showed that a decreased food intake alone could not entirely account for progressive weight loss.[38] Likewise, cachectic patients will continue to lose weight even when aggressive nutritional supplementation is used to provide adequate caloric intake. In one study, head and neck cancer patients were fed via continuous enteral alimentation under metabolic ward conditions and failed to gain significant amounts of weight.[58] Early trials in cachectic patients using nutritional supplementation in the form of total parenteral nutrition (TPN) suggested a clinical benefit.[59]

However, provision of excess calories alone did not appear to change median survival in patients with advanced cancer and many patients either maintained body weight or lost weight while receiving calories that would be predicted to result in weight gain.[60] Although TPN has decreased operative mortality and morbidity in patients with cancer,[7] it does not improve overall survival in any group studied.[9,10]

The literature regarding energy expenditure in cancer patients is contradictory, with some patients demonstrating hypermetabolism and some demonstrating hypometabolism. Resting energy expenditure (REE) has been measured in cancer patients by many different investigators in an attempt to investigate this phenomenon. Hyltander et al. measured REE in 106 cancer patients and compared them with 96 noncancer-bearing controls, finding that the cancer patients had an elevated REE compared with both weight-losing and weight-stable controls.[61] Falconer et al. determined that in 21 cachectic patients with pancreatic cancer, at least a component of weight loss was due to increased REE.[50] Despite these perceived differences, other investigators have demonstrated that these differences are abolished when levels are corrected for measurements of lean body mass.[46] In a study of patients with nonmetastatic primary sarcomas, REE was significantly higher in the sarcoma patients than in controls, even when corrected for lean body mass.[48]

This pattern of elevated energy expenditure in the face of anorexia and diminished caloric intake is one of the key features that distinguishes the cachectic syndrome from starvation alone. Healthy individuals, when confronted with reduced caloric consumption, adapt their metabolic profile so that overall energy expenditure is diminished. Body lipids become the preferential metabolic substrate, with relative preservation of lean muscle until late in the course of starvation.

Although patients with advanced cancer commonly demonstrate hypermetabolism, this abnormality is not invariably present in all cancer patients with weight loss. In a report of 200 patients with a variety of tumors, 33% had an increase in energy expenditure but almost the same number of patients demonstrated hypometabolism.[62] Differences also appear to exist between different types of malignancies. Patients with small-cell lung cancer have increased REE compared with healthy controls, but patients with colon cancer demonstrate no significant differences from control.[63] Other tumors that have been associated with hypermetabolism include sarcomas, leukemias, and bronchial carcinomas, whereas gastrointestinal tumors have been associated with decreased energy expenditure.[64] Any increase in energy metabolism is important in anorectic subjects since it accelerates weight loss. Some reports have demonstrated reduced energy expenditure in hypermetabolic cancer patients after successful antineoplastic treatment,[65] suggesting that the tumor itself is capable of increasing the metabolic rate. However, it is unlikely that the tumor itself accounts for the entire increase in energy expenditure since the tumor usually accounts for less than 5% of total body mass. A more likely explanation is the release of endogenous mediators that alter energy metabolism in the host.[66]

Causes of Cancer Cachexia

Carbohydrate metabolism

Repeated clinical and experimental observations have documented abnormal carbohydrate metabolism in cancer patients and tumor-bearing laboratory animals,[52,60,68–74] as listed in Table 5.4. Several investigators have noted increased rates of hepatic glucose production in cancer patients with weight loss. Douglas and Shaw[75] demonstrated that this increase was dependent on the tumor mass and associated with increased rates of gluconeogenesis. Hepatic gluconeogenesis via de novo production from amino acids and recycling from lactate has been measured in rats by radiolabeled tracer studies.[52,68,76,77] The rates of gluconeogenesis and glucose turnover are significantly increased in tumor-bearing animals as compared with control animals. Tumor burden also appeared to play a role, with higher rates of Cori cycling in rats with large tumor burdens compared with nontumor-bearing controls or rats with small tumor burdens.[78] However, decreased levels of serum glucose have been detected even in animals with small tumors, with levels declining as tumor burden increased.[77,79]

Serum levels of glucose were decreased even in the presence of increased gluconeogenesis and increased Cori cycle activity,[52,77] suggesting accelerated whole-body protein catabolism. This effect was not secondary to elevated insulin levels, which increased only minimally in cachectic tumor-bearing animals.[52] Increasing activity of the gluconeogenic enzyme phosphoenolpyruvate carboxykinase activity in liver tissue correlated with increasing tumor burden until the tumor was very advanced.[80] Inhibition of gluconeogenesis from amino acid precursors causes serum levels of glucose to decrease more dramatically in animals with small tumors than in nontumor-bearing controls. Some authors have even suggested that inhibition of accelerated gluconeogenesis may be an effective anticancer therapy, by depriving the tumor of glucose.[22] Others have suggested that possible reduction in Cori cycle activity in cancer patients may both inhibit tumor growth and prevent some of the cachectic effects, since this energy-consuming mechanism may be in part responsible for the increase in energy expenditure.[81]

Patients with localized esophageal cancer and without weight loss have altered forearm glucose metabolism, including increased glucose extraction and lactate release.[52,82] In humans bearing soft-tissue sarcomas of the extremities, glucose uptake is higher in the tumor-bearing limb than in the contralateral nontumor-bearing limb, with the rate of glucose uptake correlating with tumor burden.[83] These two studies have different implications. In the esophageal cancer patients, there appears to be a systemic effect by the tumor, reflected by abnormal glucose utilization by host muscle from a site distinct and remote from the tumor itself. In the study of extremity sarcomas, the tumor itself appears to utilize the glucose. These may represent two mechanisms by which abnormal glucose metabolism is established in cancer patients.

Modest increases in glucose oxidation have also been observed in cancer patients.[84] At the same time, glucose production is less sensitive to suppression by insulin. This insulin resistance of host tissues may play a role in the frequently observed glucose intolerance in patients with advanced cancer.[82,85–89] Abnormal glucose disposal has been demonstrated in several studies using glucose tolerance tests in patients with progressive cancer of various histologies.[82,90] Patients with metastatic cancer but without weight loss and noncancer controls appear to have similar serum glucose concentrations. Following an intravenous glucose infusion, there is an impaired glucose disposal rate despite an appropriate increase in serum levels of insulin, which is comparable to that seen in noncancer-bearing controls. The presence of metastases appears to make this insulin resistance more pronounced.[90] Sarcoma patients without apparent weight loss or hypophagia have also been found to have an abnormal glucose tolerance that appears to correlate with tumor burden.[82] A study by Lundhold et al.[91] suggested that there may be decreased pancreatic beta-cell receptor sensitivity leading to inadequate insulin release in response to glucose loading in cancer patients.[92]

Lipid metabolism

Elevated circulating levels of lipid and depletion of host fat reserves are the principle abnormalities of lipid metabolism seen in patients with cancer cachexia. Shaw and Wolfe[93] found that patients with advanced cancer had increased rates of glycerol and free fatty acid turnover, suggesting that the decreased fat stores are at least in part due to increased fat mobilization. This lipid mobilization may occur early in the development of the disease because of its high caloric value at a time when the metabolic demands of the host are high. This is evidenced by the fact that tumor-bearing rats may have elevated plasma levels of triglycerides and cholesterol prior to alterations in food intake or onset of weight loss.[6] Tracer studies using cachectic mice bearing MAC16 adenocarcinoma demonstrated an increased radiolabeled lipid accumulation by the tumor. This suggests that the cachectic animals have an increased utilization of fat as an energy source and that the overall energy requirements are higher in the cachectic state.[94] Other alterations in lipid metabolism that have been characterized in animal models include: increased free fatty acid (FFA) and triacylglycerol synthesis, reduction in serum lipoprotein lipase (LPL) activity, increased lipolysis, and decreased lipid clearance and immunosuppression (Table 5.4).[95–97]

LPL appears to play a central role in the abnormalities of lipid metabolism detected in the tumor-bearing condition. LPL is responsible for the movement of triglycerides from blood into adipocytes for lipid synthesis. Cachectic tumor-bearing rats exhibit hypertriglyceridemia, which is reversible with surgical removal of tumor.[95] Cancer patients with weight loss exhibit decreased levels of LPL activity in association with the elevated circulating levels of triglycerides and cholesterol. Vlassara et al.[97] measured plasma LPL activity in 28 cancer patients with varying degrees of weight loss and found a 35% decreased LPL activity in the cancer group, with the degree of reduction in enzyme activity correlating with percent body weight loss. Tumor type also correlated with the degree of reduction in LPL activity: lung cancer patients had the greatest amount of weight loss and showed the lowest enzyme activity, whereas breast cancer patients had minimal weight loss and showed normal levels of LPL activity. The mechanism of this suppression of LPL is different from that which occurs in starvation. In the latter, lipid mobilization occurs in part by decreased LPL activity but is accompanied by decreased plasma insulin levels. Vlassara et at.[97] have shown that cancer-associated reductions in plasma LPL are accompanied by normal or even increased insulin levels. Elevated insulin levels during a time of anorexia and weight loss represent a maladaptive host response, since insulin ordinarily promotes lipid storage, not fat oxidation.

Several LPL-inhibiting factors have been identified. The first factor is tumor necrosis factor (TNF; previously known as cachectin), which appears to be a prime mediator of the toxicity and cachexia associated with acute and chronic infectious disease, but whether it is involved in the development of cancer-associated cachexia[98,99] remains controversial. In addition, IL-1, IL-6, leukemia-inhibitory factor (LIF), and interferon-γ (IFN-γ) have all been shown to suppress LPL activity both in vitro and in vivo.[27,100–102]

These same cytokines have also been shown to promote lipolysis in normal adipocytes. Studies have revealed that TNF, IFN-γ, IL-1, and LIF all increase lipolysis rates in cultured murine adipocytes, whereas IL-6 has minimal effect.[103,104] However, TNF has no effect on cultured human adipocytes, making the role of TNF as a mediator of altered lipid metabolism in cancer patients less clear.[105] Other lipolysis-promoting factors have been identified as well, but they remain to be fully characterized.[106,107] Although patients with cancer cachexia exhibit elevated whole-body rates of lipolysis that have been associated with variable cytokine production, the exact mechanism by which this happens has not been clearly elucidated.[56] A proposed mechanism by which this lipolysis occurs is through increased intracellular accumulation of cAMP, a result of stimulation of adipose-cell adenylate cyclase.[108] The accumulated cAMP stimulates a cAMP-dependent protein kinase, which then activates a cellular triglyceride lipase.[108,109] Inhibition of adenylate cyclase by omega-3 polyunsaturated fatty acids (PUFAs) blocks the accumulation of cAMP. In vivo studies of mice bearing MAC16 adenocarcinomas showed reduced body weight loss, with increased body fat and muscle weight in animals fed omega-3 PUFAs.[108]

Clearly, increased lipolysis lead to depletion of host adipose reserves, as seen in cachectic cancer patients. However, the hyperlipidemia found in these patients may have further implications. Increased lipids have been found to have specific immunoregulatory effects on monocytes and macrophages,[110,111] and plasma from hyperlipidemic patients has been shown to be immunosuppressive.[110,112] Therefore, the end result of increased lipolysis and decreased lipid clearance in cancer patients may be immunosuppression and decreased survival.

Protein metabolism

Although loss of adipose tissue constitutes the majority of the weight lost in cancer cachexia, skeletal muscle mass depletion is perhaps more clinically significant in terms of the overall survival of the patient. During acute fasting, skeletal muscle is broken down to provide substrates for gluconeogenesis. However, during chronic fasting the body adapts to conserve nitrogen and maintain functional lean body mass by preferentially using adipose stores and decreasing energy expenditure. The cancer-bearing host loses this ability to adapt,[19,20,113] and depletion of vital host protein is detected clinically as skeletal muscle atrophy and myopathy, visceral organ atrophy, and hypoalbuminemia.[2,18] Complex changes in nitrogen metabolism involving inappropriate elevations in whole-body protein turnover, muscle protein synthesis and catabolism, liver protein synthesis, and plasma amino acid levels ultimately result in host protein wasting. There appears to be a positive correlation between this abnormal protein metabolism and the disease process in that the more aggressive the disease, the higher the nitrogen loss[114] and the poorer the prognosis.[115]

There are many ways to measure these abnormalities in protein metabolism, including anthropometric measurements, determination of nitrogen balance, measurement of serum proteins and/or free amino acid concentrations, urinary excretion of 3-methylhistidine (an amino acid that is released during skeletal muscle catabolism but not metabolized), and by amino acid kinetics.[116,117] Of these, tracer studies of regional and whole-body kinetics using labeled amino acids provide the best quantitative information about protein metabolism. However, the metabolism of the tumor itself will need to be taken into account when using this method.

Norton and co-workers,[118] using stable isotope tracer methodology and ^{15}N-glycine, showed that in a group of malnourished cancer patients, some patients had increased whole-body protein turnover while others had a normal turnover rate. This supports the concept that tumor-bearing patients exhibit a failure to adapt even in times of nutritional depletion. Furthermore, this increased protein turnover was not suppressed using nutritional repletion in the form of TPN.[118] Additional evidence is given by the finding that cachectic cancer patients have an elevated protein turnover based upon higher fractional synthetic rates and increased protein catabolic rates.[119] This protein turnover in cancer patients is significantly higher than that of malnourished control patients, and increased rates of whole-body protein turnover have been found in patients with a variety of tumor histologies.[112,120-124]

Why this increased protein turnover occurs remains poorly understood. Tumors appear to have an increased demand for certain amino acids and may be generating factors into the host circulation to recruit nitrogen from other tissues.[125] Because of this increased demand, investigators have demonstrated that tumors derive their necessary nitrogen and nutrients at the expense of the host, regardless of nutritional intake.[126,127] Furthermore, tumor excision appears to reverse cancer cachexia and increase nitrogen balance, although this is highly dependent on postoperative food intake.[128]

Theoretically, skeletal muscle depletion can result from accelerated degradation and/or reduced synthesis,[53,120,129] and experimental studies have shown evidence of both. Studies in human rectus abdominis muscle from cancer patients compared with age-matched controls have shown decreased muscle protein synthesis as measured by decreased incorporation of ^{14}C-leucine into muscle protein.[130] However, several animal studies suggest that protein catabolism is abnormally elevated in tumor-bearing host muscle. Emery et al.[131] reported an 80% increase in free 3-methylhistidine in the muscle of tumor-bearing mice; urinary 3-methyhistidine has been found to be significantly higher in sarcoma-bearing rats compared with controls;[53] and others have noted positive correlation between decrease in host muscle weight and increase in tumor burden.[132]

Attempts have been made to correlate plasma amino acid levels with weight loss and cachexia. Plasma amino acid levels have been measured both in experimental models and in patients. Some investigators have found comparable total plasma amino acid levels in tumor-bearing and control animals,[133] while others have found decreased levels in tumor-bearing animals.[51] Cancer patients without weight loss appeared to have plasma amino acid levels comparable to noncancer patients.[134,135] Patients with esophageal cancer and a 20% weight loss have a marked reduction in concentrations of total and individual plasma amino acids, except for branched-chain amino acids.[136] However, in general, despite large tumor burdens and weight loss, amino acid levels have been similar to controls and have not proved useful in the assessment and management of cancer cachexia.

Much research has been done in an attempt to define the mechanism of altered protein metabolism in cancer patients. In a laboratory model, mice bearing cachexia-inducing MAC16 adenocarcinomas were found to have increased levels of prostaglandin E2 (PGE2) in the gastrocnemius muscle as compared to control mice bearing noncachexia-inducing MAC13 adenocarcinomas.[137] Treatment with a prostaglandin inhibitor (indomethacin) or with eicosapentanoic acid inhibited the increase in levels of PGE2 and blocked muscle protein degradation,[137] which suggests that PGE2 plays a role in muscle catabolism and provides possible treatment strategies.

Two cytosolic proteolytic pathways exist in skeletal muscle: one is calcium-dependent and the other is ATP-ubiquitin-dependent.[138] Recent experiments suggest that the ATP-ubiquitin-dependent proteolytic pathway is responsible for the proteolysis of most skeletal muscle proteins. The atrophying muscle of cachectic rats bearing Yoshida sarcoma was found to have increased mRNA levels for ubiquitin, its carrier protein and proteosome subunits.[138] In vitro results demonstrated that depletion of ATP almost completely suppressed the increased proteolysis seen in muscles in this rat model.[138] Llovera et al.[134] demonstrated a greater than 30% decrease in mass of the gastrocnemius and extensor digitorum longus muscles of rats bearing the Yoshida AH-130 ascites hepatoma as compared with nontumor-bearing controls and found an increase in ubiquitin conjugates in the skeletal muscle of these tumor-bearing rats.

Many laboratory and clinical studies have documented an increase in hepatic protein synthesis in cancer-bearing hosts. Warren et al.[139,140] demonstrated a 2-fold increase in synthetic rates of total cellular hepatic protein in hepatocytes isolated from tumor-bearing animals versus control hepatocytes. This increase was proportional to tumor burden. Along with this increased synthesis, there appeared to be an increased degradation as well, since there was no net protein accrual. Hepatocytes isolated from cancer patients show a marked increase in protein synthesis compared with those from patients with benign disease.[135] However, in skeletal muscle, protein synthesis is decreased, whereas protein degradation is increased.[141] These findings demonstrate the markedly abnormal protein metabolism of the cancer-bearing host. The mobilization of host protein from skeletal muscle surpasses the increased hepatic protein synthesis, resulting in overall protein catabolism. Preservation of host protein is an important goal in therapies directed against cancer cachexia[4,142–146] since loss of protein stores may result in death once a critical mass has been reduced.[2,18]

Mechanisms of Cancer Cachexia

Despite an enormous amount of research, the mechanisms of cancer cachexia remain incompletely and poorly understood. Figure 5.2 is a proposed mechanism for cancer cachexia. Many of the physiologic changes seen in cancer cachexia resemble starvation.[2,18,20] However, if this were the case, exogenously supplied nutrients and calories either enterally or parentally should reverse the sequelae of cachexia, improve response to antitumor therapy and ultimately, survival. This does not happen. Few studies document improvement in lean body mass in cachectic animals or patients[4,147] and most studies using TPN fail to demonstrate any clinical benefit.[20,148,149] Certainly, decreased food intake does occur in cancer cachexia; however, these data are inconsistent with the notion that cancer cachexia is merely a result of simple starvation. In addition, a large number of laboratory and clinical studies have uniformly identified cancer-specific alterations in carbohydrate, protein, and lipid metabolism independent of starvation.[51–53]

Some have suggested that increased energy requirements of the tumor itself may explain the net loss of weight and energy by the host.[2,18] The nitrogen and substrate demands of the tumor are supplied by the host at its expense.[2,18] However, the tumor burden in humans is generally small and the basic metabolic rate of neoplastic tissue has been shown to be comparable to the tissue from which it originated[150] and cannot explain the inordinate loss of body composition

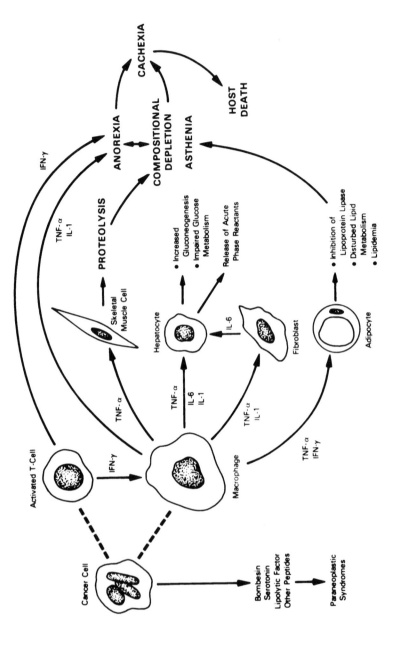

Figure 5.2. Suggested mechanism for cancer cachexia. (Reproduced with permission from Langstein, H.R., Mechanisms of Cancer Cachexia, *Hematol Oncol Clin N Am* 5: 103–123, 1991.[45])

or the other changes seen. In other conditions of excess energy expenditure or demand (such as pregnancy or exposure to cold), the host increases energy intake to meet increased metabolic demands. This adaptive behavior is absent in the cancer patient, making the increased substrate requirements of the tumor an unlikely culprit as the sole cause of cancer cachexia. Energy-losing metabolic pathways such as increased Cori cycling/gluconeogenesis, although contributing to some of the metabolic effects of the tumor, cannot fully explain the observed host depletion.

Recently, attention has focused on circulating humoral factors that are either elaborated by the tumor itself or by the host in response to the tumor. Since the 1950s, researchers have described a variety of tumor extracts that can depress liver enzyme activity, decrease protein synthesis in skeletal muscle, increase lipolysis, and kill healthy animals.[151-155] An extract from urine of patients with cancer has been reported to depress food intake, body weight, and motor activity of mice[156] and other reports have suggested the presence of anorectic and lipolytic factors from blood or urine of cancer patients.[157,158]

Compelling evidence that circulating factor(s) may mediate cancer-associated anorexia and cachexia in laboratory animals has come from Norton et al.[159] A parabiotic rat model was created in which a normal rat was surgically joined, sharing 1.5% of its circulation, with a tumor-bearing rat. Despite the fact that only one of the animals hosted a nonmetastasizing tumor, both animals developed anorexia, weight loss, and other sequelae of cancer cachexia. At necropsy there was no evidence of tumor in the coupled normal rat. Some human tumors, including small-cell lung cancer, produce humoral factors, such as serotonin or bombesin, that have the ability to suppress host appetite. However, only a minority of laboratory and clinical tumors produce such factors, not explaining the high incidence of cachexia among cancer patients. Furthermore, these peptides have no systemic effects and cannot account for the multiple metabolic abnormalities seen in cancer cachexia.

From these studies it is clear that both experimental animal and human tumors produce factors that cause some of the clinical manifestations of cancer cachexia. Presently, there is considerable interest in the possible role of the proinflammatory cytokins TNF, IL-1, IL-6, LIF, and IFN-γ in the pathogenesis of cancer cachexia. Extensive work with laboratory animal models has detected increased tissue and monocyte gene expression of IL-1, IL-6, and LIF.[27,57] Chronic administration of these cytokines in vivo has resulted in many of the classic features seen in experimental and human cancer cachexia (Table 5.5),[160] and passive immunization with antibodies against some of these cytokines has shown improvement in food intake and lean body mass.[160] However, the presence of these cytokines in the plasma and body fluids of patients with malignancy is variable and inconsistent.[119,161-163] In addition, many of these cytokines have overlapping activities, making it unlikely that any one single substance is the sole cause of cancer cachexia. These cytokines have been studied and described in detail.

Table 5.5. Evidence for cytokines as mediators of cancer cachexia

Cytokine	Source	Food intake	Body weight	Lipids Synthesis	Lipolysis	Proteins Synthesis	Proteolysis	APP	Temp	Death
TNF-α	Macrophage	↓	↓	↓	↑	↓	↑	↑	↑	Yes
IL-1(α or β)	Macrophage	↓	↓	↓	↑	↓	↑	↑	↑	Yes
IL-6	Macrophage Fibroblast	↓	↓	NA	NA	NA	NA	NA	NA	NA
IFN-γ	Activated T lymphocytes	↓	↓	↓	↑	NA	NA	NA	NA	No
D-factor	Macrophage Fibroblast T lymphocytes	↓	↓	↓	↑	↓	NA	↑	NA	Yes

Source: Reproduced with permission from McNamara et al.[160]
APP = acute phase proteins; TNF = tumor necrosis factor; IL = interleukin; IFN = interferon; NA = not available; ↑ = increased; ↓ = decreased.

Tumor necrosis factor (TNF)

Although the role of TNF in the pathophysiology of endotoxemia and gram-negative sepsis is well-understood, its role as a possible mediator in the pathogenesis of cancer cachexia is less defined. The suggestion that an inappropriate synthesis of TNF may accompany clinical malignancy and disease progression came from Cerami et al.,[164-166] who noted that rabbits infected with trypanosomiasis developed hypertriglyceridemia, reduced LPL activity, and a marked body wasting. This led to the discovery of a circulating serum LPL-suppressing factor, which was termed "cachectin." This monocyte/macrophage product was subsequently found to have the same genetic sequence as a protein previously isolated from the serum of BCG-primed mice treated with endotoxin. This factor was called "TNF" for its ability to induce hemorrhagic necrosis of tumors.[167,168] The identification of reduced plasma LPL activity in the serum of cancer patients with associated weight loss supported TNF as a possible mediator of cancer cachexia.

Stovroff's group and others reported that macrophages from tumor-bearing rats secreted more TNF in response to endotoxin than did monocytes from nontumor-bearing rats, with levels correlating with degree of cachexia and returning to normal following resection of tumor.[29,169] RNA specific for TNF is expressed by blood monocytes in a greater proportion of cancer patients than in controls.[170] Furthermore, constitutive and induced TNF expression have been noted in cell lines derived from human tumors, such as breast and ovarian carcinomas, Hodgkins disease, Kaposi's sarcoma, and acute myeloid leukemia.[171-175] Although this does not specifically identify TNF as the causative agent in cancer cachexia, it does strongly associate TNF with cancer pathophysiology.

Evidence that some of the physiological actions of TNF simulate those observed in cancer cachexia is well described at the cellular level. Cultured adipocytes incubated with medium from endotoxin-stimulated macrophages, or with recombinant TNF, show suppression of key lipogenic enzymes in fat cells, including LPL.[176] Myocytes exposed to TNF increase glucose uptake and become depleted of glycogen stores as glycogenolysis is stimulated.[177] Hepatocytes (both from cachectic cancer patients and from animals) treated with TNF develop increased rates of amino acid uptake, acute-phase protein synthesis, and gluconeogenesis.[23,178,179]

Administration of TNF to diabetic rats with reduced LPL activity produces a progressive increase in serum triglycerides secondary to de novo lipogenesis in the liver.[180] TNF has also been found to produce hyperlipidemia, lipolysis, and increased rates of fatty acid turnover in humans, which is similar to some of the physiologic changes seen in cancer patients.[181] Although TNF does not directly influence muscle catabolism in vitro, it enhances muscle degradation in experimental situations in which body weight loss is not apparent[182] and increases whole-body muscle catabolism in laboratory animals.[23,183,184] Rats exposed systemically to sublethal doses of TNF responded with increasing muscle and decreasing liver proteolysis, which is similar to that observed in inflammation and in cancer.[184] Studies using anti-TNF antibodies in rats bearing a highly cachectigenic tumor, Yoshida ascites hepatoma AH-130, support TNF-α as a mediator in the lipid and protein metabolic changes that develop in cachectic tumor-bearing rats. Anti-TNF antibody-treated animals were found to have a significant increase in LPL activity in white adipose tissue and decreased protein degradation rates in skeletal muscle, heart, and liver as compared to animals treated with nonimmune IgG.[185,186] However, recent data demonstrated that although anti-TNF antibodies were able to suppress hypertriglyceridemia, they had no effect on cholesterol metabolism, suggesting that cholesterol and lipid metabolism are regulated differently during tumor growth.[187]

Chronic administration of recombinant human TNF to laboratory animals results in marked anorexia and weight loss suggestive of cancer cachexia and the magnitude of these changes appears to be dependent on the method, dose, route, and frequency of administration.[183,188–193] Bolus intraperitoneal administration of recombinant human TNF in rodents causes a clear reduction in food intake and a loss of body weight, but after several days, animals begin to eat normally and gain weight despite continued bolus administration.[192] This tolerance to the anorectic and weight-losing effects of TNF can be overcome by continuous intravenous infusion of TNF[190] or escalating doses of TNF.[183] Administration of TNF by a subcutaneously implanted minipump caused progressive dose-dependent anorexia, loss of body weight, and carcass depletion.[189] Oliff et al.[191] found that a subcutaneously implanted tumor transfected with the TNF gene that was constitutively expressed caused progressive anorexia, weight loss, lipid depletion, and earlier death than did an identical tumor without the TNF gene.

The chronic administration of increasing sublethal doses of TNF to laboratory animals produces not only anorexia and weight loss but also inflammatory changes in tissue, diminished carcass lipid and protein stores, anemia, hypoproteinemia, and increased total body water—all characteristic of changes seen during progressive cachexia.[183] In pair-fed rats, the non-TNF-treated animal exhibited carcass lipid depletion but did not demonstrate the reduction in protein composition seen in TNF-treated rats, suggesting a direct cachetic effect of TNF on muscle protein metabolism either by decreased synthesis and/or increased breakdown.[183]

In laboratory rats with large subcutaneous, methylchlorane-induced sarcomas and marked cachexia, serum levels of TNF correlate with the degree of tumor burden.[29] Animals made tolerant to the effects of TNF by chronic administration then subsequently implanted with the methylchlorane-induced sarcoma survive longer and become less cachetic than nontolerant tumor-bearing controls, despite similar rates of tumor growth in both groups.[194]

Using this same sarcoma model, Sherry et al. prevented the development of hypophagia and cachexia observed in tumor-bearing mice by using anti-TNF antibodies.[195] In these same animals, treatment also significantly reduced the extent of carcass protein and fat loss, and reduced tumor weight, which may be partially responsible for the decreased cachexia observed. The group also showed that mice bearing Lewis lung adenocarcinoma did not appear to develop tumor-induced hypophagia or weight loss, but they did demonstrate a tumor-induced loss of carcass lipid that was partially ameliorated by anti-TNF antibody treatment. In a different study, researchers administered anti-TNF antibodies to tumor-bearing rats at a point when rats were developing clear evidence of cachexia and were unable to reverse tumor-associated hypophagia or weight loss or improve survival.[26]

Fraker et al. demonstrated that administration of insulin reversed the anorexia, weight loss, and nitrogen loss associated with TNF treatment, along with improving the histologic appearance of associated tissue injury.[196] This finding is important because insulin has been shown to increase food intake and improve body composition and decrease operative mortality in tumor-bearing animals,[28] as well as improve chemotherapy response of tumor-bearing rats receiving doxorubicin.[30]

There are many lines of evidence supporting TNF as a mediator of cancer cachexia, but there are also many inconsistencies. Phase I clinical therapy trials of TNF have failed to show weight loss as a side effect of this anticancer treatment.[166,197,198] In earlier phase I trials, systematically administered TNF caused fever, chills, anorexia, and malaise without weight loss.[197–199] However, TNF was cleared rapidly from the circulation with a half-life of about 20 minutes, and this may have prevented the development of any significant weight loss. Patients receiving repeated 5-day infusions had elevated serum levels of triglycerides and developed anorexia without weight loss, suggesting that TNF, if administered in high enough doses, could lead to the physiologic manifestations of cachexia in humans.[200]

Although circulating levels of TNF have been routinely found in patients with acute and chronic infections, such levels have been an inconsistent finding in cancer patients. Detectable levels have been found in one series of patients with cancer,[161] but not in others.[162,163] Kriegler et al.[201] suggested that TNF may circulate briefly and be undetectable at other times and also may exist as a membrane-bound protein not found in serum. Patients continuously infused with TNF until they developed systemic signs of TNF toxicity did not have detectable circulating levels of TNF in serum.[190] These explanations may account for the inconsistencies in detecting circulating levels of TNF in cachectic cancer patients. Therefore, TNF may still be a mediator of cachexia in cancer patients without its detectable presence in the serum of all cachectic cancer patients.

Interleukin-1 (IL-1)

Interleukin-1 is an inflammatory cytokine released by macrophages in response to a variety of stimuli. Although its role in the pathogenesis of cancer cachexia is not clear, IL-1 shares many properties and acts synergistically with TNF. IL-1 has also been shown to stimulate the release of IL-6 from tumor cells, and it may exert some of its cachectic effects through this manner.[202]

Several laboratories have shown that chronic, sublethal administration of IL-1 to healthy animals will induce many of the host changes reminiscent of cancer cachexia;[184,203–206] however, there is little evidence that spontaneous IL-1 production is increased in cancer.[207] IL-1 was identified in the plasma of only 1 out of 23 cancer patients, compared with 5 of 6 patients with bacterial infection, and peripheral blood monocytes from 4 of these 23 cancer patients failed to produce a normal response to endotoxin stimulation. However, plasma TNF was also undetectable in the same series of patients, suggesting that plasma levels may not necessarily reflect the degree of physiologically active IL-1 or TNF in different tissues. In fact, Jensen et al. demonstrated that gene expression of IL-1 can be markedly augmented in the liver of cachectic tumor-bearing rats, while actual IL-1 protein levels are undetectable in the serum of these rats.[57]

A single dose of IL-1 stimulates hepatic uptake of gluconeogenic amino acids, increases acute-phase protein synthesis, and decreases plasma concentrations of many amino acids.[208,209] IL-1 has been shown to suppress LPL activity in vitro and in vivo[100,101] and increases plasma levels of triglycerides. These effects are similar to those of TNF and they implicate IL-1 as a potential mediator of cancer cachexia.[25,209] IL-1 induces a rise in serum insulin associated with hypoglycemia in mice and rats.[209,210] However, in rabbits, the combination of TNF and IL-1 produces hyperglycemia and increased glucose turnover similar to that seen in cachexia.[211] Furthermore, IL-1 has a synergistic effect with TNF on muscle catabolism in vivo, although it does not appear to have any direct effect.[211,212] These effects of IL-1 on glucose, lipid, and protein metabolism are complex and may be enhanced by or expressed through other mediators.

Although it is unlikely that TNF and IL-1 directly promote tumor growth, it is possible these endogenous factors render local tissue conditions suitable for progressive tumor growth. Investigative efforts have been aimed at blocking the effects of TNF (as mentioned previously) and IL-1. When antibodies to the receptor for IL-1 are chronically administered to mice bearing growing MCA101 sarcoma, less weight loss and protein depletion is seen than in tumor-bearing controls (Table 5.4).[213] However, tumor growth is also decreased, and thus the amelioration of cachectic effects in these mice may partially be a result of smaller tumor burden. In a more recent study using colon-26 bearing mice, intratumoral injections of IL-1 receptor antagonist (IL-1ra) significantly reduced cachexia, and body composition analysis confirmed that this treatment improved lean tissue and fat, as well as hypoglycemia. In this study, the treatment did not change the tumor burden, suggesting that it affected the host directly.[214] However, Costelli et al. showed in his model using cachectic AH-130-bearing rats, that daily s.c. injections of IL-1ra was completely ineffective in either inhibiting tumor proliferation or in preventing the consequent tissue depletion and protein hypercatabolism.[208] Much like TNF, IL-1 studies show many inconsistencies, and the precise mechanisms by which they are involved in the development of cancer cachexia remain unclear.

Interleukin-6 (IL-6)

Like TNF and IL-1, this cytokine is an endogenous pyrogen and stimulates the production of acute-phase proteins.[215] However, unlike TNF and IL-1, which are rarely detected in hospitalized patients with bacterial infections, thermal injury, and surgical injury, IL-6 is found to freely circulate in the serum of these patients as well as in experimental animals with inflammation.[216] Increasing evidence for a role of IL-6 in inflammatory diseases and cancer cachexia arises from the observation that many of the tissue responses initially attributed to TNF-α and IL-1 can be reproduced by IL-6.[217] Although the role of IL-6 in cancer cachexia has not been fully established, several studies support the involvement of IL-6 in this syndrome.

Gelin et al.[218] were the first to report the presence of circulating IL-6 in mice bearing a transplantable tumor. The plasma levels appear to correlate with tumor burden and are detectable in animals with a variety of tumor types. Like TNF-α, IL-6 reduces LPL activity in vivo and in vitro,[219] and this has been suggested as contributing to the loss of body fat stores associated with cancer cachexia.

A direct role for IL-6 in cancer cachexia has been the focus of recent studies. Nude mice bearing Chinese hamster ovarian (CHO) tumors transfected with a murine gene constitutively expressing IL-6 lost approximately 33% of their body weight and had measurable circulating levels of IL-6.[123] Using a cachexia-causing murine colon-26 adenocarcinoma cell line in mice, Strassmann et al. demonstrated measurable levels of IL-6 in serum from these mice with increasing levels correlating with increasing cachexia.[220] Furthermore, monoclonal antibodies to murine IL-6 significantly suppressed the development of cachexia in this mouse model (Table 5.4).[220] However, direct administration of IL-6 to animals does not appear to cause cachexia.[221,222]

Supportive evidence for the role of human IL-6 (hIL-6) has come from studies using mice bearing Lewis lung carcinoma cells transfected with hIL-6 cDNA.[223] Mice with hIL-6-transfected tumors had high levels of hIL-6 (but not of TNF or IL-1) in the serum, marked weight loss, decreased serum albumin levels, and decreased survival. There was no effect on tumor growth rate between IL-6-producing tumors and control tumors not producing IL-6.

IL-6 levels have been found to be higher in cancer patients than those in hospitalized individuals without cancer.[221,224] Levels of IL-6 but not TNF-α in serum of cancer patients with weight loss associated with colonic adenocarcinoma and multiple hepatic metastases were also found to be elevated as compared to levels from patients with cholelithiasis and no weight loss, which correlates with hepatic synthesis of acute-phase proteins.[225] Also, immune reactive IL-6 is frequently found in human tumor specimens.

Soda et al.[226] recently measured IL-6 levels in mice injected with either cachexia-inducing or noncachexia-inducing subclones of murine colon adenocarcinoma and found them to be comparable, thereby disqualifying IL-6 as a sole inducer of cachexia. Additional studies by the same group of investigators suggested that IL-6 acts as a permissive factor for the development of cachexia; while it can induce some of the symptoms typical of cachexia, it cannot in itself induce the full cachectic syndrome.[227] Although the significance of IL-6 in cancer cachexia remains yet to be defined, it is clear that IL-6 plays a role. TNF-α increases circulating IL-6 and some of its effects may be mediated or potentiated by IL-6. Further studies are required to fully evaluate the importance of IL-6 in cancer cachexia.

Interferon-gamma (IFN-γ)

A product of activated T cells and macrophages, IFN-γ has antiviral and cell-activating capacities.[228] IFN-c has been shown to inhibit LPL and decrease the rate of fatty acid synthesis in adipocytes,[102] effects comparable to those previously described in cancer cachexia, and it can act either independently or in concert with TNF and IL-1.[26]

Langstein et al. found that exogenous administration of IFN-γ caused anorexia and weight loss in experimental animals.[26] Matthys et al. demonstrated that fat loss was enhanced by IFN-γ and antagonized by anti-IFN-γ antibody.[229] These investigators also found that anti-IFN-γ treatment to tumor-bearing mice inhibited tumor growth and its associated cachexia. Nude mice injected with genetically engineered CHO cells expressing murine IFN-γ developed severe cachexia and measurable IFN-γ in the serum as compared to control mice bearing a non-IFN-γ–producing cell line. In this model, pretreatment with monoclonal antibodies against IFN-γ prevented the development of cachexia.[230] Passive immunization of methylchlorane sarcoma-bearing rats with anti-IFN-γ antibodies at the time of established tumor growth and weight loss leads to partial reversal of cachectic changes and prolongs survival, without affecting the rate of tumor growth as compared to rats treated with control antibody. Antibodies to TNF, however, did not reverse anorexia or affect survival in this tumor model.[231] It is noteworthy that serum levels of TNF or IFN-γ were not detectable in these cachectic tumor-bearing rats. These findings suggest that IFN-γ may be an important mediator in the development of cancer cachexia and suggest a potential therapeutic role for antibodies against IFN-γ.

Leukemia-inhibitory factor (LIF)

Leukemia-inhibiting factor, also known as D-factor (differentiation factor), is a glycoprotein with a wide range of physiologic activities. In vitro, LIF produces a dose-dependent inhibition of LPL activity in 3T3-L1 adipocytes and is synergistic with TNF in this inhibition.[232] A LPL-suppressing factor isolated from the conditioned media of a human melanoma cell line that caused severe cachexia in tumor-bearing mice was found to be identical to LIF, suggesting that it may be a major factor responsible for cancer cachexia.[27,233] Furthermore, mice engrafted with CHO cells genetically engineered to produce LIF develop a fatal syndrome manifested by alterations in calcium metabolism, anorexia, and weight loss.[230] However, Metcalf et al. reported that the weight loss seen in mice injected repeatedly with LIF was due to toxicity.[234,235] Therefore, one must be careful in attributing weight loss to the effects of a possible cachectic mediator rather than to simple toxicity.

Novel cancer cachectic factor

Recently, a proteoglycan of relative molecular mass 24K which produces cachexia in vivo by inducing catabolism of skeletal muscle was identified and characterized from splenocytes of mice bearing the MAC 16 tumor. This proteoglycan is distinct from the cytokines both structurally and by its ability to accelerate breakdown of skeletal muscle in vitro and in vivo and to produce weight loss in vivo by a process not involving anorexia. The 24K material was also present in urine of cachectic cancer patients ($n = 18$), but it was absent from normal subjects ($n = 16$), patients with weight loss due to trauma ($n = 17$), and cancer patients with little or no weight loss ($n = 6$). Further research, both in experimental models and in humans, is necessary to fully establish the role of this novel proteoglycan in cancer cachexia.[66]

Management of Cancer Cachexia

Since many patients with treatable cancer are malnourished, replenishment with enteral or parenteral nutrition is intuitive and may render them better suited for aggressive therapy. However, despite many retrospective and prospective randomized trials in cancer patients undergoing surgery, radiation, or chemotherapy, total parenteral nutrition (TPN) has not been able to increase patient survival or produce any significant symptomatic improvement. In addition, TPN has a complication rate of 15% and a high cost estimated at $10,000 per patient/year.[148] Recent research, therefore, has focused on a pharmacological approach that might result in symptomatic improvement, even if no significant nutritional changes are detected. Treatment is aimed primarily at countering two of the main symptoms of cancer cachexia: anorexia and chronic nausea.

Insulin has been shown to increase food intake, decrease operative mortality, and increase response to chemotherapy in experimental animal models.[28,30] Progestational drugs have been found in a number of clinical studies to increase appetite, caloric intake, and nutritional status.[13,236] The most effective type and dose of progestational drugs have not been clearly established. Cyproheptadine, hydrazine sulfate, and cannabinoids have all been suggested to have beneficial effects on appetite; their effectiveness, however, needs to be confirmed in prospective controlled trials, some of which are currently under way.

Current data suggest that megestrol acetate or other progestational agents might be useful for their ability to increase appetite and weight gain as well as overall nutritional status.[13,236] Cyproheptadine is an antihistamine with antiserotonergic properties, usually used for the treatment of allergies.[237] Results from a randomized, placebo-controlled, double-blind clinical trial,[238] were disappointing in that although the drug stimulated patient appetite and food intake mildly, it did not significantly prevent progressive weight loss. Hydrazine sulphate has been found to have a variety of effects in humans and experimental animals, including inhibition of gluconeogenesis in rats.[239] Silverstein et al. demonstrated that hydrazine sulphate may influence carbohydrate metabolism at the level of hepatic enzymes concerned with gluconeogenesis and glucose uptake in normal and cancerous rats.[240] Trials evaluating the effectiveness of hydrazine sulphate in cancer patients have yielded conflicting results, but patients appear to have an increase in caloric intake and serum albumin levels.[241] Weight gain is a recognized feature of the use of marijuana and its derivatives. In a dose-ranging study in which patients with unresectable cancer were treated with dronabinol for up to 6 weeks, patients in all groups continued to lose weight, although the rate of weight loss decreased with therapy in all doses. Symptomatic improvement was noted in both mood and appetite at all but the lowest daily dosage.[242] Further dose escalation studies are underway.

Summary

Cachexia, manifested by anorexia, weight loss, and specific metabolic alterations, is a frequent and devastating complication of advanced cancer. Current understanding of the pathophysiology of this syndrome involves the host's production of inflammatory cytokines, including TNF, IL-1, IL-6, IFN-γ, and LIF. These endogenous mediators in turn orchestrate a series of complex interrelated steps unlimately leading to a chronic state of malnourishment, wasting, and death. Because the majority of cancer patients with advanced malignancies will develop cachexia, rendering them unable to respond effectively to aggressive anticancer therapy, further research into the management and treatment of this syndrome is mandatory. Different strategies aimed at improving the metabolic parameters or nutrition of the host have not had a dramatic influence in ameliorating cachexia. Current pharmacological approaches may be effective in providing symptomatic improvement, but these studies are too immature to yield any conclusions as of yet. Cancer cachexia remains a difficult therapeutic dilemma and innovative treatment approaches with antagonists against endogenous mediators of cachexia and towards correcting abnormal metabolic pathways may provide valuable improvements with respect to survival and response to treatment of patients with this syndrome.

References

1. DeWys WD, Begg D, Lavin PT. Prognostic effect of weight loss prior to chemotherapy in cancer patients. *Am J Med* 1980; 69:491–499.

2. Kern KA, Norton JA. Cancer cachexia. *J Pareuter Enteral Nutr* 1988; 12:286–298.

3. Daly JM, Copeland EM, Dudrick SJ. Effects of intravenous nutrition on tumor growth and host immunocompetence in malnourished animals. *Surgery* 1978; 84:655–658.

4. Bozzetti F, Migliavacca S, Pupa A, Ammatuna M, Bonalumi MG, Terno G, Facchetti G. Total parenteral nutrition prevents further nutritional deterioration in patients with cancer cachexia. *Ann Surg* 1987; 205:138–143.

5. Burt ME, Stein TP, Schwade JG, Brennan MF. Whole-body protein metabolism in cancer-bearing patients. *Cancer* 1984; 53:1246–1252.

6. Tayek JA, Bistrian BR, Hehir DJ, Martin R, Moldawer LL, Blackburn GL. Improved protein kinetics and albumin synthesis by branched chain amino acid-enriched total parenteral nutrition in cancer cachexia. *Cancer* 1986; 58:147–157.

7. Muller JM, Brenner U, Dienst C, Picklmaier H. Preoperative parenteral feeding in patients with gastrointestinal carcinoma. *Lancet* 1982; 1:68–71.

8. Ignoffo RJ. Parenteral nutrition support in patients with cancer. *Pharmacotherapy* 1992; 12:353–357.

9. Williams RL, Hilton DJ, Pease S, Willson TA, Stewart CL, Gearing DP, Wagner EF, Metcalf D, Nicola NA, Gough NM. Myeloid leukaemia inhibitory factor maintains the developmental potential of embryonic stem cells. *Nature* 1988; 336:684–687.

10. Preshaw RM, Attisha RP, Hollingworth WJ. Randomized sequential trial of parenteral nutrition in healing of colonic anastomoses in man. *Can J Surg* 1979; 22:437–439.

11. Lim STK, Choa RG, Lam KH, Wong J, Ong GB. Total parenteral nutrition versus gastrostomy in the preoperative preparation of patients with carcinoma of the oesophagus. *Br J Surg* 1981; 68:69–72.

12. Thompson BR, Julian TB, Stremple JF. Perioperative total parenteral nutrition in patients with gastrointestinal cancer. *J Surg Res* 1981; 30:497–500.

13. Loprinzi CL, Ellison MN, Schaid DJ, Krook JE, Athmann LM, Dose AM, Mailliard JA, Johnson PS, Ebbert LP, Geeraerts LH. Controlled trials of megestrol acetate for the treatment of cancer anorexia and cachexia. *J Natl Cancer Inst* 1990; 82:1127–1132.

14. Moley JF, Morrison SE, Norton JA. Insulin reversal of cancer cachexia in rats. *Cancer Res* 1985; 45:4925–4931.

15. Chlebowski RT, Heber D, Richardson B, Block JB. Influence of hydrazine sulfate on abnormal carbohydrate metabolism in cancer patients with weight loss. *Cancer Res* 1984; 44:857–861.

16. Tayek JA, Heber D, Chlebowski RT. Effect of hydrazine sulphate on whole-body protein breakdown measured by 14C-lysine metabolism in lung cancer patients. *Lancet 2:* 1987; 241–244.

17. Ng B, Wolf RF, Weksler B, Brennan MF, Burt M. Growth hormone administration preserves lean body mass in sarcoma-bearing rats treated with doxorubicin. *Cancer Res* 1993; 53:5483–5486.

18. Norton JA, Peacock JL, Morrison SD. Cancer cachexia. *Crit Rev Oncol Hematol* 1987; 7:289–327.

19. Balducci L, Hardy C. Cancer and nutrition: a review. *Compr Ther* 1987; 13:60.

20. Brennan MF. Total parenteral nutrition in the cancer patient. *N Engl J Med* 1981; 305:375–382.

21. Fearon KCH, Carter DC. Cancer cachexia. *Ann Surg* 1988; 208:1.

22. Gold J. Proposed treatment of cancer by inhibition of gluconeogenesis. *Oncology* 1968; 22:185.

23. Moldawer LL, Georgieff M, Lundholm K. Interleukin 1, tumour necrosis factor-alpha (cachectin) and the pathogenesis of cancer cachexia. *Clin Physiol* 1987; 7:263–274.

24. Bendtzen K. Interleukin 1, interleukin 6 and TNF in infection, inflammation and immunity. *Immunol Lett* 1988; 19:183–192.

25. Evans RD, Argiles JM, Williamson DH. Metabolic effects of tumour necrosis factor-α (cachectin) and interleukin-1. *Clin Sci* 1991; 77:357–364.

26. Langstein HN, Fraker DL, Norton JA. Reversal of cancer cachexia by antibodies to interferon-gamma but not cachectin/tumor necrosis factor. *Surg Forum* 1989; 15:408–410.

27. Mori M, Yamaguchi K, Honda S, et al. Cancer cachexia syndrome developed in nude mice bearing melanoma cells producing leukemia-inhibitory factor. *Cancer Res* 1991; 51:6656–6659.

28. Moley JF, Morrison SE, Norton JA. Preoperative insulin reverses cachexia and decreases mortality in tumor-bearing rats. *J Surg Res* 1987; 43:21–28.

29. Stovroff MC, Fraker DL, Norton JA. Cachectin activity in the serum of cachectic, tumor-bearing rats. *Arch Surg* 1989; 124:94–99.

30. Peacock JL, Gorschboth CM, Norton JA. Impact of insulin on doxorubicin-induced rat host toxicity and tumor regression. *Cancer Res* 1987; 47:4318–4322.

31. Sloan GM, Maher M, Brennan MF. Nutritional effects of surgery, radiation therapy, and adjuvant chemotherapy for soft tissue sarcomas. *Am J Clin Nutr* 1981; 34:1094.

32. Warren S. The immediate causes of death in the cancer. *Am J Med Sci* 1932; 184:610–615.

33. Bruera E. Clinical management of anorexia and cachexia in patients with advanced cancer. *Oncology* 1992; 49:35–42.

34. Kinsella TJ, Malcolm AW, Bothe A, Valerio D, Blackburn GL. Prospective study of nutritional support during pelvic irradiation. *Int J Radiat Oncol Biol Phys* 1981; 7:543.

35. Buzby GP, Mullen JL, Matthews DC, Hobbs CL, Rosato EF. Prognostic nutritional index in gastrointestinal surgery. *Am J Surg* 1980; 139:160–167.

36. Smale BF, Mullen JL, Buzby GP, Rosato EF. The efficacy of nutritional assessment and support in cancer surgery. *Cancer* 1981; 47:2375.

37. Nixon DW, Heymsfield SB, Cohen AE, Kutner MH. Protein calorie undernutrition in hospitalized cancer patients. *Am J Med* 1980; 68:683–690.

38. Theologides A. Pathogenesis of anorexia and cachexia in cancer. *Cancer Bull* 1982; 34:140–149.

39. Body JJ, Bokowski A. Nutrition and quality of life in cancer patients. *Eur J Cancer Clin Oncol* 1987; 23:127.

40. Kokal WA. The impact of antitumour therapy on nutrition. *Cancer* 1985; 55:273.

41. Bernstein IL, Sigmundi RA. Tumor anorexia: a learned food aversion. *Science* 1980; 209:416–418.

42. Padilla GV. Psychological aspects of nutrition and cancer. *Surg Clin North Am* 1986; 60:1121.

43. Brennan MF. Uncomplicated starvation versus cancer cachexia. *Cancer Res* 1977; 37:2359.

44. Cori CF, Cori GT. The carbohydrate metabolism of tumors. II. Changes in the sugar, lactic acid, and CO_2-combining power of blood passing through a tumor. *J Biol Chem* 1925; 66:397.

45. Langstein HN, Norton JA. Mechanisms of cancer cachexia. *Hematol Oncol Clin North Am* 1991; 5:103–123.

46. Hansell DT, Davies JW, Shenkin A, Burns HJ. The oxidation of body fuel stores in cancer patients. *Ann Surg* 1986; 204:637–642.

47. Lindmark L, Eden E, Ternell M, Bennegard K, Svaninger G, Lundholm K. Thermic effect and substrate oxidation in response to intravenous nutrition in cancer patients who lose weight. *Ann Surg* 1986; 204:628–636.

48. Peacock JL, Inculet RI, Corsey R, Ford DB, Rumble WF, Lawson D, Norton JA. Resting energy expenditure and body cell mass alterations in noncachectic patients with sarcomas. *Surgery* 1987; 102:465–472.

49. Thomson SR, Hirshberg A, Haffejee A. Resting metabolic rate of esophageal carcinoma patients: a model for energy expenditure measurement in a homogeneous cancer patient. *J Parenter Enteral Nutr* 1990; 14:119.

50. Falconer JS, Fearon KCH, Plester CE, Ross JA, Carter DC. Cytokines, the acute-phase response, and resting energy expenditure in cachectic patients with pancreatic cancer. *Ann Surg* 1994; 219:325–331.

51. Alexander HR, Chang TS, Lee JI, Stein TP, Burt ME. Amino acid and protein metabolism in the tumor bearing rat. *Proc Am Assoc Cancer Res* 1989; 30:22.

52. Burt ME, Lowry SF, Gorschboth C, Brennan MF. Metabolic alterations in a noncachectic animal tumor system. *Cancer* 1981; 47:2138–2146.

53. Norton JA, Shamberger R, Stein TP, Milne GWA, Brennan MF. The influence of tumor-bearing on protein metabolism in the rat. *J Surg Res* 1981; 30:456–462.

54. Burt ME, Aoki TT, Gorschboth CM, Brennan MF. Peripheral tissue metabolism in cancer-bearing man. *Ann Surg* 1983; 198:685–691.

55. Legaspi A, Malayappa J, Starnes HF Jr, Brennan MF. Whole body lipid and energy metabolism in the cancer patient. *Metabolism* 1987; 36:958–963.

56. Eden E, Edstrom S, Bennegard K, Lindmark L, Lundholm K. Glycerol dynamics in weight-losing cancer patients. *Surgery* 1985; 97:176–184.

57. Jensen JC, Buresh CM, Fraker DL, Langstein HN, Doherty GD, Alexander HR, Norton JA. Enhanced hepatic cytokine gene expression in cachectic tumor bearing rats. *Surg Forum* 1990; 41:469–472.

58. Heber D, Byerly LO, Tchekmedyian NS. Hormonal and metabolic abnormalities in the malnourished cancer patient: effects on host tumor interaction. *J Parenter Enteral Nutr* 1992; 16:605–645.

59. Copeland EM, Macfayder BV, Dudrick SJ. Effect of hyperalimentation in established delayed hypersensitivity in the cancer patient. *Ann Surg* 1976; 184:60–64.

60. Heber D, Byerley LO, Chi J, et al. Pathophysiology of malnutrition in the adult cancer patient. *Cancer* 1988; 58:1867–1873.

61. Hyltander A, Drott C, Körner U, Sandstrom R, Lundholm K. Elevated energy expenditure in cancer patients with solid tumors. *Eur J Cancer* 1991; 27:9–15.

62. Fearon KCH, Hansell DT, Preston T, et al. Influences of whole body protein turnover rate on resting energy expenditure in patients with cancer. *Cancer Res* 1988; 48:2590–2595.

63. Fredrix EWHM, Soefers PB, Wonters EFM, et al. Energy balance in relation to cancer cachexia. *Clin Nutr* 1990; 9:319–324.

64. Dempsey DT, Feurer ID, Knox LS, et al. Energy expenditure in malnourished gastrointestinal cancer patients. *Cancer* 1984; 53:1265–1273.

65. Bozzetti F, Pagnoni AM, Del Becchio M. Excessive caloric expenditure as a cause of malnutrition in patients with cancer. *Surg Gynecol Obstet* 1980; 150:229–234.

66. Todorow P, Cariuk P, McDevitt T, Coles B, Fearon K, Tisdale M. Characterization of a cancer cachectic factor. *Nature* 1996; 379:739–742.

68. Arbeit JM, Burt ME, Rubinstein LV, Gorschboth CM, Brennan MF. Glucose metabolism and the percentage of glucose derived from alanine: response to exogenous glucose infusion in tumor-bearing and non-tumor-bearing rats. *Cancer Res* 1982; 42:4936–4942.

69. Waterhouse C, Jeanpretre N, Keilson J. Gluconeogenesis from alanine in patients with progressive malignant disease. *Cancer Res* 1979; 39:1968–1972.

70. Holroyde CP, Reichard GA. Carbohydrate metabolism in cancer cachexia. *Cancer Treat Rev* 1981; 65:55.

71. Kahn CR. The riddle of tumour hypoglycemia revisited. *J Clin Endocrinol Metab* 1980; 9:335–360.

72. Papaioannou AN. Tumours other than insulinomas associated with hypoglycemia. *Surg Gynecol Obstet* 1966; 123:1093–1099.

73. Strain AJ. Cancer cachexia in man: a review. *Invest Cell Pathol* 1979; 2:181.

74. Shaw JHF, Wolfe RR. Glucose and urea kinetics in patients with early and advanced gastrointestinal cancer: the response to glucose infusion, parenteral feeding and surgical resection. *Surgery* 1986; 101:181–191.

75. Douglas RG, Shaw JHF. Metabolic effects of cancer. *Br J Surg* 1990; 77:246–254.

76. Lowry SF, Foster DM, Norton JA, Berman M, Brennan MR. Glucose disposal and gluconeogenesis from alanine in tumor-bearing Fischer 344 rats. *J Natl Cancer Inst* 1981; 66:653–658.

77. Inculet RI, Peacock JL, Gorschboth CM, Norton JA. Gluconeogenesis in the tumor-influenced rat hepatocyte: importance of tumor burden, lactate, insulin, and glucagon. *J Natl Cancer Inst* 1987; 79:1039–1046.

78. Torosian MH, Bartlett DL, Chatzidakis C, Stein TP. Effect of tumor burden on futile glucose and lipid cycling in tumor-bearing animals. *J Surg Res* 1993; 55:68–73.

79. Alexander HR, DePippo P, Rao S, Burt ME. Substrate alterations in a sarcoma-bearing rat model: effect of tumor growth and resection. *J Surg Res* 1990; 48:471–475.

80. Gutman A, Thilo E, Biran S. Enzymes of gluconeogenesis in tumor-bearing rats. *Isr J Med Sci* 1969; 5:998–1001.

81. Dills WL, Jr. Nutritional and physiological consequences of tumour glycolysis. *Parasitology* 1993; 107:S177–S186.

82. Norton JA, Maher M, Wesley R, White D, Brennan MF. Glucose intolerance in sarcoma patients. *Cancer* 1984; 54:3022–3027.

83. Norton JA, Burt ME, Brennan MF. In vivo utilization of substrate by human sarcoma-bearing limbs. *Cancer* 1980; 45:2934–2939.

84. Hansell DT, Davies JWL, Burns HJG. The relationship between resting energy expenditure and weight loss in benign and malignant disease. *Ann Surg* 1986; 203:240.

85. Marks PA, Bishop JSA. The glucose metabolism of patients with malignant disease and normal subjects as studied by means of an intravenous glucose tolerance test. *J Clin Invest* 1956; 35:254–260.

86. Holroyde CP, Skutches CL, Boden G, Reichard GA. Glucose metabolism in cachectic patients with colorectal cancer. *Cancer Res* 1984; 44:5910–5913.

87. Schein PS, Kisner DD, Hatter D, Blecher M, Hamosh M. Cachexia of malignancy: potential role of insulin in nutritional management. *Cancer* 1979; 43:2070.

88. Jasani B, Donaldson LK, Ratcliff ED, et al. Mechanism of impaired glucose tolerance in patients with neoplasia. *Br J Cancer* 1978; 38:282–287.

89. Bishops JS, Marks PA. Studies on carbohydrate metabolism in patients with neoplastic disease: II. Response to insulin administration. *J Clin Invest* 1959; 38:668–672.

90. Copeland GP, Al-Sumidaie AM, Leinster SJ, Davis JC, Hipkin LH. Glucose metabolism in patients with gastrointestinal malignancy but without excessive weight loss. *Eur J Surg Oncol* 1987; 13:11–16.

91. Lundholm K, Holm G, Schersten T. Insulin resistance in patients with cancer. *Cancer* 1978; 38:4665–4670.

92. Lundholm K, Bylund AC, Schersten T. Glucose tolerance in relation to skeletal muscle enzyme activities in cancer patients. *Scand J Clin Lab Invest* 1977; 37:267–272.

93. Shaw JHF, Wolfe RR. Fatty acid and glycerol kinetics in septic patients and in patients with gastrointestinal cancer: the response to glucose infusion and parenteral feeding. *Ann Surg* 1987; 205:368–376.

94. Mulligan HD, Beck SA, Tisdale MJ. Lipid metabolism in cancer cachexia. *Br J Cancer* 1992; 66:57–61.

95. Younes RN, Vydelingum NA, Noguchi Y, Brennan MF. Lipid kinetic alterations in tumor-bearing rats: reversal by tumor excision. *J Surg Res* 1990; 48:324–328.

96. Lanza-Jacoby S, Lansey SC, Miller EE, Cleary MP. Sequential changes in the activities of lipoprotein lipase and lipogenic enzymes during tumor growth in rats. *Cancer Res* 1984; 44:5062–5067.

97. Vlassara H, Spiegel RJ, Doval DS, et al. Reduced plasma lipoprotein lipase activity in patients with malignancy associated weight loss. *Horm Metab Res* 1992; 18:698–703.

98. Beutler B, Cerami A. Tumor necrosis factor in cachexia, shock, and inflammation: a common mediator. *Annu Rev Biochem* 1988; 57:505–518.

99. Moldawer LL, Sherry B, Lowry SF, Cerami A. Endogenous cachectin/tumour necrosis factor-alpha production contributes to experimental cancer-associated cachexia. *Cancer Surv* 1989; 8:854–859.

100. Price SR, Mizel SB, Pekala PH. Regulation of lipoprotein lipase synthesis and 3T3-L1 adipocyte metabolism by recombinant interleukin 1. *Biochim Biophys Acta* 1986; 889:374–381.

101. Argiles JM, Lopez-Soriano FJ, Evans RD, Williamson DH. Interleukin-1 and lipid metabolism in the rat. *Biochem J* 1989; 259:673–678.

102. Patton JS, Shepard HM, Wilking H. Interferons and tumor necrosis factor have similar catabolic effects on 3T3LI cells. *Proc Natl Acad Sci USA* 1986; 83:8313–8317.

103. Feingold KR, Doerrler W, Dinarello CA, Fiers W, Grunfeld C. Stimulation of lipolysis in cultured fat cells by tumor necrosis factor, interleukin-1, and the interferons is blocked by inhibition of prostaglandin synthesis. *Endocrinology* 1992; 130:10–16.

104. Marshall MK, Doerrler W, Feingold KR, Grunfeld C. Leukemia inhibitory factor induces changes in lipid metabolism in cultured adipocytes. *Endocrinology* 1994; 135:141–147.

105. Kern PA. Recombinant human tumor necrosis factor does not inhibit lipoprotein lipase in primary cultures of isolated human adipocytes. *J Lipid Res* 1988; 29:909–914.

106. Taylor DD, Gercel-Taylor C, Jenis LG, Devereux DF. Identification of a human tumor-derived lipolysis-promoting factor. *Cancer Res* 1992; 52:829–834.
107. Beck SA, Mulligan HD, Tisdale MJ. Lipolytic factors associated with murine and human cancer cachexia. *J Natl Cancer Inst* 1990; 82:1922–1926.
108. Tisdale MJ. Mechanism of lipid mobilization associated with cancer cachexia: interaction between the polyunsaturated fatty acid, eicosapentaenoic acid, and inhibitory guanine nucleotide-regulatory protein. *Prostaglandins Leukot Essent Fatty Acids* 1993; 48:105–109.
109. Dempsey DT, Knox LS, Mullen JL, Miller C, Fdeurer ID, Buzby GP. Energy expenditure in malnourished patients with colorectal cancer. *Arch Surg* 1986; 121:789–795.
110. Ladisch S, Poplack DG, Holiman B, et al. Immunodeficiency in familial erythroplagocytic lymphohistiocytosis. *Lancet* 1978; 1:581–583.
111. Chapman HA, Hibbs JF. Modulation of macrophage tumouricidal capability by components of normal serum: a central role of lipid. *Science* 1970; 197:282–285.
112. Spiegel RJ, Schaefer EJ, Magrath IT, et al. Plasma lipid alterations in leukemia and lymphoma. *Am J Med* 1982; 72:775–782.
113. Kurzer M, Meguid MM. Cancer and protein metabolism. *Surg Clin North Am* 1986; 66:969.
114. Koea JB, Shaw JF. The effect of tumour bulk on the metabolic response to cancer. *Ann Surg* 1992; 3:282–288.
115. Shaw JHF, Humberstone DM, Wolfe RR. Energy and protein metabolism in sarcoma patients. *Ann Surg* 1988; 207:283–289.
116. Pisters PWT, Brennan MR. Amino acid metabolism in human cancer cachexia. *Annu Rev Nutr* 1990; 10:107–112.
117. Pisters PWT, Pearlstone DB. Protein and amino acid metabolism in cancer cachexia: investigative techniques and therapeutic interventions. *Crit Rev Clin Lab Sci* 1993; 30:223–272.
118. Norton JA, Stein TP, Brennan MF. Whole body protein synthesis and turnover in normal man and malnourished patients with and without known cancer. *Ann Surg* 1981; 194:123–128.
119. Waring P, Wycherley K, Cary D, Nicola N, Metcalf D. Leukemia inhibitory factor levels are elevated in septic shock and various inflammatory body fluids. *J Clin Invest* 1992; 90:2031–2037.
120. Heber D, Chlewbowski TR, Ishibachi DE, Herrold JN, Block JB. Abnormalities in glucose and protein metabolism in non-cachectic lung cancer patients. *Cancer Res* 1982; 42:4815–4819.
121. Jeevanandam M, Horowitz GD, Lowry SF, Brennan MF. Cancer cachexia and protein metabolism. *Lancet* 1984; 1:1423–1426.
122. Kien CL, Camitta BM. Increased whole-body protein turnover in sick children with newly diagnosed leukemia or lymphoma. *Cancer Res* 1983; 43:5586–5592.
123. Kien CL, Camitta BM. Close association of accelerated rates of whole body protein turnover (synthesis and breakdown) and energy expenditure in children with newly diagnosed acute lymphocytic leukemia. *J Parenter Enteral Nutri* 1987; 11:129–134.
124. Eden E, Ekman L, Lindmark L, et al. Whole-body tyrosine flux in relation to energy expenditure in weight-losing cancer patients. *Metabolism* 1984; 33:1020–1027.

125. Stein RP, Oram-Smith JC, Leskiw MF, et al. Tumour caused changes in host protein synthesis under different dietary situations. *Cancer Res* 1976; 36:3936.

126. Reilly JJ, Goodgame JT, Jones DC, et al. DNA synthesis in rat sarcoma and liver: the effect of starvation. *J Surg Res* 1977; 22:281–286.

127. Lowry SF, Goodgame JR, Norton JA, et al. Effect of chronic protein malnutrition on host-tumour composition and growth. *Surg Forum* 1977; 23:143–145.

128. Le Bricon T, Cynober L, Baracos VE. Protein metabolism in cachectic tumour-bearing rats: effect of tumour excision. *J Surg Res* 1996; 60:207–215.

129. Goodlad GAJ, Clark CM. Leucine metabolism in skeletal muscle of the tumour-bearing rat. *Eur J Cancer* 1980; 16:1153.

130. Lundholm K, Bylund AC, Holm J. Skeletal muscle metabolism in patients with malignant tumor. *Eur J Cancer* 1976; 12:465–473.

131. Emery PW, Lowvell L, Rennie MJ. Protein synthesis measured in vivo in muscle and liver of cachectic tumour-bearing rat. *J Surg Res* 1987; 42:43–50.

132. Norton JA, Lowry SF, Brennan MF. Effect of work-induced hypertrophy on skeletal muscle of tumor and non-tumor bearing rats. *J Appl Physiol* 1979; 46:654–657.

133. Arbeit JM, Gorschboth CM, Brennan MF. Basal amino acid concentrations and the response to incremental glucose infusion in tumor bearing rats. *Cancer Res* 1985; 45:6296.

134. Llovera M, Garcia-Martinez C, Agell N, Lopez-Soriano FJ, Argiles JM. Muscle wasting associated with cancer cachexia is linked to an important activation of the ATP-dependent ubiquitin-mediated proteolysis. *Int J Cancer* 1995; 61:138–141.

135. Clarke EF, Lewis AM, Waterhouse C. Peripheral amino acid levels in patients with cancer. *Cancer* 1978; 42:2909–2913.

136. Norton JA, Gorschboth CM, Wesley RA, Burt ME, Brennan MF. Fasting plasma amino acid levels in cancer patients. *Cancer* 1985; 56:1181–1186.

137. Smith KL, Tisdale MJ. Mechanism of muscle protein degradation in cancer cachexia. *Br J Cancer* 1993; 68:314–318.

138. Temparis S, Asensi M, Taillandier D, Aurousseau E, Larbaud D, Obled A, Béchet D, Ferrara M, Estrela JM, Attaix D. Increased ATP-Ubiquitin-dependent proteolysis in skeletal muscles of tumor-bearing rats. *Cancer Res* 1994; 54:5568–5573.

139. Warren RS, Jeevanandam M, Brennan MF. Comparison of hepatic protein synthesis in vivo versus in vitro in the tumour-bearing rat. *J Surg Res* 1987; 42:43–50.

140. Warren RS, Jeevanandam M, Brennan MF. Protein synthesis in the tumour-influenced hepatocyte. *Surgery* 1979; 98:281–285.

141. Smith KL, Tisdale MS. Increased protein degradation and decreased protein synthesis in skeletal muscle during cancer cachexia. *Br J Cancer* 1993; 67:680–685.

142. Beck SA, Tisdale MJ. Nitrogen excretion in cancer cachexia and its modification by a high fat diet in mice. *Cancer Res* 1989; 49:3800–3904.

143. Buss CL. Nutritional support of the cancer patient. *Primary Care* 1987; 14:317.

144. Holmes S, Dickerson JWT. Malignant disease: nutritional implications of disease and treatment. *Cancer Metastasis Rev* 1987; 6:357.

145. Holroyde CP, Reichard GA. General metabolic abnormalities in cancer patients: anorexia and cachexia. *Surg Clin North Am* 1986; 66:947.

146. Jeevanandam M, Legaspi A, Lowry SF, et al. Effect of total parenteral nutrition on whole body protein kinetics in cachectic patients with benign or malignant disease. *J Parenter Enteral Nutr* 1988; 12:229.

147. Bozzetti F. Effects of artificial nutrition on the nutritional status of cancer patients. *J Parentar Enteral Nutr* 1989; 13:406.

148. Koretz RL. Parenteral nutrition: is it oncologically logical. *J Clin Oncol* 1984; 2:534–538.

149. McGeer AJ, Detsky AS, O'Rourke K. Parenteral nutrition in patients receiving cancer chemotherapy. *Ann Intern Med* 1989; 110:734–736.

150. Morrison SD, Moley JF, Norton JA. Contribution of inert mass to experimental cancer cachexia in rats. *J Natl Cancer Inst* 1984; 73:991.

151. Kitada S, Hays EF, Mead JF. A lipid mobilizing factor in the serum of tumor-bearing mice. *Lipids* 1980; 15:168.

152. Masumo H, Yamasak N, Okuda H. Purification and characterization of a lipolytic factor (toxohormone-L) from cell free fluid of ascites sarcoma 180. *Cancer Res* 1981; 41:284–288.

153. Liebelt FA, Gehring G, Delmonte L, et al. Paraneoplastic syndromes in experimental animal model systems. *Ann N Y Acad Sci* 1974; 230:547–564.

154. Costa G, Holland JF. Effects of Krebs-2 carcinoma on the lipid metabolism of male Swiss mice. *Cancer Res* 1962; 22:1081–1083.

155. Chalmer TM, Kekwick A, Pawan GLS. On the fat-mobilizing activity of human urine. *Lancet* 1958; 1:866–869.

156. Borai B, DeWys W. Assay for presence of anorexic substance in urine of cancer patients. *Proc AACR* 1980; 21:378.

157. Knoll J. Satietin: a highly potent anorexogenic substance in human serum. *Physiol Behav* 1979; 23:497–502.

158. Reichelt KL, Foss I, Trygstad O, et al. Humoral control of appetite. II. Purification and characterization of an anorexigenic peptide from human urine. *Neuroscience* 1978; 3:1207.

159. Norton JA, Moley JF, Green MV, Carson RE, Morrison SD. Parabiotic transfer of cancer anorexia/cachexia in male rats. *Cancer Res* 1985; 45:5547–5552.

160. McNamara MJ, Alexander HR, Norton JA. Cytokines and their role in the pathophysiology of cancer cachexia. *J Parenter Enteral Nutr* 1992; 16:505–535.

161. Balkwill F, Osborne R, Burke F, et al. Evidence for tumor necrosis factor/cachectin production in cancer. *Lancet* 1987; 2:1229–1232.

162. Socher SH, Martinez D, Craig JB, Kuhn JG, Oliff A. Tumor necrosis factor not detectable in patients with clinical cancer cachexia. *J Natl Cancer Inst* 1988; 80:595–598.

163. Moldawer LL, Lundholm CD, Lundholm K. Monocytic production and plasma bioactivities of interleukin-1 and tumour necrosis factor. *Eur J Cell Biol* 1988; 18:486–492.

164. Beutler B, Cerami A. Cachectin and tumour necrosis factor as two sides of the biological coin. *Nature* 1986; 320:584–588.

165. Beutler B, Cerami A. The common mediator of shock, cachexia and tumor necrosis. *Adv Immunol* 1988; 42:213–217.

166. Oliff A. The role of tumor necrosis factor (cachectin) in cachexia. *Cell* 1988; 54:141–142.

167. Beutler B, Mahoney J, Le Trang N, Pekala P, Cerami A. Purification of cachectin, a lipoprotein lipase-suppressing hormone secreted by endotoxin-induced RAW 264.7 cells. *J Exp Med* 1985; 161:984–995.

168. Carswell EA, Old LJ, Kassell RL, Green S, Fiore N, Williamson B. An endotoxin-induced serum factor that causes necrosis of tumors. *Proc Natl Acad Sci USA* 1975; 72:3666–3670.

169. Stovroff MC, Fraker DL, Travis WD, et al. Altered macrophage activity and tumor necrosis factor: tumor necrosis and host cachexia. *J Surg Res* 1989; 46:462–469.

170. Aderka D, Fisher S, Levo Y, et al. Cachectin/tumor necrosis factor production by cancer patients. *Lancet* 1985; 2:1190–1192.

171. Oster W, Cicco NA, Klein H, Hirano T, Kisimolto T, Lindemann A, Mertelsmann RH, Herrmann F. Participation of the cytokines interleukin 6, TNF-alpha, and interleukin 1 beta secreted by acute myelogenous leukemia blasts in autocrine and paracrine leukemia growth control. *J Clin Invest* 1989;84:451–457.

172. Spriggs D, Imamura K, Rodriguez M, Horiguchi J, Kufe DW. Induction of TNF expression and resistance in a human breast tumour cell line. *Proc Natl Acad Sci USA* 1987; 84:6563–6566.

173. Spriggs D, Imamura K, Rodriguez M, Sariban E, Kufe DW. TNF expression in epithelial tumour cell lines. *J Clin Invest* 1988; 81:455–460.

174. Hsu PL, Hsu SM. Production of TNF-alpha and lymphotoxin by cells of Hodgkin's neoplastic cell lines HDLKM-1 and KM-H2. *Am J Pathol* 1989; 135:735–745.

175. Corbeil J, Evans LA, Vasak E, Cooper DA, Penny R. Culture and properties of cells derived from Kaposi's sarcoma. *J Immunol* 1991; 146:2972–2976.

176. Tori FM, Dieckmann B, Beutler B, Cerami A, Ringold GM. A macrophage factor inhibits adipocyte gene expression: an in vitro model of cachexia. *Science* 1985; 229:867–869.

177. Lee MD, Zentella A, Pekala PH, Cerami A. Effect of endotoxin-induced monokines on glucose metabolism in the muscle cell line L6. *Proc Natl Acad Sci USA* 1987; 84:2590–2594.

178. Starnes HF, Jr, Warren RS, Brennan MF. Protein synthesis in hepatocytes isolated from patients with gastrointestinal malignancy. *J Clin Invest* 1987; 80:1384–1390.

179. Warren RS, Donner DB, Starnes HF, Jr, Brennan MF. Modulation of endogenous hormone action by recombinant human tumor necrosis factor. *Proc Natl Acad Sci USA* 1987; 84:8619–8622.

180. Feingold KR, Grunfeld C. Tumor necrosis factor-alpha stimulates lipogenesis in the rat in vivo. *J Clin Invest* 1987; 80:184–190.

181. Brobeck JR. Food and temperature. *Recent Prog Horm Res* 1960; 16:439.

182. Llover M, Lopez-Soriano FJ, Argiles JM. Effects of TNF-alpha on muscle-protein turnover in female Wistar rats. *J Natl Cancer Inst* 1993; 85:1334–1339.

183. Tracey KJ, Wei H, Manogue KR, Fong Y, Hesse DG, Nguyen HT, Kuo GC, Beuhler B, Cotran RS, Cerami A, Lowry SF. Cachectin/tumor necrosis factor induces cachexia, anemia, and inflammation. *J Exp Med* 1988; 167:1211–1227.

184. Flores EA, Bistrian BR, Pomposelli JJ, Dinarello CA, Blackburn GL, Istfan NW. Infusion of tumor necrosis factor/cachectin promotes muscle catabolism in the rat. A synergistic effect with interleukin 1. *J Clin Invest* 1989; 83:1614–1622.

185. Carbo N, Costelli P, Tessitore L, Bagby GJ, Lopez-Soriano FJ, Baccino FM, Argiles JM. Anti-TNF-alpha treatment interferes with changes in lipid metabolism in a tumour cachexia model. *Clin Sci* 1994; 87:349–355.

186. Costelli P, Carbó N, Tessitore L, Bagby GJ, Lopez-Soriano FJ, Argilés JM, Baccino FM. Tumor necrosis factor-α mediates changes in tissue protein turnover in a rat cancer cachexia model. *J Clin Invest* 1993; 92:2783–2789.

187. Dessi S, Batetta B, Spano O, Bagby FJ, Tessitore L, Costelli P, Baccino FM, Pani P, Argile JM. Perturbations of triglycerides but not of cholesterol metabolism are prevented by anti-TNF treatment in rats bearing an ascites hepatoma (Yoshida AH-130). *Br J Cancer* 1995; 72:1138–1143.

188. Warren RS, Starnes HF, Alcock N, Calvano S, Brennan MF. Hormonal and metabolic response to recombinant human tumor necrosis factor in rat: in vitro and in vivo. *Am J Physiol* 1988; 255:E206–E212.

189. Socher SM, Friedman A, Martinez D. Recombinant human tumor necrosis factor induces acute reductions in food intake and body weight in mice. *J Exp Med* 1988; 167:1957.

190. Darling G, Fraker DL, Jensen JC, Gorschboth CM, Norton JA. Cachectic effects of recombinant human tumor necrosis factor in rats. *Cancer Res* 1990; 50:4008–4013.

191. Oliff A, Defeo-Jones D, Boyer M, Martinez D, Kiefer D, Vuocolo G, Wolfe A, Socher SH. Tumors secreting human TNF/cachectin induce cachexia in mice. *Cell* 1987; 50:555–563.

192. Fraker DL, Stovroff MC, Merino MJ, Norton JA. Tolerance to tumor necrosis factor in rats and the relationship to endotoxin tolerance and toxicity. *J Exp Med* 1988; 168:95–105.

193. Tracey KJ, Morgello S, Koplin B, Fahey TJ, III, Fox J, Aledo A, Monogue KR, Cerami A. Metabolic effects of cachectin/tumor necrosis factor are modified by site of production. *J Clin Invest* 1990; 86:2014–2024.

194. Stovroff MC, Fraker DL, Swedenborg JA, Norton JA. Cachectin/tumor necrosis factor: a possible mediator of cancer anorexia in the rat. *Cancer Res* 1988; 48:4567–4572.

195. Sherry BA, Gelin J, Fong Y, Marano M, Wei H, Cerami A, Lowry SF, Lundholm KG, Moldawer LL. Anticachectin/tumor necrosis factor-α antibodies attenuate development of cachexia in tumor models. *FASEB J* 1989; 3:1956–1962.

196. Fraker DL, Merino MJ, Norton JA. Reversal of the toxic effects of cachectin by concurrent insulin administration. *Am J Physiol* 1989; 256:E725–E731.

197. Abbruzzese JL, Levin B, Ajani JA. Phase I. Trial of recombinant human gamma interferon and recombinant human tumor necrosis factor in patients with advanced gastrointestinal cancer. *Cancer Res* 1989; 49:4057.

198. Fraker DL, Alexander HR, Pass HI. Biologic therapy with TNF: systemic administration and isolation-perfusion. In: DeVita V, Hellman S, Rosenberg SA, eds. *Biologic Therapy of Cancer.* Philadelphia: J.B. Lippincott; 1995: 329–345.

199. Blick M, Sherwin SA, Rosenblum M, Gutterman J. Phase I study of recombinant tumor necrosis factor in cancer patients. *Cancer Res* 1987; 47:2986–2989.

200. Sherman ML, Spriggs DR, Arthur KA, Imamura K, Frei E, III, Kufe DW. Recombinant human tumor necrosis factor administered as a five-day continuous infusion in cancer patients: phase I toxicity and effects of lipid metabolism. *J Clin Oncol* 1988; 6:344–350.

201. Kriegler M, Perez C, DeFay K, et al. A novel form of TNF/cachectin is a cell surface cytotoxic trans-membrane protein: ramifications for the complex physiology of TNF. *Cell* 1988; 53:45–53.

202. Strassmann G, Jacob C, Evans R, Beell D, Fong M. Mechanisms of experimental cancer cachexia interaction between mononuclear phagocytes and colon 26 carcinoma and its relevance to IL-6 mediated cancer cachexia. *J Immunol* 1992; 148:3674–3678.

203. Fong Y, Moldawer LL, Marano M, Wei H, Barber A, Manogue K, Tracey KJ, Kuo G, Fischman DA, Cerami A, Lowry SF. Cachectin/TNF or IL-1a induces cachexia with redistribution of body proteins. *Am J Physiol* 1989; 256:R659–R665.

204. Moldawer LL, Andersson C, Gelin J, et al. Regulation of food intake and hepatic protein synthesis by recombinant derived cytokines. *Am J Physiol* 1988; 254:6450–6456.

205. Hellerstein MC, Meydani SN, Meydani M, Wu K, Dinarello CA. Interleukin-1-induced anorexia in the rat. *J Clin Invest* 1989; 84:228–235.

206. Tocco-Bradley R, Georgieff M, Jones CT, Moldawer LL, Dinarello CA, Blackburn GL, Bistrian BR. Changes in energy expenditure and fat metabolism in rats infused with interleukin 1. *Eur J Clin Invest* 1987; 17:504–510.

207. Gemlo BT, Palladino MA, Jaffe HS, Espevik TP, Raynor AA. Circulating cytokines in patients with metastatic cancer treated with recombinant interleukin-2 and lymphokine-activated killer cells. *Cancer Res* 1988; 48:5864–5867.

208. Costelli P, Llover M, Carbo N, Garcia-Martinez C, et al. Interleukin-1 receptor antagonist (IL-1ra) is unable to reverse cachexia in rats bearing an ascites hepatoma (Yowhida AH-130). *Cancer Lett* 1995; 95:33–38.

209. Argiles JM, Lopez-Soriano FJ, Wiggins D, Williamson DH. Comparative effects of tumour necrosis factor a (cachectin), interleukin-1-β and tumour growth on amino acid metabolism in the rat in vivo. Absorption and tissue uptake of a-amino [^{14}C] isobutyrate. *Biochem J* 1989; 261:357–362.

210. Del Rey A, Besedovsky H. Interleukin-1 affects glucose homeostasis. *Am J Physiol* 1987; 253:R794–R798.

211. Tredget EE, Yu YM, Zhong S, Burini R, Okusawa S, Gelfand JA, Dinarello CA, Young VR, Burke JF. Role of interleukin-1 and tumor necrosis factor in energy metabolism in rabbits. *Am J Physiol* 1988; 255:E760–E768.

212. Pomposelli JJ, Flores EA, Bistrian BR. Role of biochemical mediators in clinical nutrition and surgical metabolism. *J Parenter Enteral Nutr* 1988; 12:212–218.

213. Gelin J, Moldawer LL, Lonnroth C, Sherry B, Chizzonite R, Lundholm K. Role of endogenous tumor necrosis factor α and interleukin 1 for experimental tumor growth and the development of cancer cachexia. *Cancer Res* 1991; 51:415–421.

214. Strassmann G, Masui Y, Chizzonite R, Fong M. Mechanisms of experimental cancer cachexia. *J Immunol* 1993; 150:2341–2345.

215. Heinrich PC, Castell JV, Andus T. Interleukin-6 and the acute phase response. *Biochem J* 1990; 265:621–636.

216. Fong Y, Moldawer LL, Marano M, et al. Endotoxemia elicits circulating beta$_2$-interferon/interleukin-6 in man. *J Immunol* 1989; 142:2321–2325.

217. Akira S, Hirano T, Taga T, et al. Biology of multifunctional cytokines: IL-6 and related molecules. *FASEB J* 1990; 4:2860–2967.

218. Gelin J, Moldawer LL, Engless I, et al. Appearance of hybridoma growth factor/interleukin-6 in the serum of mice bearing a methylcholanthrene-induced sarcoma. *Biochem Biophys Res Commun* 1988; 157:575–580.

219. Greenberg AS, Nordan RP, McIntosh J, Calvo JC, Scow RO, Jablons D. Interleukin 6 reduces lipoprotein lipase activity in adipose tissue of mice in vivo and in 3T3-L1 adipocytes: a possible role for interleukin 6 in cancer cachexia. *Cancer Res* 1992; 52:4113–4116.

220. Strassmann G, Fong M, Kenney JS, Jacob CO. Evidence for the involvement of interleukin 6 in experimental cancer cachexia. *J Clin Invest* 1992; 89:1681–1684.

221. Jablons DM, McIntosh JK, Mulé JJ. Induction of interferon-2/interleukin-6 by cytokine administration and detection of circulating interleukin-6 in the tumor bearing state. *Ann N Y Acad Sci* 1989; 557:157–160.
222. Mule JJ, McIntosh JK, Jablons DM, Rosenberg SA. Antitumor activity of recombinant interleukin-6 in mice. *J Exp Med* 1990; 171:629–636.
223. Ohe Y, Podack ER, Olsen KJ, Miyahara Y, Miura K, Saito H, Koishihara Y, Ohsugi Y, Ohira T, Nichio K, Saijo N. Interleukin-6 cDNA transfected Lewis lung carcinoma cells show unaltered net tumour growth rate but cause weight loss and shorten survival in syngenic mice. *Br J Cancer* 1993; 67:939–944.
224. McIntosh JK, Jablons DM, Mulé JJ, et al. In vivo induction of IL-6 by administration of exogenous cytokines and detection of de novo serum levels of IL-6 in tumorbearing mice. *J Immunol* 1989; 143:162.
225. Fearon KCH, McMillan DC, Preston T, Winstanley FP, Cruickshank AM, Shenkin A. Elevated circulating interleukin-6 is associated with an acute-phase response but reduced fixed hepatic protein synthesis in patients with cancer. *Ann Surg* 1991; 213:26–31.
226. Soda K, Kawakami M, Kashii A, Miyata M. Characterization of mice bearing subclones of colon 26 adenocarcinoma disqualifies interleukin-6 as the sole inducer of cachexia. *Jpn J Cancer Res* 1994; 85:1124–1130.
227. Soda K, Kawakami M, Kashii A, Miyata M. Manifestations of cancer cachexia induced by colon 26 adenocarcinoma are not fully ascribable to interleukin-6. *Int J Cancer* 1995; 62:332–336.
228. Matthys P, Dukmans R, Proost P, et al. Severe cachexia in mice inoculated with interferon-gamma-producing tumor cells. *Int J Cancer* 1991; 49:77–82.
229. Matthys P, Heremans H, Opdenakker G, Billiau A. Anti-interferon-gamma antibody treatment, growth of Lewis lung tumors in mice and tumor-associated cachexia. *Eur J Cancer* 1991; 27:182–187.
230. Metcalf D, Gearing DP. Fatal syndrome in mice engrafted with cells producing high levels of the leukemia inhibitory factor. *Proc Natl Acad Sci USA* 1989; 86:5948–5952.
231. Langstein HN, Doherty GM, Fraker DL, Buresh CM, Norton JA. The roles of interferon-gamma and tumor necrosis factor in an experimental rat model of cancer cachexia. *Cancer Res* 1991; 51:2302–2306.
232. Berg M, Fraker DL, Alexander HR. Characterization of differentiation factor/leukaemia inhibitory factor effect on lipoprotein lipase activity and mRNA in 3T3-L1 adipocytes. *Cytokine* 1994; 6:425–432.
233. Mori M, Yamaguchi K, Abe K. Purification of a lipoprotein lipase-inhibiting protein produced by a melanoma cell line associated with cancer cachexia. *Biochem Biophys Res Comm* 1989; 160:1085–1092.
234. Metcalf D. The leukemia inhibitory factor (LIF). *Int J Cell Cloning* 1991; 9:95–108.
235. Metcalf D, Nicola NIA, Gearing DP. Effects of injected leukemia inhibitory factor on hematopoietic and other tissues in mice. *Blood* 1990; 76:50–56.
236. Tchekmedyian S, Tait N, Moody M, et al. High dose megestrol acetate: a possible treatment for cachexia. *JAMA* 1987; 257:1195–1199.
237. Anonymous. Cyproheptadine. *Lancet* 1978; 1:368.
238. Kardinal CG, Loprinzi CL, Schaid DJ, Hass AC, Dose AM, Athmann LM, Mailliard JA, McCormack GW, Gerstner JB, Schray MF. A controlled trial of cyproheptadine in cancer patients with anorexia and/or cachexia. *Cancer* 1990; 65:2657–2662.

239. Ray PD, Hanson RL, Lardy HA. Inhibition by hydrazine of gluconeogenisis in the rat. *J Biol Chem* 1970; 5:690–696.

240. Silverstein R, Bhatia P, Svoboda DS. Effect of hydrazine sulfate on glucose-regulating enzymes in the normal and cancerous rat. *Immunopharmacology* 1989; 17:37–43.

241. Chlebowski RT, Bulcavage L, Grosvenor M, Oktay E, Block JB, Chlebowski JS, Ali I, Frashoff R. Hydrazine sulfate influence on nutritional status and survival in non-small-cell lung cancer. *J Clin Oncol* 1990; 8:9–15.

242. Wadleigh R, Spaulding GM, Lumbershky B, et al. Dronabinol enhancement of appetite and cancer patients (Abstract). *Proc Am Soc Oncol* 1990; 9:331.

6

The Pharmacological Manipulation of Appetite

CHARLES L. LOPRINZI

Cancer anorexia/cachexia is clearly a major clinical problem for many patients who die from cancer. Anorexia and asthenia have been identified as more common symptoms in patients entering hospice programs than are pain or dysphagia.[1] In addition, it is felt that a large number of patients dying from cancer die from asthenia.[2] Anorexia appears to cause suffering for both patients themselves and for their family members as the patients appear to waste away without even trying to eat. In response to this substantial clinical problem, a number of drugs have been evaluated as potential means for reversing cancer anorexia/cachexia.

Before discussing specific drugs, it is worth discussing study design issues. While there are sophisticated methodologies for determining changes in body composition among different body compartments (fluid, lean tissue, and adipose tissue), the methodologies available are relatively cumbersome and few large clinical trials have utilized this technology. As a surrogate, body weight has been frequently used in clinical trials. This can be problematic for patients who develop edema or ascites, common problems in patients with advanced cancer. Nonetheless, weight changes in those patients who do not develop clinical evidence of edema or ascites can be a helpful measure of whether patients are actually gaining true body mass on a particular trial.

Although body weights may be an objective measurement of whether a patient is increasing true body mass and thus presumably caloric intake, it is probably more important in most patients to try to reverse anorexia, as opposed to trying to reverse cachexia. This is because anorexia is probably a more potent cause of suffering in advanced patients than is cachexia. Although anorexia is clearly a subjective symptom (as is pain), it is something that can be objectively measured (as can pain) by the use of relatively simple questionnaire instruments.

As a rule, the anorexia questionnaires that have been utilized in clinical trials have not undergone formal validity testing, a process that might take years in and of itself. Nonetheless, there are several pieces of information which demonstrate that the information obtained on these questionnaires is reliable and valid. These reasons are as follows: *(1)* several related questions on individual questionnaires provide similar data;[3-5] *(2)* multiple trials using different questionnaires have come to the same conclusion regarding a single drug and its effect on anorexia/cachexia;[3,6-9] and *(3)* measurements of appetite changes directly correlate with changes in nonfluid body weight gains.[5] These data, and the clinical experience with evaluating thousands of patients on randomized clinical trials, substantiate that there is appropriate methodology available for studying means of inhibiting cancer anorexia/cachexia. However, a few words of caution are in order here. First, uncontrolled clinical trials are to be interpreted with a large dose of wariness. This is because a "stimulation of appetite" appears to be present in approximately 40% of patients receiving a placebo, as illustrated in several controlled trials.[3,4,10]

In addition to the requirement for control arms in randomized clinical trials, relatively large patient numbers are necessary for the following reasons. *(1)* There is a relatively large diversity of patients with cancer anorexia/cachexia, with varying primary tumor sites and varying degrees of anorexia/cachexia. *(2)* There are a number of other treatments, such as chemotherapy and radiation therapy, that patients with cancer anorexia/cachexia are concurrently receiving. *(3)* A relatively large dropout of patients occurs within weeks of entering a cancer anorexia/cachexia trial, given the relatively poor overall prognosis of this patient group; the median time that patients might continue on such a clinical trial is on the order of approximately 6 weeks.[3,4] Despite these limitations, however, valuable information can be provided by large, controlled clinical trials.

Proven Antidotes for Cancer Anorexia/Cachexia

Progestational agents

Progestational analogues such as megestrol acetate or medroxyprogesterone acetate are the most thoroughly studied and appear to be the most powerful appetite stimulants available for clinical practice. The vast bulk of information regarding these drugs has been generated with the use of megestrol acetate. Nonetheless, the small amount of data generated from the study of medroxyprogesterone acetate[11] suggests that similar findings are seen with both of these progestational agents.

These drugs were initially noted to cause appetite stimulation and weight gain when they were utilized in patients with advanced breast or endometrial cancer.[12,13] Pilot evaluations of megestrol acetate in patients with cancer other than breast or endometrial cancer suggested that these drugs stimulated appetite and led to nonfluid weight gain. In these pilot trials there was a suggestion of a dose–response effect.[14] On the basis of these preliminary data, a number of placebo-controlled, double-blinded, randomized clinical trials were performed in patients with cancer anorexia/cachexia. The first published report of such a trial appeared in 1990. This trial demonstrated a substantial increase in appetite and fluid intake in patients receiving 800 mg per day of megestrol acetate compared with a placebo.[3] Subsequent to this came publications of independently conducted, placebo-controlled trials comparing various doses (ranging from 240 mg to 1600 mg per day) of megestrol acetate, consistently demonstrating an appetite stimulation for this drug.[6–8] In addition to these trials in patients with cancer anorexia/cachexia, randomized, placebo-controlled clinical trials have also demonstrated that megestrol acetate stimulates appetite and causes weight gain in patients with AIDS anorexia/cachexia.[9,15] It is reasonable to hypothesize that the etiologies behind cancer anorexia/cachexia and its therapy are quite similar to that of AIDS anorexia/cachexia.

The multiple, positive placebo-controlled trials of various doses of megestrol acetate for cancer anorexia/cachexia set the stage for a trial to address the dose–response question. To this end, a four-arm randomized trial, involving a total of approximately 320 patients, evaluated megestrol acetate doses of 160, 480, 800, and 1280 mg per day as a single daily dose. This trial demonstrated a positive dose–response effect as doses increased from 160 mg to 800 mg per day.[5] No further appetite stimulation was seen at doses of 1280 mg per day.

In addition to the multiple trials evaluating the effect of megestrol acetate on appetite and body weight, a few trials have evaluated body composition changes with this drug. These trials demonstrate that megestrol acetate leads to an increase in true body mass as opposed to just fluid accumulation.[9,16,17] Much of this weight gain is adipose tissue, as opposed to lean body mass, but this can have a favorable impact upon patients with marked anorexia/cachexia.

Given the knowledge that megestrol acetate improves appetite and leads to nonfluid weight gain in patients with advanced cancer, and that anorexia and cachexia can cause suffering and may lead to death by inanition in advanced cancer patients, the question has arisen as to whether megestrol acetate could improve the quality of life and/or survival of patients with advanced incurable cancers. Pursuant to this, a relatively large, placebo-controlled clinical trial was developed to study megestrol acetate versus placebo in a relatively uniform group of newly diagnosed cancer patients. Chosen for this study were patients with previously untreated, extensive-stage small-cell lung cancer. All patients were assigned to receive four cycles of etoposide and cisplatin chemotherapy and subsequently to receive tailored radiation therapy. Patients were randomly assigned to receive 800 mg per day of megestrol acetate or an identical-appearing placebo. This study did not support the prestudy hypothesis, as it demonstrated that there was no substantial difference in quality of life measurements or survival among the groups of patients randomized to megestrol acetate versus placebo.[18]

With regard to the toxicity of megestrol acetate, this drug is generally well tolerated by most patients. Early trials evaluating whether it caused nausea or vomiting paradoxically demonstrated that megestrol acetate has anti-emetic properties. In fact, it appears to decrease the nausea and vomiting that is seen in patients with advanced cancer by approximately two-thirds.[3,8,18] There are some data to suggest that megestrol acetate causes peripheral edema, but this is usually a very mild problem that can be readily alleviated by mild diuretics.[19] This drug appears to mildly increase the incidence of thromboembolic phenomenon, probably more so in patients receiving concomitant chemotherapy.[18,19] Megestrol acetate has been reported to cause reversible impotence in some men[9] and withdrawal menstrual bleeding within 2 or 3 weeks of discontinuing it in some women.[20]

Megestrol acetate clearly decreases serum cortisol levels and appears to do this through an inhibition of the pituitary–adrenal axis.[21] In most patients this appears to be an asymptomatic clinical phenomenon. Nonetheless, it is important that physicians be aware of this situation. In one placebo-controlled clinical trial of patients receiving concomitant chemotherapy[18] there was a trend toward more septic deaths in the patients receiving megestrol acetate, despite less myelosuppression in this group. It has been hypothesized that this is because of an inability of patients to generate a physiologic steroid boost during periods of stress.[18] Thus it is recommended that patients receiving megestrol acetate get stress doses of corticosteroids during periods of substantial trauma, infection, or surgery. In clinical practice, for decades we have stopped megestrol acetate without a taper and have not noted any clinically apparent detriment in the overwhelming majority of patients. Nonetheless, rare reports of Addisonian signs and symptoms have recently been reported in patients who had megestrol acetate abruptly stopped.[22] If patients develop such symptoms, they should be treated with corticosteroids and subsequently have the corticosteroids tapered in a usual manner for patients who have been on long-term corticosteroids.

Corticosteroids

Corticosteroids are the next most thoroughly studied drug for treatment of cancer anorexia/cachexia. Placebo-controlled trials of this drug were conducted well before any trials were conducted with progestational drugs. Four placebo-controlled clinical trials have all demonstrated that corticosteroids can temporarily stimulate appetite in patients with advanced cancer.[23–26] None of them have shown a positive effect on body weight. The primary potential advantage of corticosteroids, over progestational agents, is that they can be much less expensive in terms of drug delivery. The potential disadvantages are that their appetite-stimulatory properties do not appear to be as potent as those of progestational agents, and they appear to have more clinically apparent toxicities. A clinical trial is currently taking place to prospectively compare corticosteroids and progestational agents (see below).

Potentially Useful Medications Undergoing Evaluation for Treatment of Cancer Anorexia/Cachexia

Dronabinol

Dronabinol is a derivative of marijuana that is available in a tablet form. Small pilot evaluations have provided preliminary information suggesting that this drug might be helpful as an appetite stimulant in patients with anorexia/cachexia.[27-30] To date, placebo-controlled clinical trials have not been done in patients with cancer anorexia/cachexia. Nonetheless, on the basis of a single placebo-controlled, clinical trial of this drug in patients with AIDS anorexia/cachexia,[31] dronabinol has been FDA-approved for treatment of AIDS anorexia/cachexia. More definitive evaluation of this drug in patients with cancer anorexia/cachexia is ongoing.

Metaclopromide

Metaclopromide is a medication that has been used for treatment of gastric paresis, chemotherapy-associated nausea and vomiting, and for narcotic-induced constipation. A pilot trial has suggested that this drug might have some efficacy for the treatment of cancer anorexia/cachexia.[32] But because of the hazards of small pilot trials in this situation and the substantial "placebo effect," more definitive clinical evaluation of this drug is needed before recommending it for treatment of cancer anorexia/cachexia.

Anabolic steroids

Anabolic steroids can lead to an increase in muscle mass.[33] This has resulted in the use of these drugs for athletes, despite this practice being discouraged because of the side effects that can be associated with them. With this background, pilot experience has suggested that anabolic steroids might have some effect on cancer anorexia/cachexia.[34] An anabolic steroid is currently being tested in a comparative clinical trial (see below) in patients with cancer anorexia/cachexia, but it is not recommended for routine use, pending the results of this trial.

Branched-chain amino acids

Preliminary studies suggested that branched-chain amino acids might be efficacious in patients for treatment of cancer anorexia/cachexia.[35] It has been hypothesized that this therapy might overcome alterations in host protein and amino acid metabolism associated with malignant cachexia. More definitive work is necessary to better understand the potential pros and cons of using this approach for treatment of cancer anorexia/cachexia.

Medications Definitively Tested but Which Do Not Appear to Be Helpful

Cyproheptadine

Cyproheptadine is an antiserotinergic antihistamine that has been demonstrated to have appetite-stimulatory properties in healthy patients and in some patients with anorexia nervosa. Based upon studies from the 1970s which illustrated this property, a large placebo-controlled clinical trial was conducted in approximately 300 patients with cancer anorexia/cachexia. This trial demonstrated very mild appetite stimulatory properties of cyproheptadine in patients with cancer anorexia/cachexia, but the effect was minimal and did not translate into any nonfluid weight gain. It was thus concluded that this drug was not a potent enough appetite stimulant to recommend for reversing cancer anorexia/cachexia.[4] An exception to this rule applies to patients with the carcinoid syndrome in which, presumably, a direct antiserotonergic effect counterbalances the excess serotonergic activity of carcinoid tumors. In these patients, cyproheptadine can lead to substantial weight gain.[36]

Pentoxyfilline

On the basis of promising preliminary information demonstrating that pentoxyfilline could inhibit RNA expression of tumor necrosis factor,[37] a prospective, placebo-controlled clinical trial was conducted. Unfortunately, this clinical trial did not demonstrate any suggestion of appetite stimulation or weight gain in patients with advanced cancer anorexia/cachexia.[10]

Hydrazine sulfate

Hydrazine sulfate is a controversial drug that has been around in various testing modalities for approximately two decades.[37-42] Because preliminary evidence suggested that it might have beneficial properties for patients with cancer anorexia/cachexia, three relatively large, placebo-controlled, double-blinded clinical trials were conducted. None of these trials was able to demonstrate any benefit for hydrazine sulfate in patients with advanced cancer.[43-45]

Recommendations for Clinical Practice

The current clinical knowledge of cancer anorexia/cachexia indicates that patients should not be treated prophylactically for this disorder, just as they should not be treated prophylactically with narcotics, despite pain being a common problem in patients with advanced cancer. Nonetheless, it is reasonable to treat those patients for whom anorexia/cachexia is a prominent clinical problem, as it causes suffering for patients and/or their families. The drug of choice for this situation is megestrol acetate because it appears to be the most powerful appetite stimulant available, has undergone dose-response testing, and has relatively few toxicities. I recommend a starting dose of 400–800 per day over a 2-week period. If there is no appreciable benefit in terms of appetite stimulation or antiemetic properties by the end of the 2-week period, this medication should cease. If there is evident benefit, the drug should be continued. It may be able to be titrated down to 400 or 200 mg per day. The drug is then continued as long as there is evident clinical benefit. An alternative to megestrol acetate is to use a corticosteroid, such as dexamethasone, with a dosage of 3.0 mg per day.

Ongoing Clinical Trials

A randomized North Central Cancer Treatment Group clinical trial involving a total of 450 patients evaluated megestrol acetate versus the anabolic steroid, fluoxymesterone, versus the corticosteroid, dexamethasone, in patients with advanced cancer anorexia/cachexia. The final results of this trial should be available in 1998. Another similar-sized clinical trial is accruing patients to compare megestrol acetate with dronabinol to the combination of these two drugs in a similar population of patients. This trial is also being conducted by the North Central Cancer Treatment Group.

References

1. Bruera E, MacDonald RN. Asthenia in patients with advanced cancer. *J Pain Symptom Manage* 1988; 3:9–14.
2. DeWys WD, Begg C, Lavin PT, et al. Prognostic effect of weight loss prior to chemotherapy in cancer patients. *Am J Med* 1980; 69:491–497.
3. Loprinzi CL, Ellison NM, Schaid DJ, et al. Controlled trial of megestrol acetate for the treatment of cancer anorexia and cachexia. *J Natl Cancer Inst* 1990; 82:1127–1132.
4. Kardinal CG, Loprinzi CL, Schaid DJ, et al. A controlled trial of cyproheptadine in cancer patients with anorexia and/or cachexia. *Cancer* 1990; 65:2657–2662.
5. Loprinzi CL, Michalak JC, Schaid DJ, Mailliard JA, Athmann LH, Goldberg RM, Tschetter LK, Hatfield AK, Morton RF. Phase III evaluation of four doses of megestrol acetate as therapy for patients with cancer anorexia and/or cachexia. *J Clin Oncol* 1993; 11:762–767.
6. Bruera E, Macmillan K, Kuehn N, et al. A controlled trial of megestrol acetate on appetite, caloric intake, nutritional status, and other symptoms in patients with advanced cancer. *Cancer* 1990; 66:1279–1282.
7. Feliu J, Gonzalez-Baron M, Berrocal A, Artal A, Ordonez A, Garrido P, Zamora PO, Garcia de Paredea ML, Montero JM. Usefulness of megestrol acetate in cancer cachexia and anorexia. *Am J Clin Oncol CCT* 1992; 15:436–440.

8. Tchekmedyian NS, Hickman M, Siau J, Greco FA, Keller J, Browder H, Aisner J. Megestrol acetate in cancer anorexia and weight loss. *Cancer* 1992; 69:1268–1274.

9. Von Roenn JH, Armstrong D, Kotler DP, Cohn DL, Klimas NG, Tchekmedyian NS, et al. Megestrol acetate in patients with AIDS-related cachexia. *Ann Intern Med* 1994; 121:393–399.

10. Goldberg RM, Loprinzi CL, Mailliard JA, O'Fallon JR, Krook JE, Ghosh C, Hestorff RD, Chong SF, Reuter NF, Shanahan TG. Pentoxifylline for treatment of cancer anorexia/cachexia? A randomized double-blinded, placebo-controlled trial. *J Clin Oncol* 1995; 13:2856–2859.

11. Downer S, Joel S, Allbright A, Plant H, Stubbs L, Talbot D, Slevin M. A double blind placebo controlled trial of medroxyprogesteorne acetate (MPA) in cancer cachexia. *Br J Cancer* 1993; 67:1102–1105.

12. Gregory EJ, Cohen SC, Oines DW, et al. Megestrol acetate therapy for advanced breast cancer. *J Clin Oncol* 1985; 3:155–160.

13. Bonomi P, Pessis D, Bunting N, et al. Megestrol acetate used as primary hormonal therapy in stage D prostatic cancer. *Semin Oncol* 1985; 12:36–39.

14. Tchekmedyian NS, Tait N, Moody M, et al. High-dose megestrol acetate: a possible treatment for cachexia. *JAMA* 1987; 257:1195–1198.

15. Oster MH, Enders SR, Samuels SJ, Cone LA, Hooton TM, Browder HP, et al. Megestrol acetate in patients with AIDS and cachexia. *Ann Intern Med* 1994; 121:400–408.

16. Loprinzi CL, Schaid DJ, Dose AM, Burnham NL, Jensen MD. Body-composition changes in patients who gain weight while receiving megestrol acetate. *J Clin Oncol* 1993; 11:152–154.

17. Reitmeier M, Hartenstein RC. Megestrol acetate and determination of body composition by bioelectral impedance analysis in cancer cachexia (Abstract). *Proc Am Soc Clin Oncol* 1990; 9:325.

18. Rowland KM, Jr, Loprinzi CL, Shaw EG, Maksymiuk AW, Kuross SA, et al. Randomized double blind placebo controlled trial of cisplatin and etoposide plus megestrol acetate/placebo in extensive stage small cell lung cancer. A North Central Cancer Treatment Group Study. *J Clin Oncol* 1996; 14:135–141.

19. Loprinzi CL, Johnson P, Jensen M. Megestrol acetate for anorexia and cachexia. *Oncology* 1992; 49 (Suppl 2):46–49.

20. Loprinzi CL, Michalak JC, Quella SK, O'Fallon JR, Hatfield AK, Nelimark RA, Dose AM, Fischer T, Johnson C, Klatt NE, Bate W, Rospond RM, Oesterline JE. Megestrol acetate for the prevention of hot flashes. *N Engl J Med* 1994; 33:347–352.

21. Loprinzi CL, Jensen MD, Jiang NS, Schaid DJ. Effect of megestrol acetate on the human pituitary-adrenal axis. *Mayo Clin Proc* 1992; 67:1160–1162.

22. Leinung MC, Liporace R, Miller CH. Induction of adrenal suppression by megestrol acetate in patients with AIDS. *Ann Intern Med* 1995; 122:843–845.

23. Moertel CG, Schutt AJ, Reitemeier RJ, Hahn RG. Corticosteroid therapy of preterminal gastrointestinal cancer. *Cancer* 1974; 33:1607–1609.

24. Bruera E, Roca E, Cedaro L, et al. Action of oral methylprednisolone in terminal cancer patients: a prospective randomized double-blind study. *Cancer Treat Rep* 1985; 69:751–754.

25. Popiela T, Lucchi R, Giongo F. Methylprednisolone as an appetite stimulant in patients with cancer. *Eur J Cancer Clin Oncol* 1989; 25:1823–1829

26. Wilcox J, Corr J, Shaw J, et al. Prednisolone as an appetite stimulant in patients with cancer. *Br Med J* 1984; 288:27.

27. Nelson K, Walsh D, Deeter P, Sheehan F. A phase II study of delta-9-tetrahydrocannabinol for appetite stimulation in cancer-associated anorexia. *J Palliat Care* 1994; 19:14–18.

28. Sacks N, Hutcheson JR, Watts JM, Webb RE. Case report: the effect of tetrahydrocannabinol on food intake during chemotherapy. *J Am Coll Nutr* 1990; 9:630–632.

29. Plasse TF, Gorter RW, Krasnow SH, Lane M, Shepard KV, Wadleight RG. Recent clinical experience with dronabinol. *Pharmacol Biochem Behav* 1991; 40:695–700.

30. Regelson W, Butler JR, Schulz J, Kirk T, Peek L, Green ML, Zalis MO. q[9]-tetrahydrocannabinol as an effective antidepressant and appetite-stimulating agent in advanced cancer patients. In: Brauda MC, Szxara S, eds. *The Pharmacology of Marihuana*. New York: Raven Press; 1976:763–776.

31. Beal JE, Olson R, Laubenstein L, Morales JO, Bellman P, Yango B, Lefkowitz L, Plasse TFD, Shepard KV. Dronabinol as a treatment for anorexia associated with weight loss in patients with AIDS. *J Pain Symptom Manage* 1995; 10:89.

32. Nelson KA, Walsh A. Metoclopramide in anorexia caused by cancer-associated dyspepsia syndrome (CADS). *J Palliat Care* 1993; 9:14–18.

33. Freed DJ, Banks AJ, Longson D, Burley DM. Anabolic steroids in athletics: crossover double-blind trial on weight lifters. *Br Med J* 1975; 5:471–473.

34. Chlebowski RT, Herrold J, Ali I, Ioktay E, Chelbowski JS, et al. Influence of nadrolone decanoate on weight loss in advanced non-small cell lung cancer. *Cancer* 1986; 58:183–186.

35. Pisters PW, Perlstone DB. Protein and amino acid metabolism in cancer cachexia: investigative techniques and therapeutic interventions. *Crit Rev Clin Lab Sci* 1993; 30:223–272.

36. Moertel CG, Kvols LK, Rubin J. A study of cyproheptadine in the treatment of metastatic carcinoid tumor and the malignant carcinoid syndrome. *Cancer* 1991; 67:33–36.

37. Dezube BJ, Fridovbich-Keil JL, Bouvard I, Lange RF, Pardee AB. Pentoxifylline and well-being in patients with cancer. *Lancet* 1990; I 335:662.

38. Lerner HJ, Regelson W. Clinical trial of hydrazine sulfate in solid tumors. *Cancer Treat Rep* 1976; 60:959–960.

39. Ochua Megace Jr, Wittes RE, Krakoff LC. Trial of hydrazine sulfate (NSC-150014) in patients with cancer. *Cancer Chemother Rep* 1975; 59:1151–1153.

40. Spremulli E, Wampler GL, Regelson W. Clinical study of hydrazine sulfate in advanced cancer patients. *Cancer Chemother Pharmacol* 1979; 3:121–124.

41. Filov VA, Danova LA, Gershanovich ML, et al. Hydrazine sulfate: experimental and clinical results, mechanism of action. In: Filov VA, Ivin BA, Dementyeva NP, et al., eds. *Medical Therapy of Tumors*. Leningrad, USSR: USSR Ministry of Health; 1983:92–139.

42. Chelbowski RT, Bulcavage L, Grosvenor M, et al. Hydrazine sulfate influence on nutritional status and survival in non-small cell lung cancer. *J Clin Oncol* 1990; 8:9–15.

43. Loprinzi CL, Goldberg RG, Su JOI, Mailliard J, Maksymiuk A, Kugler J, Jett J, Ghosh C, Pfeifle D, Wender D, Burch P. Placebo-controlled trial of hydrazine sulfate in patients with newly diagnosed non-small cell lung cancer. *J Clin Oncol* 1994; 12:1126–1129.

44. Loprinzi CL, Kuross SA, O'Fallon JR, Gesme DH, Gerstner JB, Rospond RM, Cobau CD, Goldberg RM. Randomized placebo-controlled evaluation of hydrazine sulfate in patients with advanced colorectal cancer. *J Clin Oncol* 1994; 12:1121–1125.
45. Kosty MPO, Fleishman SB, Herndon JE, Couglin K, Kornblith AB, Scalzo A, Morris JC, Mortimer J, Green MR. Cisplatin, vinblastine, and hydrazine sulfate in advanced, non-small cell lung cancer: a randomized placebo-controlled, double-blind phase III study of the cancer and leukemia group B. *J Clin Oncol* 1994; 12:1113–1120.

7

Practical Considerations in the Management of Anorexia/Cachexia: What Do We Say and What Do We Do?

ROBIN L. FAINSINGER

Cachexia and anorexia are both highly prevalent problems in advanced cancer patients. Anorexia generally refers to loss of appetite and a poor food intake, while cachexia refers to the weight loss suffered by these patients. Eighty to ninety percent of patients with advanced malignant disease have been reported to suffer from cachexia and anorexia.[1,2] While the ideal clinical management would be to remove the underlying cause, this is clearly not possible with the majority of these patients.

Dietary counseling, enteral and parenteral nutrition, and various pharmacological managements have all been suggested as possible treatment modalities. There have been many different reports of patients receiving all variations of these suggested therapies. These reports in turn have generated many reviews on the topic of cancer cachexia/anorexia, which, not surprisingly, have often referenced essentially the same available literature.[3–12] These many literature reports have been supplemented with frequent presentations at conferences around the world.

To the average practitioner looking after advanced cancer patients, these reports, reviews, and presentations may prove difficult to translate into a practical approach. The sometimes conflicting conclusions of different reviews and uncertain or unproven value of the different treatment options and costs of treatment, the likelihood of benefit to the individual patient, and varying circumstances of palliative care groups around the world are all problems that the practitioner has to consider.

As a result, this chapter will attempt to highlight the areas of agreement and controversy in the literature. Important lessons can also be learned from reports of practical experience in implementing treatment recommendations for managing cancer cachexia/anorexia. As MacDonald et al.[8] have pointed out: "At present, a 'heap of facts' garnered by research workers working in disparate areas is available to the clinical investigator concerned with cancer cachexia. The web connecting these observations in a coherent mosaic, however, remains to be fully woven." This chapter will attempt to create some coherence for the clinical practitioner.

Establishing the Purpose of Treatment

Various researchers have investigated the purpose of palliative treatment. Their views are summarized below.

Tchekmedyian[3] states that the intervention goals should be defined prior to instituting treatment. Symptom control and patient comfort are the major issues to evaluate in advanced cancer. Loprinzi[5] notes that it is unlikely that any of the therapeutic options will have much impact on patient survival. However, effective therapy could increase the quality of life just as effective analgesics and antiemetics do.

Bruera and colleagues[2,6,7] have been hopeful that successful treatment may result in improvements in both life expectancy and quality of life. However, as cure of the underlying cancer is not possible in the majority of advanced cancer patients, the main goal becomes improving quality of life. To achieve this goal, cachexia must be addressed. The four clinical manifestations of cachexia targeted by palliative interventions are decreased food intake, chronic nausea, asthenia, and changes in body image.

MacDonald et al.[8] note that because family studies demonstrate that problems associated with cachexia rank at the top of physical causes of suffering and psychosocial distress, cancer research outcome measures should emphasize improvement in function and satisfaction with therapy. Nelson et al.[9] state further that because there is no evidence that this problem can be cured or reversed, treatment should emphasize improving quality of life. The main target symptoms would be improving appetite and food intake.

Ottery[10,11] takes a more comprehensive approach to the goals of treatment in the cancer patient, maintaining that such goals are to support nutritional status, body composition, functional status, and quality of life. Emphasis is placed on early intervention, as attempts to reverse severe nutritional depletion are often as unsuccessful as chemotherapeutic approaches in advanced cancer patients.

The common theme of treatment purpose is clearly quality of life. This translates into treatment aimed at relieving nausea; improving appetite and maintaining or gaining weight; and psychosocial support and education to assist the patient and family in understanding and accepting the benefits and limits of treatment intervention.

Role of the Dietitian

Not surprisingly, reports written by dietitians strongly advocate for their role in the management of cancer patients with anorexia/cachexia.[12,13] Emphasis is made on the skills of dietitians in assessing nutritional status, dietary needs, and advice required by patients and their families. Dietitians can enhance comfort, food safety, and economic considerations, while continuing to maximize nutrition.

Loprinzi et al.[4] state that dietary counseling by a dietitian is a frequently used and reasonable approach in the management of cancer anorexia/cachexia. However, "the limitations of dietary counselling in this clinical situation are glaringly evident."[4] Tchekmedyian[3] notes, however, that a dietitian is useful not only in assessing nutritional needs but in providing patient education, counseling, and follow-up in an attempt to stabilize weight and improve food intake.

Bruera and colleagues[2,6,7] maintain that dietary counseling of patients and families is important in alleviating the anxiety and conflict that sometimes develops around the patient's inability to consume what would normally be considered an adequate diet. Nutrition counseling contributed to an increase in daily calorie intake by a mean of 450 calories in a series of 50 patients.[2] However, caloric intake fell to base line levels after 3 weeks of follow-up.

Ottery[10,11] advocates a formal clinic to address nutritional related issues. Their service offers a multidisciplinary nutritional clinic consisting of a dietitian, a physician, and an oncology clinical nurse specialist. Nutritional intervention is generally aimed at oral and enteral support, with most patients receiving only oral intake intervention. More than 70% of referred patients have apparently maintained or gained weight, and they have improved or maintained visceral protein status.

The inclusion of a dietitian in the interdisciplinary palliative care team is widely accepted and is included by many palliative care programs when describing the nature of their team.[14,16] However, there are also examples in the literature of descriptions of interdisciplinary palliative care teams that do not list a dietitian.[17–19]

The lack of formal prospective trials evaluating the benefit of nutritional support and dietitians in the management of cancer cachexia/anorexia has been recognized.[10,11] Prospective nutritional trials are being designed and a Society for Nutritional Oncology Adjuvant Therapy has been organized.[10,11]

Enteral and Parenteral Nutrition

What do we say?

Most health care professionals working in palliative care would probably concur with Shaw[12] that parenteral feeding is not appropriate for advanced cancer patients. The high cost, potential complications, and ethical considerations exclude use for all but extremely rare clinical situations.

Bozzetti[20] notes that in certain circumstances, enteral nutrition might help cancer patients with weight loss exacerbated by fistulas, short bowel obstruction, and vomiting or malabsorbtion caused by the tumor or the treatment. Nevertheless, data suggest that metabolic abnormalities besides simple starvation play a part in cancer malnutrition, which are difficult to reverse by nutritional support alone. The nutritional benefits of enteral nutrition are limited, with some evidence suggesting that the main benefit to anticipate is prevention of further nutritional deterioration rather than restoration to normal nutritional status.

Loprinzi[5] notes that because cancer anorexia/cachexia has been associated with decreased caloric intake, study has been undertaken to determine whether enteral or parenteral hyperalimentation would be beneficial. Extensive investigations have not supported the use of hyperalimentation as a helpful modality for these patients.

Bruera and colleagues[2,6,7] claim that enteral nutrition is far less expensive than parenteral nutrition and that parenteral nutrition has shown no benefit over enteral nutrition in patients with a functional bowel. Nevertheless, enteral nutrition is associated with significant morbidity, such as aspiration pneumonia and diarrhea. Enteral nutrition may be useful particularly for patients with advanced head and neck cancer or esophageal cancer because they are unable to swallow but are still disturbed by appetite and hunger. Studies of parenteral nutrition have not demonstrated that this treatment has a significant impact on tumor response to radiation or chemotherapy, treatment toxicity, or survival; these studies also have not assessed quality-of-life issues such as strength, performance status, and psychological issues. Given the high cost of parenteral nutrition, the difficulty of maintaining this treatment in the home, and significant associated morbidity, this treatment modality should continue to have a role only in highly selected cases.

Tchekmedyian[3] maintains that enteral nutrition can be helpful with partial obstruction or dysfunction of the gastrointestinal tract. Parenteral nutrition may be helpful for patients whose gastrointestinal function does not allow enteral feeding. However, in advanced cancer patients, parenteral nutrition does not appear to be of benefit and survival is not prolonged. As a result, routine use of enteral or parenteral nutrition is not recommended unless a symptomatic benefit is anticipated.

MacDonald et al.[8] caution that clinicians must diagnose the situations in which cancer patients are losing weight simply because of starvation. These may be corrected with enteral or parenteral nutrition. All changes in weight should not be automatically assumed to be due to the cachexia–anorexia syndrome. Examples of patients who may benefit from enteral and parenteral nutrition include patients with head and neck cancer, and some patients with ovarian carcinoma with intermittent small bowel obstruction. Nevertheless, the majority of cancer patients losing weight suffer from a complex metabolic aberration that will not respond to the replacement of calories via the enteral or parenteral route.

Nelson et al.[9] have found that when voluntary food intake is inadequate in the presence of a normal gastrointestinal tract, additional nutritional support can be provided by the enteral route. This has the advantage of being less expensive than parenteral nutrition, as well as providing stimulation of normal enzymes and mucosal activity. They are critical, however, of the consensus that parenteral nutrition is unhelpful, as their analysis of the reported trials reveals some important defects. These include small patient numbers, varying degrees of nutritional deficits and duration of parenteral nutrition, and variations in the cancer diagnosis. Mattox[21] concurs that studies evaluating the use of parenteral nutrition in cancer patients suffer from inadequacies. Nelson et al.[9] conclude that the current lack of enthusiasm for parenteral nutrition may be due to inappropriate use, whereas the possible benefit in subgroups may simply reflect the primary cause as a lack of food intake, rather than metabolic changes due to the cancer anorexia–cachexia syndrome. They believe there is still a need to evaluate parenteral nutrition, perhaps alongside other treatment modalities such as megestrol acetate.

Klein and Koretz[22] reviewed 70 prospective randomized clinical trials evaluating the clinical efficacy of parenteral and enteral nutrition support in cancer patients. They concluded that the available data suggest that if nutritional support has a theraputic benefit in cancer patients, it is very small or limited to only a small subset of patients. The beneficial effects reported with specialized nutrition formulas is intriguing and requires further study. Further clinical trials are needed to determine the efficacy of nutritional support in defined cancer populations and the possible benefit to quality of life.

Bloch's editorial[23] on the review by Klein and Koretz[22] expresses disappointment that despite all the technologic advances, we are still unable to successfully provide nutritional support to malnourished cancer patients. Nevertheless, Bloch concludes that "although we have been unable to solve the fundamental problem of how best to nutritionally support those cancer patients who become wasted, we should continue to seek answers to these elusive questions."[23]

Although the many health care professionals working with advanced cancer patients appear to agree on the limitations of enteral and parenteral nutrition, there are other reports advocating relatively common use of enteral and parenteral nutrition for cancer patients.

Daly et al.[24] report a study evaluating long-term enteral nutrition support in postoperative cancer patients. Sixty patients with upper gastrointestinal cancer undergoing major abdominal operations were entered into the study. Patients were randomized to receive four variations of jejunostomy tube feedings. They concluded that they were able to demonstrate that supplemental enteral feeding significantly increased biochemical measurements, decreased postoperative complications, and decreased the need for rehospitalization. Grant[25] believes that this study clearly challenges the practice of limited nutritional support for perioperative cancer patients. The relatively small patient numbers were noted, but Grant concludes that larger prospective randomized trials are necessary because the potential benefit for surgical cancer patients may well be worth the effort.

In a further contradiction of the palliative care literature, Grant[25] notes that although cancer cachexia may account for some wasting in the postoperative cancer patient, most malnutrition results from inadequate dietary intake. It has been proposed that up to 40% of cancer patients die prematurely from complications of wasting, and this statistic may be even higher today.

King et al.[26] reviewed their experience with gynecologic cancer patients receiving home parenteral nutrition to determine improvements on nutritional parameters, survival, and quality of life. Sixty-one cancer patients treated with parenteral nutrition over a 10-year period were reviewed retrospectively. Fifty-six percent of the patients had ovarian cancer, and 25% had cervical cancer. The major indication for parenteral nutrition was inoperable mechanical bowel obstruction (72%). The mean length of parenteral nutrition in all patients was 108.6 days; the median was 66.5 days; and the range 14–479 days. Mean survival from the date of parenteral nutrition initiation was 167.5 days; the median was 60 days; and the range, 2–780 days. The quality-of-life data is difficult to interpret, given the retrospective nature of this review. The authors note that there are no prospective, randomized studies on the benefit of parenteral nutrition in patients with incurable disease. They conclude that because parenteral nutrition may provide significant palliation in selected cancer patients, it may prove difficult to proceed with such a study. They believe parenteral nutrition is a viable option in some of their advanced gynecologic cancer patients, with the potential for significant improvement of symptoms and quality of life.

What do we do?

Bruera and MacDonald[2] reported their experience with the use of enteral nutrition in a cancer patient population that included those with head and neck tumors, testicular tumors, and lymphomas, all of whom were undergoing aggressive chemotherapy for symptomatic or curative intent. In this group of 106 consecutive patients, 25 continued to lose weight after nutritional counseling, and as a result, received enteral nutrition via a gastric tube. Outcome and success of treatment were not reported.

Maltoni et al.[27] reported a case that demonstrates some of the difficulty in discontinuing enteral nutrition in patients with advanced cancer. The patient described had prolonged and apparently irreversible cognitive failure, which raised doubts about maintenance of the enteral feeding. The main arguments against continuing nutrition were the lack of evidence of improvement in quality of life, and prolongation of the dying process by an artificial means. The patient presented subsequently recovered, had the enteral nutrition discontinued, and continued to live for a protracted period of time.

Mercadante[28] has investigated the limitations of parenteral nutrition in patients with advanced cancer and the need to limit use to occasional, well-selected cases. Decision-making may be complicated by the inability of the patient or family to accept the lack of an alternative when the oral route is not available, by the difficulty in discontinuing parenteral nutrition started in the hospital when a home discharge is planned, and by the adverse psychological impact of treatment withdrawal for some patients and families. The difficulty in estimating survival time can also complicate decisions regarding parenteral nutrition. Mercadante's study followed the experience of the palliative care group in Palermo, Italy. During a 5-year period, 13/1150 patients (1.1%) cared for at home by a palliative care program received parenteral nutrition. All patients had advanced cancer. The survival time of these patients after institution of parenteral nutrition ranged from 3 to 121 days. Of the 13 patients, 11 survived for 33 days or less. Mercandante notes that while parenteral nutrition is not their usual palliative care practice, there may be special circumstances when use is appropriate. These decisions should be made on an individual basis and should include patients able to maintain a reasonable level of activity. Other factors to be considered in using parenteral nutrition are whether use may prevent hospital admissions, patients and families clearly understand the advantages and disadvantages, and a skilled team is able to continue to provide support.

Bruera and MacDonald[2] report that at the Cross Cancer Institute in Edmonton, Canada, parenteral nutrition was used in only 3% of 106 consecutive malnourished patients. From 1990 to 1995 at the Palliative Care Unit of the Edmonton General Hospital, approximately 1000 patients were admitted and none received parenteral nutrition (unpublished data). The potential advantages and use of parenteral nutrition in specific individual cases was discussed.[29] Nevertheless, this treatment modality was not used for any of the patients.

During a 1-year period from October 1994 to October 1995, 278 in-patients were seen in consultation by the Palliative Care Program at the Royal Alexandra Hospital, Edmonton. Only two of these patients received parenteral nutrition (0.7%) (unpublished data). A 59-year-old man with disseminated gastric cancer received parenteral nutrition for a 29-day period, during which he continued to deteriorate steadily. The parenteral nutrition was discontinued 36 hours before the patient died. The lack of anticipated benefit was fully explained to the patient; however, he could not accept this explanation and continued to request parenteral nutrition despite intermittent treatment-related complications and obvious deterioration. The second patient was a 65-year-old woman with a carcinoid tumor, with widespread peritoneal disease and a nonfunctional gastrointestinal tract. This patient was felt to be appropriate for total parenteral nutrition because she had a very slow growing tumor. She has continued to do well at home and has maintained her weight 6 months after being discharged on home parenteral nutrition.

Enteral and parenteral nutrition is used more frequently in the United States than in other countries. Howard[30] documented the clinical study of 2168 patients with active cancer who received home nutritional support. Of these patients, 1672 patients received home parenteral nutrition, and 1296 patients received home enteral nutrition. It should be noted that in Europe, parenteral nutrition is used in about 2 persons per million, whereas in the United States the figure is 80 persons per million. A possible explanation for this discrepancy is more regulation and restraint of health care costs in other countries than in the United States.

Survival figures showed that at 1 year, 28% of the cancer patients on parenteral nutrition and 32% of the patients on enteral nutrition were still alive. Ninety percent of the deaths were attributed to the primary diagnosis, 9% to other medical conditions, and less than 1% were felt to be due to complications related to enteral or parenteral nutrition. Howard concludes that patients with "cured" cancer with problems such as severe radiation enteritis would clearly benefit from parenteral nutrition. The subgroup of 20% of patients noted to survive 1 year with "active" cancer are probably those with slow-growing or potentially curable diseases. Clearly in this group parenteral nutrition can be justified. Finally, given that the majority of "active" cancer patients receiving enteral or parenteral nutrition died in 6–9 months, the appropriateness of treatment for this group of patients is less clear. Howard notes that the increased use of parenteral nutrition in the United States, particularly in the home, may be due to increased public awareness of treatment availability. This in turn has resulted in patient and family demand, increased training of health care professionals in providing this treatment, and the willingness of health insurers to pay for it, particularly if it shortens a more expensive hospital admission.

These conflicting views on the benefits of parenteral nutrition for advanced cancer patients highlight the ethical problems for the clinician.[31] Will parenteral nutrition do more good than harm (beneficence)? Does the patient have the right to a medically futile treatment (autonomy)? How is access to health care and treatment costs impacted by the wider issue of the limitations of the society (justice)?

Drug Therapy

What do we say?

A number of drugs have been proposed as therapies in the management of cachexia and anorexia. These include corticosteroids, progestational agents, cyprophetadine, hydrazine sulfate, cannabinoids, and pentoxifylline.[3–7,9–11] As previously noted, the various reports of these agents have been extensively reviewed and the conclusions of these reviews are worth noting for their similarities and differences.

Loprinzi[45] concludes that there are placebo-controlled, double-blind, clinical trials showing appetite improvement with both progestational hormones and corticosteroids in cancer patients with anorexia/cachexia. Thus both agents could be useful in clinical practice for these patients. Future trials are needed to compare the abilities of these two treatments on appetite stimulation and weight gain. At present, it would appear that more weight gain will occur with the use of drugs such as megestrol acetate. A reasonable starting dosage would be 160–800 mg per day. The dose of 800 mg per day requires the ingestion of 20 tablets at a cost of $15–$20 per day in the United States. Recently, a liquid preparation has become available, allowing more convenience with decreased cost.

Ottery[10,11] believes that megestrol acetate is the most promising agent available and also notes the benefits of the recent availability of the oral suspension. The recommended starting dosage is 800 mg daily for 24 days, followed by a decreasing dosage if appetite is improved. Steroids are also often prescribed for improved appetite and sense of well-being, however Ottery does not recommend them because of the potential exacerbation of muscle deterioration.

Nelson et al.[9] consider metoclopramide the first-line agent for appetite stimulation for patients with cancer-associated anorexia and cachexia because it treats delayed gastric emptying and gastroparesis in advanced cancer patients. The recommended dosage is 10 mg four times per day before meals and at bedtime. Megestrol acetate is used in patients with less advanced cancer who do not require rapid or dramatic results. The recommended starting dosage is 160 mg per day, titrating upwards as necessary. Dexamethasone is used when a more rapid effect is required, in doses of 4–8 mg per day. Cannabinoids are used in patients who have experience with the drug and are comfortable with the possible neurological side effects. Attempts have been made to use the drug that offers other secondary benefits with an acceptable side-effect profile, e.g., using dexamethasone in a patient with anorexia and bone pain rather than megestrol acetate.

Bruera and Fainsinger[7] recommend adequate management of chronic nausea when this is the main symptom by the use of gastric stimulant agents such as metoclopramide. Megestrol acetate is suggested for patients with profound anorexia who are expected to survive for weeks to months. Patients with a shorter prognosis or difficulty tolerating progestional agents may benefit from a brief course of corticosteroids. Progestional agents appear to have the advantage of increasing caloric intake and improving nutritional status, whereas the benefits of corticosteroids are short-lasting and symptomatic.

Davis and Hardy[32] caution that although the published results of some drug therapies such as megestrol acetate and corticosteroids are encouraging, patients with advanced cachexia, poor performance status, and limited prognosis are unlikely to have been recruited for clinical trials. Thus, an unrealistic and overoptimistic view of theraputic benefits may have been presented.

What do we do?

There have been a few reports from some palliative care groups documenting their prescribing patterns.

Curtis and Walsh[33] describe the drugs prescribed for an outpatient population followed by the palliative care service of the Cleveland Clinic Foundation. Records of 81 patients with advanced cancer were reviewed. Metoclopramide (28%), dexamethasone (23%), and prednisone (5%) were included in the 15 most commonly prescribed drugs. The information presented does not provide information on symptoms, and as a result, it is impossible to determine how many of these patients received these medications for the management of anorexia or cachexia. Megestrol acetate or cannabinoids do not appear to have been prescribed for any of these patients.

Twycross et al.[34] in Oxford, England, reported their experience with 385 inpatients and outpatients, followed for at least 3 weeks over a 5-year period. Dexamethasone (28%), metoclopramide (20%), and prednisone (10%) are included in the 16 most commonly prescribed medications. No patients appear to have been prescribed megestrol acetate or a cannabinoid for cancer-associated anorexia or cachexia.

The Palliative Care Unit at the Edmonton General Hospital, Edmonton, has documented the medication profile of patients prior to admission and compared this with the drug profile during admission.[35] One hundred consecutive patients admitted over a 9-month period during 1993 were reviewed. Metoclopramide was prescribed for 45% of patients on admission and was prescribed for 96% of patients at least once during the admission. Dexamethasone had been prescribed for 33% of patients on admission, compared with 71% of patients during admission, whereas prednisone was prescribed for 6% and 3% of patients, respectively. Megestrol acetate was prescribed for 2% of patients on admission, compared with 4% of patients during admission. The mean duration of admission was 31 ± 28 days. The information reviewed does not show differentiation of how many of these medications were prescribed for cancer-related anorexia and cachexia alone.

The Palliative Care Consulting Service at the Royal Alexandra Hospital in Edmonton followed 278 patients for an average of 20 days during the period October 1994 to September 1995. Megestrol acetate and cannabinoids were not recommended by the consulting service for any of these patients, although metoclopramide and dexamethasone were used for the management of nausea in some patients (unpublished data).

The charts of 83 advanced cancer outpatients seen at the Pain and Symptom Control Clinic at the Cross Cancer Institute, Edmonton, were also reviewed. Of these patients, 6/83 (7%) were started on megestrol acetate for anorexia/cachexia. No patients were prescribed cannabinoids.

Documentation on pharmacological practice of palliative care groups for symptoms related to cancer anorexia/cachexia is sketchy. Nevertheless, the evidence would suggest that this common problem is seldom managed by megestrol acetate or cannabinoids.

Conclusion

There is some consensus that quality of life is the main goal of treatment of cancer anorexia/cachexia. There is also some variation in the issues included under this umbrella.

Inclusion of a dietitian within an interdisciplinary palliative care team is widely recognized as useful and helpful. Dietitians need to do research documenting the benefits of their nutritional support role.

Enteral and parenteral nutrition can help well-selected patients. The selection of patients appears to vary widely in different settings; such decisions are driven by local social, financial, and medical circumstances.

The literature on the benefits of pharmacological management of cancer anorexia/cachexia does not appear to have been translated into widespread clinical use. Possible explanations are: *(1)* cachexia may become a lesser issue for palliative care groups seeing advanced cancer patients with other major symptom problems: *(2)* the better candidates for pharmacological management may be seen more often by oncologists or family physicians; and *(3)* available drugs may be underused or too expensive, or clinicans may have found too little clinical benefit to justify their common use.

References

1. Grant JP. Preventing complications of surgery: emphasis on nutritional factors. In: Laszlo J, Daken N, eds. *Physicians Guide to Cancer Care Complications: Prevention and Management.* New York: Dekker; 1986:48–52.
2. Bruera E, MacDonald RN. Nutrition in cancer patients: an update and review of our experience. *J Pain Symptom Manage* 1988; 3:133–140.
3. Tchekmedyian NS. Clinical approaches to nutritional support in cancer. *Curr Opin Oncol* 1993; 5:633–638.
4. Loprinzi CL, Goldberg RM, Burnham NL. Cancer-associated anorexia and cachexia. *Drugs* 1992; 43:499–506.
5. Loprinzi CL. Management of cancer anorexia/cachexia. *Support Care Cancer* 1995; 3:120–122.
6. Bruera E. Is the pharmacological treatment of cancer cachexia possible? *Support Care Cancer* 1993; 1:298–304.
7. Bruera E, Fainsinger RL. Clinical management of cachexia and anorexia. In: Doyle D, Hanks G, MacDonald N, eds. *Oxford Textbook of Palliative Medicine.* Oxford: Oxford University Press; 1993:4.3.6:330–337.
8. MacDonald N, Alexander R, Bruera E. Cachexia-anorexia-asthenia. *J Pain Symptom Manage* 1995; 10:151–155.
9. Nelson K, Walsh D, Sheehan FA. The cancer anorexia-cachexia syndrome. *J Clin Oncol* 1994; 12:213–255.
10. Ottery FD. Cancer cachexia. *Cancer Practice* 1994; 2:123–131.
11. Ottery FD. Supportive nutrition to prevent cachexia and improve quality of life. *Semin Oncol* 1995; 22:98–111.
12. Shaw C. Nutritional aspects of advanced cancer. *Palliat Med* 1992; 6:105–110.
13. Maillet JO, King D. Nutritional care of the terminally ill adult. In: Gallagher-Allred C, Amenta MO, eds. *Nutrition and Hydration In Hospice Care.* New York: Haworth Press; 1993:37–54.
14. Fainsinger R, Bruera E, Miller MJ, Hanson J, MacEachern T. Symptom control during the last week of life on a palliative care unit. *J Palliat Care* 1991; 7:5–11.
15. Ajemian I. The interdisciplinary team. In: Doyle D, Hanks G, MacDonald N, eds. *Textbook of Palliative Medicine.* Oxford: Oxford University Press; 1993;2.2:17–28.

16. Coyle N. Supportive care program, pain service, Memorial Sloan-Kettering Cancer Centre. *Support Care Cancer* 1995; 3:161–163.

17. Meier ML, Neuenschwander H. Hospice—A home care service for terminally ill cancer patients in southern Switzerland. *Support Care Cancer* 1995; 3:389–392.

18. de Stoutz N, Glaus A. Supportive and palliative care of cancer patients at Kantonsspital St. Gallen, Switzerland. *Support Care Cancer* 1995; 3:221–226.

19. Stuart-Harris R. Sacred Heart Hospice: An Australian centre of palliative medicine. *Support Care Cancer* 1995; 3:280–284.

20. Bozzetti F. Is enteral nutrition a primary therapy in cancer patients? *Gut* 1994; 1:S65–S68.

21. Mattox TW. Drug use evaluation approach to monitoring use of total parenteral nutrition: a review of criteria for use in cancer patients. *Nutr Pract* 1993; 8:233–237.

22. Klein S, Koretz RL. Nutrition support in patients with cancer: what do the data really show? *Nutr Clin Pract* 1994; 9:91–100.

23. Bloch AS. Feeding the cancer patient: where have we come from, where are we going? *Nutri Clin Pract* 1994; 9:87–89.

24. Daly JM, Weintraub FN, Shou J. Enteral nutrition during multimodality therapy in upper gastrointestinal cancer patients. *Ann Surg* 1995; 221:327–338.

25. Grant JP. On enteral nutrition during multimodality therapy in upper gastrointestinal cancer patients. *Ann Surg* 1995; 221:325–326.

26. King LA, Carson LS, Konstantinides N, et al. Outcome assessment of home parenteral nutrition in patients with gynecologic malignances: what have we learned in a decade of experience? *Gynecol Oncol* 1993; 51:377–382.

27. Maltoni M, Franco JJ, Bruera E. Case report: enteral nutrition in a severely sedated, confused terminal cancer patients. *J Palliat Care* 1992; 8(4):49–51.

28. Mercadante S. Parenteral nutrition at home in advanced cancer patients. *J Pain Symptom Manage* 1995; 10:476–480.

29. Fainsinger R, Chan K, Bruera E. Total parenteral nutrition for a terminally ill patient? *J Palliat Care* 1992; 8(2):30–32.

30. Howard N. Home parenteral and enteral nutrition in cancer patients. *Cancer* 1993; 72:3531–3541.

31. Sharp JW, Roncagli T. Home parenteral nutrition in advanced cancer. Ethical and psychosocial aspects. *Cancer Pract* 1993; 1:119–24.

32. Davis CL, Hardy JR. Palliative care. *BMJ* 1994; 308:1359–1362.

33. Curtis EB, Walsh TD. Prescribing practices of a palliative care service. *J Pain Symptom Manage* 1993; 8:312–316.

34. Twycross RG, Bergl S, John S, Lewis K. Monitoring drug use in palliative care. *Palliat Med* 1994; 8:137–143.

35. Watanabe S, Fainsinger RL, Bruera E. Commonly prescribed medications in advanced cancer patients. *J Palliat Care* 1995; 11(3):70.

8

Ethical Issues in Hydration and Nutrition

NEIL MacDONALD

Science creates new ethical issues, but it also leads to a re-evaluation of existing standards. Offering food and drink to the dying is intimately tied with compassionate care. Today, we can extend this offer through the employment of technical means of sustenance. Under commonly encountered circumstances, we now know that forcing nutrition on patients with advanced cancer may actually harm them, while controversy swirls around the hydration of patients in their final days.

One should distinguish matters of principle from matters of fact, for both are involved and related in the ethics of hydration and nutrition. Controversies relating to matters of fact require evidence for their resolution, and that evidence comes from observation and research. The principles governing clinical decisions about hydration and nutrition relate to the rights of patients to make their own informed choices and refusals about medical treatment. In the case of Robert Corbeil, the judge of the Quebec Superior Court declared that Mr. Corbeil had the right to refuse to eat and to be fed, even if he died as a result. The critical issue was whether the patient was sufficiently lucid and balanced of mind to make a decision on his own behalf. That others may have found his decision unreasonable was irrelevant.

It is also a matter of principle that doctors are not obliged by law or by ethics to begin or continue with treatments that are therapeutically useless and not in the patient's best interests. This principle comes particularly into play when patients cannot make decisions on their own behalf. Whether and in what conditions hydration and nutrition are therapeutically useless, or even possibly harmful, is largely a matter of fact, a matter to be settled by observation. So clinical ethics requires a judicious combination of both principles and facts to arrive at clinical decisions that respect both the needs of a patient's body and the choices of the patient's mind.

In this chapter we explore ethical issues related to hydration and nutrition in patients with advanced chronic illness. The model considered is the patient with advanced cancer, but many of the principles are relevant to patients with other advanced chronic, ultimately fatal disorders. The central theme of the chapter is the impact of scientific studies on ethics, with consequent need to maintain basic principles of morality and to constantly review the interpretation of these principles in light of one's current understanding of biology.

Table 8.1[1] outlines the ethical issues that arise at the end of life; a number of them encompass questions on nutrition and hydration:

1. *Resource allocation.* The patient who cannot eat requires relatively expensive enteral or parenteral therapy in order to maintain calorie intake. Is this a justified expense?

2. *Prolonging futile therapy.* In the final scene of King Lear, one of his attendants says about the dying Lear: "Vex not his ghost—Oh let him pass; he hates him that would upon the rack of this tough world stretch him out longer."[2] Meaningful prolongation of life is unlikely to occur with enteral or parenteral nutrition and hydration in patients with advanced cancer. If this is the case, is it morally acceptable to maintain these therapies?

3. *Withholding or withdrawing or therapy.* Perhaps the prolongation of life achieved with nutrition and hydration is trivial, but will we not die if these are removed? What is the difference between these acts and active euthanasia?

Current ethical thinking categorizes technical sustaining of hydration or nutrition as medical procedures. As such, decisions to forego these interventions should carry the same ethical weight as decisions to withdraw transfusion therapy or dialysis. Ethics and law are not always bedfellows, but the modern views of ethicists and judges on this point appear to be consonant.

Although ethicists, palliative care physicians, and nurses may share this view, it is not widespread among broader groups of North American physicians. A sizable minority of physicians regard maintenance of hydration and nutrition as essential features of medical care and as somehow distinct from other technical processes such as transfusion or dialysis.[3,4]

Part of this dilemma may relate to the maintenance of the concept of "ordinary" and "extraordinary" care as factors in decision making. Rather than establishing a "cut-off line" related to the complexity of therapy or its weight as a cultural totem, the emphasis should be on patient–family choice or the rational assessment of therapeutic benefit. The terms "ordinary" and "extraordinary" were frequently used in Catholic ethical discussions; they are now commonly replaced by the more apt terms "proportionate" and "disproportionate."

Against this background of current thought, I hold the view that decisions to maintain hydration and nutrition will depend upon the informed decision of the patient or the patient's surrogates. Presumably, their decisions must be influenced by the advice they receive from medical attendants, advice which

Table 8.1. Ethical issues in palliative care

Resource allocation

Can we afford to maintain our values? Is there evidence that the increasing lack of resources may cause selection of second-rate health care options with consequent compromise of patient care?

Life-prolonging treatment

Issues related to the costs (human and fiscal) of using aggressive therapies in situations in which the risk of adverse effects is high and beneficial outcome problematic.

Do Not Resuscitate (DNR) regulations. Are they often irrelevant? Is there a risk that health professionals may conclude that DNR discussions satisfy the requirement for discussing death and dying issues with the patient and family?

Problem priority

Do we often ignore pain or other aspects of suffering while addressing more trivial elements of illness?

Pain and symptom control

Is not relief of relievable suffering a fundamental patient–family right?

Communication, consent, and competence

Do we ensure that all patients have access to the most competent care?

Do patients understand relative levels of health care competence and are they in a position to make a decision based on this information?

Do patients have the necessary information for making logical choices?

Do they fully comprehend the information we provide?

Do we sometimes use relentless therapeutic exercises as a substitute for conducting difficult supportive conversations?

Confidentiality

How do we exchange privileged information within a team while preserving patient–family rights and dignity?

Research

In situations in which cognitive failure is common, do we ensure that patients are competent to give informed consent?

Does participation in a research study alter the covenant of the physician to look after a patient?

What are the responsibilities for continuing care when the study is over?

Are some studies by their very nature impossible to carry out in a fragile population of dying patients and their families?

Are principles relevant to informed consent in research studies applicable to obtaining informed consent in the nonresearch setting?

Sponsorship of research: does private research support drive the public research agenda, and subsequently influence resource allocation, fueling futile efforts with increased cost in suffering and waste of resources?

Education

The principles of palliative care are fundamental components of medical practice. Does our current medical educational system recognize and reflect this tenet?

(continued)

Table 8.1. Ethical issues in palliative care   *(continued)*

Issues related to withholding or withdrawal of therapy

Do we, and do our patients and families understand the difference between these acts and physician-assisted suicide or euthanasia?

Palliative care standards

Should palliative care programs be expected to demonstrate a basic standard of care and competence so as not to delude the community, damage the credibility of palliative care, and waste scarce public and private support?

Media influences

Public views of medical care are shaped by media priorities and the accuracy and balance of reportage. Is the public properly informed on medical issues?

Cultural issues

Truth-telling is only one example of cultural differences in the management of dying patients. How do we respect cultures yet maintain a consistent ethical approach?

Dual ethical standards

Many patients are in their current situation because they are influenced by the blandishments of advertisements for lethal products. Why should business people hold different ethical standards than health professionals? Why should one group regard it as ethical to do whatever is legally allowed for profit when health professional groups regard the promotion of illness for gain as a fundamentally amoral activity?

Responsibilities of health professionals to:

Patient

Patient and family

Institution

Society

Own family

Ethical resolution of conflicting demands

Euthanasia and physician-assisted suicide

Source: Adapted and reprinted with permission from MacDonald N. From the front lines. *J Palliat Care* 1994; 10(3):44–47.

stems from knowledge of pathophysiologic abnormalities and their effects on patient well-being.

Decisions on Hydration

As stated in another forum,[5] the arguments for and against hydration can be summarized as presented in Table 8.2. In looking at the scientific aspects of these arguments, one is struck by the paucity of evidence to sustain sometimes vigorously espoused views. Indeed, dehydration will result in decreased urine output, but the beneficial effects of fluid restriction on vomiting, pulmonary symptoms,

Table 8.2. Arguments for and against hydration

Arguments against

1. Comatose patients do not experience pain, thirst, etc.

2. Fluid may prolong the dying process.

3. Less urine output means less need for bed pan, urinal, commode, or catheter.

4. Less gastrointestinal fluid and less vomiting.

5. Less pulmonary secretions and less cough, choking, and congestion.

6. Minimize edema and ascites.

7. Decreased fluids and electrolyte imbalance act as natural anesthetics for the central nervous system with decreased levels of consciousness and decreased suffering.

Arguments for

1. Dying patients are more comfortable if they receive adequate hydration.

2. There is no evidence that fluids alone prolong life to any meaningful decree.

3. Dehydration and electrolyte imbalance can cause confusion, restlessness, and neuromuscular irritability.

4. Water is administered to dying people who complain of thirst, so why not give parenteral hydration.

5. Arguments regarding poor quality of life detract from efforts to find ways to improve comfort and life quality.

6. Parenteral hydration is the minimum standard of care and discontinuing this treatment is to break a bond with the patient.

7. Withholding fluid to the dying patient sets a precedent for withholding therapies to other compromised patient groups.

---

and, particularly, edema and ascites, are not well established. Evidence relating fluid and electrolyte imbalance to improved pain control rests on animal work.

Conversely, the correlation between control of thirst and hydration status in patients at the end of life is modest.[6] Well-hydrated patients can experience severe thirst, presumably because of the influence of oral factors such as mouth breathing and infection. Thirst can be controlled with small amounts of oral fluids, as can be attested by any of us who, thirsty after physical exertion, note rapid relief after our first few liquid gulps—relief occurring long before our fluid and electrolyte status could be appreciably corrected. This observation in healthy individuals is mirrored by the consensus views of most palliative care physicians and nurses who similarly note control of thirst with small amounts of fluids and maintenance of a clean mouth.

In the author's opinion, the most critical physiologic argument relating to the hydration controversy concerns mentation and the relationship between polypharmacy, so common in dying patients, and their hydration status. Fainsinger and Bruera believe that adoption of a more vigorous hydration posture in their unit in part is responsible for the diminished incidence of delirium that they have noted in recent years.[7] They are concerned that the benefits of reduced urine output in dehydrated patients is more than balanced by the risk of adverse drug reactions secondary to failure to clear the primary agent or toxic drug metabolites. Aligned to their view is the concern that the touted benefits of dehydration in the patient in the last days of life may be a specious argument if the patient's semicomatose or sedated status (secondary to the need to control delirium), now used to justify withholding fluids, was caused by earlier diminished fluid intake.

Changes in mental status are among the most devastating symptoms experienced by dying patients. While the degree of anguish felt by the delirious patient is hard to define in terms of suffering (patients who recover from delirious states usually do not remember the incident),[8] their behavior is a source of great distress to family members and may generate conflict between the family and similarly concerned health professionals. The waves of conflict often spread as nurses in immediate contact with the patient may feel that physicians are not taking sufficient steps to control the delirium. Is a laissez-faire attitude towards hydration correlated with an increased incidence of delirium in dying patients? The provocative observations of Bruera and Fainsinger[7,8] should be followed up with more definitive studies.

Cancer control programs must include four preventive strategies, starting with prevention of the disease, if possible; prevention of invasive disease (through early diagnostic programs); prevention of mortality in patients with invasive disease (anticancer therapy); and prevention of suffering.[9] We now believe that we can control much of the suffering associated with pain through early identification and management of the problem. Similarly, if delirium and other central nervous system effects can be prevented through earlier consideration of hydration problems in association with drug therapy, given new scientific considerations, our current view on the ethics of hydration in patients with advanced illness would shift.

Pending further information, the author believes that the following guidelines for hydration are reasonable.

Patient choice*

1. Competent patients can accept or refuse hydration when given pertinent information.
2. For incompetent patients, a balancing of advantages and disadvantages should be undertaken. The patient's interests are paramount in decisions. Incompetent patients may be represented by a legal guardian or health care agent.

*Modeled upon guidelines on enteral feeding published by the Bioethics Centre of the University of Alberta.

Decision-making process

1. Patients, families and friends, and caregivers should know that hydration can be ethically withheld and withdrawn.
2. Hydration may be initiated on a time-limited basis to allow an assessment of the advantages and disadvantages.
3. A time-limited trial of hydration is always recommended if there is doubt about the advantages or disadvantages of hydration.
4. After a decision has been made to initiate or stop hydration, the emotional impact of the decision on caregivers, family members, and others must be recognized.
5. The advantages and disadvantages of hydration for family members, close friends, caregivers, and society may influence the decisions made by competent patients or made for incompetent patients.
6. Unless there is a contraindication, patients who are not otherwise cognitively impaired and who are receiving pharmacologic agents that could cause delirium should receive adequate hydration to ensure reasonable drug metabolism and excretion.

Hypodermoclysis

Most articles discussing drawbacks of hydration in dying patients refer to the difficulties of maintaining hydration using intravenous techniques. Here is an example where recent clinical research skews the hydration argument somewhat in the direction of rehydration. Primarily because of the work of Schen and Singer-Edelstein,[10] Gluck,[11] Hays,[12] and subsequently, Fainsinger, Bruera, and their colleagues in Edmonton,[13] hypodermoclysis (subcutaneous infusion of fluids) is now widely used in palliative care programs. Clysis is not a new technique. Although subcutaneous clysis was once accepted, it fell into disuse because of the injudicious use of nonelectrolyte solutions (which are poorly absorbed when administered subcutaneously) and the improvement in intravenous techniques and fluid sources. We now know that, with the assistance of modest doses of hyaluronidase, solutions containing normal saline can be infused into patients in doses up to 120 ml/hour (small studies report patients tolerating boluses of even larger amounts).[14]

The use of hypodermoclysis to hydrate patients has many advantages over the intravenous route.[13] These may be stated as follows:

1. The problem of difficult and painful intravenous access is obviated.
2. Physicians or specially skilled nurses are not required to commence a subcutaneous infusion.
3. Hospitalization is not necessary and clysis, either continuous or intermittent, can be maintained in a home setting for long periods of time.

4. Subcutaneous sites can normally be sustained for many days without
   change. Thrombosis is not a problem whereas local cellulitis is normally
   not a substantial problem in the absence of associated administration of
   drugs. Even in these situations, careful observation of the subcutaneous
   site and rotation of site will prevent major complications.

Nutrition

"Dis-moi ce que tu manges, je te dirai ce que tu es."

Brillat-Savarin, *Physiologie du Goût*

Poor appetite, weight loss, and alterations in bowel function (e.g., chronic nausea and constipation) are common problems in patients with advanced cancer.
Ultimately, malnutrition may actually result in a patient's demise, possible ac-
counting for 25% of patient deaths.[15] While the defining qualities of the
cachexia–anorexia syndrome remain imprecise, clinicians recognize that most
weight loss in cancer patients, and associated metabolic abnormalities, is caused
by a cascade of cytokines and/or tumor products generated as products of
tumor–host interaction. Successful control of this problem will depend upon
reversal of the aberrant metabolic pattern. In the interim, some patients may
have temporary reversal of weight loss, and improvement in appetite following
therapy with pharmacologic agents such as megestrol. Commonly employed
enteral and parenteral nutritional aids may temporarily improve weight loss,
but they do not significantly influence the overall course of illness. Unlike hydration, the use of enteral and parenteral feeding is associated with significant
cost and the risk of adverse effects.

In contrast with hydration, less controversy surrounds decisions to withhold
enteral or parenteral nutrition in the last days of life. At least this is the case
among palliative care physicians who may hold varying views on the importance
of hydration but tend to think as one with respect to technical approaches to
feeding dying patients. These views are not uniform among physicians, as patients
on general hospital wards may still die with an enteral tube in place or with
parenteral feeding only recently discontinued. As discussed earlier in the section
on hydration, physicians appear to rank order the technical means of delaying
death and, like the community from which they arise, find great difficulty in
withdrawing sustenance. Decisions on artificial nutrition can be a focal point for
family disputes. Family members do not appreciate the biology of the
cachexia–anorexia syndrome; they only know that a loved one is losing weight and
strength, cannot eat, and appears to be starving to death.

Nevertheless, ethical issues concerning decisions on nutrition are more
straightforward today than those involving hydration. There is no evidence that
current techniques prevent asthenia or prolong life for cancer patients with the
cachexia–anorexia syndrome. Three factors must, however, be kept in mind:

1. As easier techniques for hydration, such as the use of hypodermoclysis, influence the arguments for and against hydration, it may be that a clearer understanding of the cachexia–anorexia syndrome and the introduction of more specific nutritional aids will change current approaches.

2. Not all cancer patients who are losing weight and cannot eat have the cachexia–anorexia syndrome. Some are, indeed, starving to death and would benefit from enteral or parenteral nutrition. Often included in this group are patients with head and neck cancer, or cancer of the esophagus who cannot swallow, patients with malabsorption disorders, and patients with ovarian cancer and intermittent bowel obstruction. As the definition of the cachexia–anorexia syndrome is not exact, absolute criteria for identifying patients who will benefit from parenteral nutrition are not in place. When in doubt, it is reasonable to offer a time-limited trial of enteral or parenteral nutrition, keeping in mind that there is no ethical distinction between offering a therapy, with subsequent withdrawal, if it appears to be futile, and not starting a therapy in the first place.

3. Asthenia and cachexia are the major problems limiting patient mobility and creating dependence upon families and institutions. This symptom constellation should be selected for a task force research initiative. The basic science foundation must be expanded and integrated, but sufficient information is at hand to sustain a multidisciplinary research drive.[16]

Earlier in this chapter a decision process for hydration in patients with terminal illness was outlined (see Table 8.2). The first five points also apply to enteral and parenteral nutritional decisions. Adoption of a purely clinical analysis of nutritional benefit, while scientifically valid, may not fully satisfy our ethical obligations to patients and families. In every culture in the world through recorded time rituals surrounding food and drink are powerful components of community and family life. To be near a loved one in their last hours and to offer them sustenance remains a commonly held view of the obligation of family and friends. Like Brillat-Savarin, they may link a loved one's food intake with their fundamental human qualities.

It may be difficult for family and friends to address the existential distress of a loved one or to communicate fully and clearly at the end of life when patterns of communication were not well established earlier in relationships. Family members will need a gentle, careful explanation of why assisted nutrition is no longer necessary. The maintenance of technical links, if this substitutes for speaking to family members, is ethically questionable.

Few patients with advanced cancer complain of hunger towards the end of their lives.[17] When present, it is normally readily alleviated with modest amounts of oral food intake. Therefore, anguish associated with unrelieved hungers is a rare event in dying patients. When present, it clearly must be relieved with whatever means are available, natural or artificial.

Although a technically difficult, potentially dangerous, and expensive artificial feeding strategy may be abjured, health professionals remain obligated to further, not to discourage, the symbolic links that patients, families, and friends share. Physical symbolic links are important in such circumstances; the benefits of a drink of water extend far beyond its effect on osmolarity, and the value of a morsel of food, beyond its caloric count. Therefore, decisions to withhold technical approaches to nourishing a patient must be accompanied by a set of practical approaches to maintain, as much as possible, natural means of intake of food and drink. These include the following.

1. Patients who may have difficulty with oral feeding because of neurologic impairment or partial obstruction may be able to take certain types of food frequently and in small amounts , when nursing support is available and when the feedings are skillfully administered. Withdrawal of artificial feeding, except in the very last days of life, creates an obligation to assess the possibility of small oral feedings and to.teach proper techniques for maintaining oral nutrition to responsible family members.

2. As with hydration, if the patient is sentient, the patient's desires, hold primacy. Food should never be forced upon patients who do not wish to be fed. Exceptions to this principle require justification.

3. Oral feeding is sometime difficult because of associated correctable gastrointestinal problems. Unresolved nausea, severe constipation, abdominal cramping, heartburn, depression, or a dirty mouth should not contribute to the inability to take oral nourishment. The skillful use of appetite stimulants may modestly increase a patient's interest in food and assist in family–patient interactions. Time-limited trials of steroids and progestational agents may sometimes be indicated.

4. Hospital environments are often not conducive to communal repasts. Correctable factors include serving appetizing food that meets the patient's desires, served at the right temperature, in the right amount, in the most attractive way; removal of adverse cues, such as unpleasant odors; and addition of positive reinforcements. These may include music, a restful setting, and, if it was previously the patient's custom, the provision of small amounts of alcohol.

In conclusion, the use of assisted nutrition and hydration has to be judged in light of the current understanding of pathophysiology and the governing realizable clinical goals for *this* patient *now*. These goals will change as the patient's condition changes. It makes little clinical or ethical sense to go all the way with a treatment that made sense when started, but no longer has clinical meaning now.

Acknowledgments

I am grateful to Dr. David J. Roy for his review of this chapter and his helpful comments. Sections of this chapter are adapted, with permission, from Indications and ethical considerations in the hydration of patients with advanced cancer. In: Bruera E. Higginson I, eds. *Cachexia–Anorexia Syndrome in Cancer Patients*. New York: Oxford University Press. 1996.

References

1. MacDonald N. From the front lines. *J Palliat Care* 1994; 10(3):44–47.
2. Shakespeare W. *King Lear* Speech of Kent, Act V, Scene III.
3. Solomon MZ, O'Donnell L, Jennings B, et al. Decisions near the end of life: professional views on life-sustaining treatments. *Am J Public Health* 1993; 83(1):14–23.
4. Christakis NA, Asch DA. Biases in how physicians choose to withdraw life support. *Lancet* 1993; 342:642–646.
5. MacDonald N, Fainsinger R. Indications and ethical considerations in the hydration of patients with advanced cancer. In: Bruera E, Higginson I, eds. *Cachexia–Anorexia Syndrome in Cancer Patients.* New York: Oxford University Press, 1996.
6. Musgrave C, Bartal N, Opstad J. The sensation of thirst in dying patients receiving IV hydration. *J Pallia Care* 1995; 11(4):17–21.
7. Bruera E, Franco JJ, Maltoni M, Watanabe S, Suarez-Almazor M. Changing pattern of agitated impaired mental status in patients with advanced cancer: association with cognitive monitoring, hydration, and opioid rotation. *J Pain Symptom Manage* 1995; 10(4):287–291.
8. Bruera E, Fainsinger RL, Miller MJ, Kuehn N. The assessment of pain intensity in patients with cognitive failure: a preliminary report. *J Pain Symptom Manage* 1992; 7(5):267–270.
9. MacDonald N. Palliative care—the fourth phase of cancer prevention. *Cancer Detect Prevent* 199; 15(3):253–255.
10. Schen RJ, Singer-Edelstein M. Subcutaneous infusions in the elderly. *J Am Geriatr Soc* 1981; 24:583–585.
11. Gluck SM. Advantages of hypodermoclysis. *J Am Geriatr Soc* 1984; 32:691–692.
12. Hays H. Hypodermoclysis for symptom control in terminal cancer. *Can Family Phys* 1985; 31:1253–1256.
13. Fainsinger R, MacEachern T, Miller MJ, et al. The use of hypodermoclysis for rehydration in terminally ill cancer patients. *J Pain Symptom Manage* 1994; 9(5):298–302.
14. Bruera E, de Stoutz ND, Fainsinger RL, Spachynski K, Suarez-Almazor M, Hanson J. Comparison of two different concentrations of hyaluronidase in patients receiving one-hour infusions of hypodermoclysis. *J Pain Symptom Manage* 1995; 10(7):505–509.
15. Warren RS. The immediate causes of death in cancer. *Am J Med Sci* 1932: 184:610.
16. MacDonald N, Alexander R, Bruera E. Cachexia-anorexia-asthenia. *J Pain Symptom Manage* 1995; 10(2):151–155.
17. McCann RM, Hall WJ, Groth-Juncker A. Comfort care for terminally ill patients. The appropriate use of nutrition and hydration. *JAMA* 1994; 272(16):1263–1266.

III

ASTHENIA

Introduction: Asthenia: Definitions and Dimensions

RUSSELL K. PORTENOY

Patients with chronic medical diseases commonly report a distressing lack of vitality. This phenomenon is characterized by a range of descriptors, which together suggest both physical and mental aspects. The physical aspects may be characterized by weakness or tiredness, which suggests dysfunction in muscles, or by lethargy or sleepiness, which indicates difficulties in maintaining alertness. Other descriptors, such as apathy, lassitude, inattention, difficulty concentrating, or loss of motivation, recognize a prominent mental (usually cognitive) aspect.

Two commonly used terms, asthenia and fatigue, capture these characteristics more broadly. Either can refer to a sense of diminished vitality in physical or mental functioning, or both, that occurs in the setting of medical disease. Although an asthenia–anorexia–cachexia syndrome has been appreciated in patients with far-advanced diseases, including cancer, the empirical data now available do not provide a basis for distinguishing the asthenia component of this syndrome from a constellation of symptoms generally described as fatigue. For now, progress in understanding and managing the lack of vitality that commonly afflicts the medically ill would be facilitated by considering fatigue and asthenia together.

Asthenia, or fatigue, is a symptom. Like other symptoms, it is fundamentally subjective. This subjectivity implies that the "weakness" often reported as part of the symptomatology does not require an objective correlate. Although some patients who report fatigue have demonstrable muscle weakness, most do not. Some patients experience easy fatigability with physical activity, but this, too, does not require a correlate on physical examination or electrophysiologic testing. Although objective evidence of a physical problem can help the clinician understand the origins of the complaint and maybe choose a therapy, such evidence is not required to confirm or quantitate the patient's report.

The symptom of asthenia, or fatigue, is also multidimensional.[1,2] As suggested previously, the most useful construct divides the phenomenon broadly into physical and mental aspects. There is no empirical basis to this or any other division, however, and careful descriptive studies in the future may encourage other distinctions.

The physical dimension of asthenia or fatigue is usually described as a perception of muscle weakness or a tendency to fatigue rapidly. Physical activity is difficult to sustain, and in some cases, dyspnea accompanies even minimal exertion. Rest or sleep does not return perceived strength or stamina to normal.

The mental component, like the physical aspect, is also diverse in presentation. Some patients describe a lack of motivation or interest in objects or activities. Others report difficulty in concentrating or maintaining attention. Mood may be flat or depressed. Lethargy or a tendency to somnolence may be noted; there may or may not be a need for excessive sleep. Again, rest or sleep may lessen the problem but does not eliminate it.

Guided by the multidimensional construct, future investigations may be able to identify subtypes of asthenia, which will be characterized by a specific set of patient complaints and suggest a specific group of underlying etiologies or mechanisms. The value of this approach is evident in the management of pain, another multidimensional symptom, which is now commonly classified on the basis of verbal descriptors into categories of inferred mechanisms (e.g., so-called nociceptive pain vs. neuropathic pain).

The need for empirical studies of asthenia or fatigue is highlighted by its prevalence and adverse consequences. In one recent survey, for example, more than 70% of a mixed cancer population responding to a cross-sectional survey reported fatigue during the prior week and more than half of these patients perceived it as highly distressing.[3] This high prevalence reflects the coalescence of varied factors that may contribute to the phenomenon. Largely on the basis of clinical observation, asthenia or fatigue can be linked to the following conditions:

1. The disease itself, perhaps through host response (such as cytokine production)
2. Any primary treatment for the disease, including surgery, chemotherapy, or radiotherapy
3. Associated metabolic disturbances, including anemia or leukopenia, hypoxia, renal or hepatic insufficiency, or malnutrition
4. Intercurrent systemic disorders, such as infection
5. The use of centrally acting drugs, including those for symptom control (such as opioids, sedative-hypnotics, antidepressants, anticonvulsants, or others)
6. A primary sleep disorder
7. A depressive disorder

Recognition of these varied potential etiologies already encourages an approach to the treatment of asthenia or fatigue based on a comprehensive assessment of disease-related and treatment-related phenomena, and associated medical and psychiatric morbidity. The treatment strategy first should attempt to reverse contributing factors when possible. Given the limited data now available, a more targeted approach (for example interventions focused on the physical aspects over the mental aspects, or vice versa), is not possible.

The high prevalence and aversive impact of asthenia in the medically ill is a strong impetus for further research. Descriptive studies are needed to refine a definition, clarify criteria for diagnosis, and determine relationships among symptom constellations and the many factors that may predispose patients to asthenia or fatigue, or sustain symptoms once they begin. Systematic surveys may be able to suggest discrete syndromes that relate etiology to phenomenology. Basic and clinical research is needed to elucidate the specific mechanisms responsible for the varied types. Intervention trials, which can be targeted to specific clinical subtypes or mechanisms, are needed to improve management. Current knowledge about asthenia or fatigue is very limited, and progress is likely if the symptom is accorded the attention it clearly deserves.

References

1. Jacobs LA, Piper BF. The phenomenon of fatigue and the cancer patient. In: McCorkle R, Grant M, Frank-Stromborg M, Baird S, eds. *Cancer Nursing. A Comprehensive Textbook.* 2nd ed. Philadelphia: W.B. Saunders; 1996; 1193–1210.
2. Winningham ML, Nail LM, Burke MB, et al. Fatigue and the cancer experience: the state of the knowledge. *Oncol Nursing Forum* 1994; 21:23–36.
3. Portenoy RK, Thaler HT, Kornblith AB, et al. Symptom prevalence, characteristics and distress in a cancer population. *Qual Life Res* 1994; 3:183–189.

9

Pathophysiology of Cancer Asthenia

HANS NEUENSCHWANDER AND EDUARDO BRUERA

Pathophysiology of Asthenia in Noncancer Populations

Fatigue, a normal response during or after a physical or a strenous mental effort, has to be considered a physiological phenomenon. It may have a beneficial, protective function to prevent exhaustion and overexertion. Sometimes fatigue can even be experienced as a pleasant feeling if it is of reasonable duration. On the other hand, fatigue as a pathological condition is always experienced as an unpleasant sensation.

Asthenia is perceived as an unpleasant sensation whenever it exceeds one's physiological resources, such as rest that must be recuperated. In a number of nontumor-associated conditions, asthenia, experienced as fatigue and/or weakness, is definitely a component or even a leading symptom (Table 9.1).

Although asthenia-inducing mechanisms may differ from one condition to another, some similarities can be identified. Traditionally, exercise-induced fatigue has been related to the occurrence of final states of the metabolism, such as the depletion of muscle glycogen, the decrease in plasma glucose, and the increase in free fatty acids in the plasma. Recently, attention has turned to the mechanisms of central fatigue, and fatigue has been studied in clinical conditions other than cancer. Depending on the situation, the mechanisms and the pathophysiology have been shown to be different, and can thus not be applied to all cases. Patients undergoing major abdominal surgery are known to experience postoperative fatigue. Schroeder et al., in a carefully conducted trial, found increased fatigue for the first two weeks following the operation and muscle strength recovered within 1–3 months. Fatigue after surgery in this trial was not accompanied by any muscular defect, thus the apparent muscular weakness might be a secondary phenomenon to central fatigue.[1] On the other hand, Minotti et al. found that increased muscle fatigue in patients with congestive heart failure is not caused by an impaired central motor drive or an abnormality in neuromuscular junctions transmissions (see also

Table 9.1 Clinical conditions associated with asthenia

Chronic fatigue syndrome
Depression
Acute infection, chronic infection (such as tuberculosis, brucellosis, mononucleosis etc.), postinfectious status
Endocrinologic disease such as morbus Addison, poorly controlled diabetes mellitus, etc.
Chronic heart failure
Chronic pulmonary disease with a partial or total respiratory insufficiency
Chronic inflammatory rheumatic disease
AIDS

section on Muscle, below, and Table 9.2) but rather by an abnormality in the muscle itself.[2] For didactic reasons it therefore makes sense to focus on the two important target organs or tissues: the brain and the muscle.

Nervous system

Brasil-Neto et al. showed in 1993 and 1994 that the amplitudes of motor-evoked potentials elicited by transcranial magnetic stimulation were transiently decreased after exercise.[3,4] This finding indicates that the motor pathways of the central nervous system (CNS) are involved in the generation of physiological fatigue. The responsible mechanism is probably a decreased efficiency in the generation of descending volleys in the motor cortex. It is assumed that local (probably cortical) neurotransmitter depletion and mobilization are responsible

Table 9.2 Physiological classification of fatigue

Type of fatigue	Definition	Possible mechanism
Central	Strength- or heat-generated by voluntary effort less than that by electrical stimulation	Failure to sustain recruitment and/or frequency of motor units
Peripheral	Same strength loss or heat generation with voluntary and stimulated contractions	
High-frequency fatigue	Selective loss of strength at high stimulation frequency	Impaired neuromuscular transmission and/or propagation of muscle action potential
Low-frequency fatigue	Selective loss of strength at low stimulation frequency	Impaired excitation–contraction coupling

Source: Reproduced with permission from Sahlin.[13]

for this phenomenon and ultimately, at least in part, for the central fatigue experienced by normal subjects.

It is now accepted that fatigue during prolonged exercise is also influenced by the brain serotonergic system.[5] Prolonged exercise results in increased availability of tryptophan and increased brain 5-HT activity. A causal relationship between fatigue and 5-HT activity has been hypothesized but has yet to be established.[6] There is evidence that increased 5-HT activity influences both brain dopamine synthesis and brain dopamine effect.[7] In an accurate trial on rats, Bialey et al. have shown that physical exhaustion is affected by drugs that change the brain's 5-HT activity.[8] Furthermore, in this experiment, these effects did not appear to be substrate-dependent. Animals that were treated with a 5-HT antagonist, and consequently were able to maintain higher brain dopamine concentrations during prolonged effort, exercised longer. These data suggest that pharmacologically altered brain 5-HT activity may change dopamine concentration in the brain and lead to an alteration of fatigue perception or may at least be involved in determining the onset of fatigue in prolonged exercise.

The example of chronic fatigue syndrome (CFS) illustrates the difficulty in increasing the pathophysiologic understanding of fatigue generation. CFS was described several decades ago. It may arise sporadically, but several clustered outbreaks had already been reported in the 1930s, 40s, and 50s, suggesting an infectious cause.[9] Although the etiology of CFS is obviously different from cancer fatigue, a similar evolution might be identified in both diseases. The Centers for Disease Control (CDC) has made considerable efforts to better define CFS and to understand the mechanisms by which it functions. However, neurological involvement is only recently beginning to be confirmed by documentation of abnormalities in cerebral perfusion, hypothalamic function, and especially, neurotransmitter regulation.[10] Gibson et al.[11] found normal muscle functions at rest and during recovery in CFS patients. However, CFS patients had higher perceptions of exertion *during* exercise compared with the norm. This suggests that central factors are limiting the exercise capacity in some of these patients. Recently, a strong association between CFS and neurally mediated hypotension has been postulated. In a study carried out by Bou-Holaigah et al., 70% of 23 patients with CFS were found to have severe orthostatic syndrome as expression of a failure of the autonomic nervous system.[12]

Muscle

Muscle weakness can be classified in three groups:

1. The problem may be located in *neuromuscular transmission*. A typical example of such a mechanism is represented by myasthenia gravis.
2. *Energy sources* are inadequate. Short activities that require only brief muscular contractions are possible with the presence of ATP and creatin. Longer activities lead to increased use of local glycogen and to an accu-

mulation of lactate. Both the anaerobic, and subsequently, the aerobic process, induce an increased proton flux. The tissue pH decreases and interferes with the intracellular energetic process and lowers the rate of ADP-rephosphorylation. Recent studies indicate that in many cases, muscle fatigue is directly related to the incapacity to regenerate ATP.[13]

3. There is loss of the *contractile machinery*. This condition is usually due to a destructive process such as atrophy caused by disuse or in metabolic myopathies, in which an atrophy of type 2 fibers can often be found.

It must be established whether failure to exert effort is caused by a failure in the neural drive (fatigue in the mind, or at least in the nervous system) or in the muscle[14] (Table 9.2). For research purposes, central fatigue can be differentiated from peripheral fatigue by comparing voluntary with electrically stimulated contractions.

Pathophysiology of Cancer-Related Asthenia

In most cancer patients, the etiology of asthenia is unknown or at least there is no golden rule to properly define one or several major mechanisms leading to this symptom. To an even greater extent than other frequent symptoms, such as pain or mood disorders, asthenia may be a major symptom as such and/or accompany or be induced by other symptoms. Furthermore, the evolution of cancer asthenia might be influenced by other disorders and their therapeutic approaches. Thus we are dealing with a typical multidimensional and multicausal symptom. Sometimes one predominant abnormality can be identified, but often there is an aggregate of less prevalent abnormalities.[15]

A number of causes in different fields are consistently associated with cancer asthenia. The three main mechanisms causing these changes are direct tumor effects, tumor-induced products, and tumor-accompanying factors. This includes side effects of both tumor-directed and palliative therapeutic measures. (Fig. 9.1)

Although little is known in this field, it is accepted that the cancer itself is able to release a number of substances capable of significantly altering the intermediary metabolism of the host. These substances were termed "asthenins" by Theologides.[16] On the other hand, cancer induces the host macrophages and lymphocytes to produce a number of cytokines such as tumor necrosis factor (TNF), interleukin-1 (IL-1), IL-6, and IL-2. This inflammatory reaction, also known in other clinical conditions such as sepsis, can in some cases be considered the main mechanism leading to anorexia and cachexia. Experiments with parabiotic pairs of rats (one of them tumor-bearing) showed that the healthy partner experienced anorexia and cachexia mediated by circulating substances. There is some evidence that a similar mechanism can be postulated for asthenia as well. This assumption may be supported by the fact that tumor-free muscle tissue from tumor-bearing animals shows alterations in the activity of various enzymes, distri-

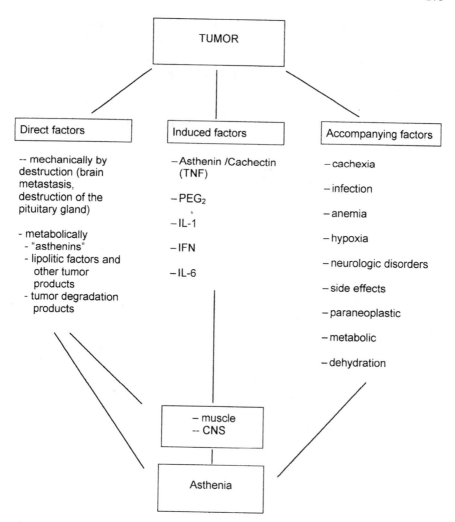

Figure 9.1. Mechanisms causing tumor asthenia.

bution of isoenzymes and synthesis and the breakdown of myofibrillar and sarco-plasmic proteins.[16]

As in nontumorous conditions, the muscle and CNS have to be considered the principal target tissues or organs involved in the generation of cancer asthenia (fatigue and weakness). For reasons of clarity, we could attribute fatigue more to the mechanisms occurring in the brain and general weakness to what happens in the muscles. As mentioned previously, research on animal models (fatigue in-duced by exertion during overactivity) and the model of chronic infectious disease (CFS and others) and depressive disorders have produced greater knowledge of central fatigue. Whether this knowledge can be applied to the situation of tumor asthenia has yet to be established. Because cancer asthenia does not lend itself to laboratory conditions comparable to those in the two models of research mentioned above, but represents a typical multidimensional pattern, a proper definition of the mechanisms is much more difficult to attain. It can probably be approached clinically by therapeutic/pharmacological measures that interfere with the tryptophan–serotonin–dopamine metabolism. Recent findings in CFS patients suggest an important involvement of the central and peripheral autonomic nervous system in general asthenia. Future research must assess whether these mechanisms are also present in tumor asthenia. More than 50% of patients with CFS-associated orthostasis improve significantly when treated with agents directed at neurally mediated hypotension. Clinical studies are needed to verify whether these findings are applicable to cancer-related asthenia and thus present a promise for therapy.[12] While our knowledge of the brain mechanisms is limited and can only be hypothesized on the basis of findings obtained in conditions not related to cancer, it is well recognized that some muscular alterations do occur in tumor-bearing patients.

In the literature there is a strong tendency to correlate asthenia with the cachexia–anorexia complex. This is supported by findings in the geriatric noncancer population in which malnutrition is a major issue. Nevertheless, it is important to stress that cachexia is not a requisite condition for asthenia to occur. Patients with advanced cancer also have muscle abnormalities that could occur in the absence of decreased food intake and/or weight loss.[16] A typical finding is the atrophy of type-2 muscle fibers (responsible for high anaerobic glycolytic metabolism) and an increased production of lactic acid. Bruera et al.[17] tested the muscle function in a group of patients with breast cancer and asthenia. The muscle function was electrically stimulated on the adductor pollicis muscle, via the ulnar nerve. Compared with the control group, the asthenic, noncachectic tumor patients showed decreased strength, decreased relaxation speed, and increased muscle fatigue after sustained stimulation. The result was corrected for the ultrasonographic muscle size. These results suggest that impaired muscle function in these cases may be an important underlying mechanism of asthenia.[17] In another group of patients with breast cancer no correlation was found between asthenia and nutritional status or weight.[18]

Our limited knowledge of central fatigue is drawn from research on animal models, which for the most part were not affected by cancer but overexerted by physical overactivity or by infection. The extent to which these findings can be applied to the situation of cancer patients has yet to be determined.

The Relationship Between Asthenia and Cachexia

The relationship between asthenia and cachexia is complex (Fig. 9.2).[19] As already shown, there are conditions in which asthenia exists without cachexia. However,

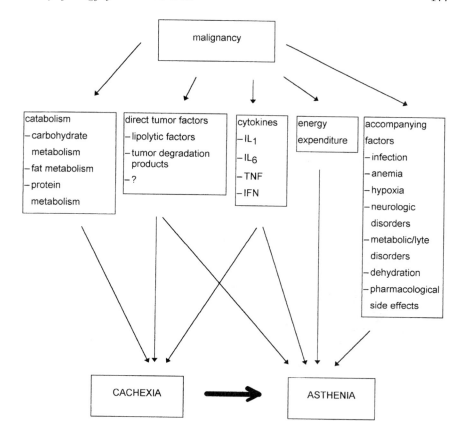

Figure 9.2. Mechanisms involved in the cachexia–asthenia complex.

in most advanced tumor situations, both are present and in a number of cases, there is probably a strong link between the two, or asthenia might be an epiphenomenon of the cachexia syndrome rather than an isolated, autonomous symptom (Fig. 9.3).

A number of metabolic abnormalities present in cancer patients may intervene in the cachexia–asthenia relationship. Thus it is important to focus on issues such as energy expenditure and fat metabolism, especially pathologic lipolyses and muscle protein degradation associated with gluconeogenesis. The pathophysiology of these processes is discussed in detail in Chapter 5 of this book.

The available data regarding energy expenditure are controversial. Under physiological conditions, the basal metabolic rate decreases as a response to chronic starvation. In malignant disease, the findings are even more controversial, although there is increasing evidence that at least some patients with advanced tumors present increased rates of metabolism and energy expenditure compared with control groups with similar weight loss.[20,21]

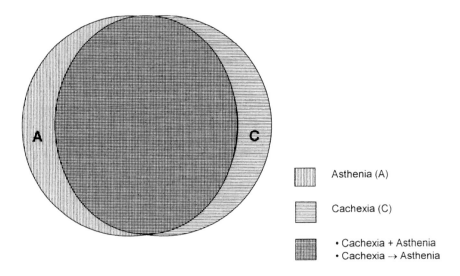

Figure 9.3. Cachexia–asthenia: cause-and-effect relationship?

An increased rate of gluconeogenesis from amino acids has been recognized and is partially related to the tumor burden. Furthermore, increased Cori cycling as an energy-consuming mechanism may contribute to raising energy expenditure.[22] We have frequently encountered glucose intolerance associated with hyperinsulinism.

Free fatty acids and amino acids are the principal products resulting from muscle and adipose tissue catabolism. Lipids are important substrates for cellular membranes and have an important function as intracellular mediators (eicosanoids, phospholipids), yet tumors are unable to synthesize their own lipids. Nutritional conditions leading to catabolism of host fat tissue (e.g., an acute fast) result in a stimulation of tumor growth, which suggests that products from host fat stores may be a limiting factor for tumor growth.[23]

During starvation of healthy subjects, a decrease in protein turnover can be observed.[24] Tumor-bearing subjects show an increased need for amino acids, resulting in a protein breakdown throughout the body. Cancer cachexia might thus reflect a state of inappropriate adaptation to a state of fasting.

Some data support the hypothesis that wasting is induced by direct catabolism of host components by tumor products, especially with regard to lipid mobilization.[25] On the other hand, cachexia is not strictly dependent on the stage and burden of the tumor. Indeed, it can be an early effect, and a simple competition between host and tumor is unlikely to be responsible for cachexia. An important role is attributed to a number of mediators such as TNF, IL-1, IL-6, or IFN.

Cachexia leads to loss of muscle mass. This may partially explain cachexia-related asthenia. Even in the presence of normal protein and caloric intake and normal body weight, structural and biochemical muscle abnormalities are found in cancer patients.[26–28] Some metabolic abnormalities related to cachexia are specifically responsible for muscle breakdown. Among these is an increased concentration of cathepsin-D (a lysosomal enzyme involved in the intracellular degradation of macromolecules).[29] The administration of substances, such as eicosapentaenolic acid (EPA), that are capable of inhibiting protein degradation might be a promising alternative for therapeutic intervention in these patients.[30]

Tumor-free muscle tissue of cancer patients shows excessive lactate production.[26] It is unclear whether lactate is part of the pathogenetic mechanism of weakness or just an epiphenomenon of it. The atrophy of type-2 muscle fibers has been suggested as a systemic effect of cancer even during early and nonmetastatic stages.[31] Loss of the contractile machinery of muscle is common in pathological processes such as dystrophy, atrophy, inactivity, and metabolic myopathies (treatment with corticosteroids, hypothyroidism, vitamin-D-deficiency). In these conditions there is also evidence of atrophy of type-2 fibers.

Our knowledge of malnutrition and its highly significant implications for the well-being of the elderly is more consistent in gerontology than in the study of malignant disease. Geriatricians have developed a number of preclinical instruments and tests (especially blood tests) that may allow us to prevent rather than treat malnutrition-associated asthenia by complementing food intake both qualitatively and quantitatively.

Unfortunately, these new findings in geriatric noncancer patients are probably not directly applicable to the cancer patient. There is no evidence that cachexia–anorexia and the related asthenia are reversible through nutritional manipulations since the etiology might be different in each case.

Conclusion

Our knowledge of the mechanisms and pathophysiologic courses of cancer-associated asthenia are still limited. For pragmatic clinical issues it seems reasonable to address the two major target organs: the brain (for fatigue) and the muscle (for weakness). However, in a number of cases, the failure of the autonomic nervous system is a consistant mechanism contributing to asthenia. Recent findings in the field of the CFS support this hypothesis, and it should be verified in the cancer population by clinical trials.

There is general agreement that cachexia is a major condition leading to asthenia even though clinical situations exist in which the relationship is not as closeknit as assumed. Clinical research, with the aim of better understanding and finally correcting the symptom, should be done on the same groups that would eventually benefit from positive results, and no rapid conclusions should be drawn from analogies in similar but not identical clinical situations. Furthermore, results from clinical investigations should be the results of trials in which asthenia was the main question and endpoint—not a side issue.

References

1. Schroeder D, Hill GL. Postoperative fatigue: a prospective physiological study of patients undergoing major abdominal surgery. *Aust N Z J Surg* 1991; 61(10):774–779.

2. Minotti JR, Pillay P, Chang L, Wells L, Massie BM. Neurophysiological assessment of skeletal muscle fatigue in patients with congestive heart failure. *Circulation* 1992; 86(3):903–908.

3. Brasil-Neto JP, Pascual-Leone A, Valls-Solé J, Cammarota A, Cohen LG, Hallett M. Postexercise depression of motor evoked potentials: a measure of central nervous system fatigue. *Exp Brain Res* 1993; 93:181–184.

4. Brasil-Neto JP, Cohen LG, Hallett M. Central fatigue as revealed by postexercise decrement of motor evoked potentials. *Muscle Nerve* 1994; 17:713–719.

5. Newsholme EA, Acworth IN, Bloomstrand E. Amino acids, brain neurotransmitters, and functional link between muscle and brain that is important in sustained exercise. In: Benzi G, ed. *Advances in Myochemistry*. London: Libbey Eurotext; 1987:127–133.

6. Chaouloff F, Lande D, Elghozi JL. Physical exercise: evidence for differential consequences of tryptophan on 5-HT synthesis and metabolism in central serotonergic cell bodies and terminals. *J Neural Transm* 1989; 78:121–130.

7. Korsgaard S, Gerlach J, Christensson E. Behavioral aspects of serotonine-dopamine interaction in the monkey. *Eur J Pharmacol* 1985; 118:245–252.

8. Bailey SP, Davis JM, Ahlborn EN. Neuroendocrine and substrate response to altered brain 5-HT activity during prolonged exercise to fatigue. *J Appl Physiol* 1993; 74:3006–3012.

9. Straus SE. Chronic fatigue syndrome. In: Isselbacher KJ, Braunwald E, Wilson JD, Martin JB, Fauci AS, Kasper DL, ed. *Harrison's Principles of Internal Medicine*. 13th ed. New York: McGraw Hill; 1993:2398–2400.

10. Kent-Braun JA, Sharna KR, Weiner MW, et al. Central basis of muscle fatigue in chronic fatigue syndrome. *Neurology* 1993; 43:125–131.

11. Gibson H, Carroll N, Chague JE, Edwards RH. Exercise performance and tatiguability in patients with chronic fatigue syndrome. *J Neurol Neurosurg Psychiatry* 1993; 56(9):993–998.

12. Bou-Holaigah I, Rowe PC, Kan J, Calkins H. The relationship between neurally mediated hypotension and the chronic fatigue syndrome. *JAMA* 1995; 274:(12):961–967.

13. Sahlin K. Acid-base balance during high intensity exercise. In: Harries, Williams, Stanish, Micheli, ed. *Oxford Textbook of Sportsmedicine*. New York: Oxford University Press; 1994:45–52.

14. Edwards RHT. New techniques for studying human muscle function, metabolism and fatigue. *Muscle Nerve* 1984; 7:599–609.

15. Neuenschwander H, Bruera E. Asthenia. In: Doyle D, Hanks GW, MacDonald N, ed. *The Oxford Textbook of Palliative Medicine*. 2nd. ed. New York: Oxford University Press; 1998:573–582.

16. Theologides A. Anorexins, astehnins, and cachectins in cancer. *Am J Med* 1986; 81:696–698.

17. Bruera E, Brenneis C, Michaud M, Jackson F, MacDonald RN. Association between involuntary muscle function and asthenia, nutritional status, lean body mass, psychometric assessment and tumor mass in patients with advanced breast cancer. *Proc Am Soc Clin Oncol* 1987; 6:261.

18. Bruera E, Brenneis C, Michaud M, Raft J, Magnan A, Tennant A, Hanson J, MacDonald RV. Association between asthenia and nutritional status, lean body mass, anemia, psychometrical status and tumor mass in patients with advanced breast cancer. *J Pain Symptom Manage* 1989; 4(2):59–63.

19. Neuenschwander H, Bruera E. Asthenia cachexia. In: Bruera E, Higginson I, eds. *Cachexia–Anorexia Syndrome in Cancer Patients*. New York: Oxford University Press; 1996:57–75.

20. Legaspi A, Jeevanadam M, Starnes HF, Brennan MF. Whole body lipid and energy metabolism in the cancer patient. *Metabolism* 1987; 10:958–963.

21. Nelson KA, Walsh D, Sheehan FA. The cancer anorexia–cachexia syndrome. *J Clin Oncol* 1994; 12:213–225.

22. Douglas RG, Shaw JHF. Metabolic effects of cancer. *Br J Surg* 1990; 77:246–254.

23. Tisdale MJ. Cancer cachexia. *Br J Cancer* 1991; 63:337–342.

24. Rose D, Horowitz GD, Jeevanadam M, Brennan MF, Shives GT, Lowry SF. Whole body protein kinetics during acute starvation and intravenous refeeding in normal man. *Federation Proc* 1983; 42:1070.

25. Beck SA, Tisdale MJ. Lipid mobilising factors specifically associated with cancer cachexia. *Br J Cancer* 1991; 63:846–850.

26. Holroyde R, Axelrod RS, Skutchers CL, Haff AC, Paul P, Reichard SA. Lactate metabolism in patients with metastatic colorectal cancer. *Cancer Res* 1979; 39:4900–4904.

27. Beck S, Mulligan H, Tisdale M. Lipolytic factors associated with murine and human cancer cachexia. *J Natl Cancer Inst* 1990; 82:1922–1926.

28. Smith KL, Tisdale MJ. Mechanism of muscle protein degradation in cancer cachexia. *Br J Cancer* 1993; 68:314–318.

29. Beck SA, Tisdale MJ. Production of lipolytic and proteolytic factors by a murine tumor producing cachexia in the host. *Cancer Res* 1987; 47:5919–5923.

30. Beck SA, Smith KL, Tisdale MJ. Anticachectic and antitumor effect of eicosapentaenolic acid and its effect on protein turnover. *Cancer Res* 1991; 51:6089–6093.

31. Warmolts JR, Re PK, Lewis RJ, Engel WK. Type II muscle fibre atrophy (II-Atrophy): an early sistemic effect of cancer. *Neurology* 1975; 2:374.

10

The Reversible Causes of Asthenia in Cancer Patients

JAMES F. CLEARY

Although asthenia is a relatively new term in oncology, the symptoms that it encompasses have long been recognized as part of the clinical presentation of cancer. Asthenia is derived from the Greek: a (absence) thenia (strength) and is defined as a lack of strength, diminution of vital power, weakness, debility (Oxford English Dictionary). For many years, "asthenia" has been considered to be a natural concomitant of malignant neoplasms and it was suggested that asthenia may be a form of carcinomatous myopathy.[1]

Myopathies are primarily associated with weakness, but Theologides[2] expanded the definition of asthenia to incorporate more than the absence of strength. He defined asthenia as "a systemic disability characterized physically by generalized weakness, loss of strength, and easy fatigability of the muscles and mentally by the diminished capacity for intellectual endeavors and an emotional lability or apathy."[2]

Of these symptoms, muscle weakness and easy fatigability are the most obvious clinical features of cancer-associated asthenia. Together with the concept of asthenia, Theologides also postulated the concept of asthenins, or substances postulated to provoke metabolic and functional alterations in host muscles that lead collectively to marked weakness.[3] He commented that the pathogenesis of weakness, easy fatigability of muscles, and the asthenia syndrome in general was unclear,[2] a situation that persists to this day.

Bruera and colleagues have done much to address the issue of asthenia and have stated that asthenia is a combination of the symptoms of fatigue and weakness.[4] Fatigue or lassitude were defined as "easy tiring and decreased capacity to maintain adequate performance" and generalized weakness was defined as "the anticipatory subjective sensation of difficulty in initiating an activity."[4] Asthenia, according to Bruera et al., does not include the localized or regional weakness resulting from neurological (nerve or muscle) disorders. In their experience, the incidence of asthenia in a population of cancer patients ranged up to 90%.[4] Coyle and colleagues[5] interviewed 90 advanced cancer patients in the Supportive Care Program of the Memorial Sloan-Kettering Cancer Center (MSKCC) 4 weeks prior to death. Fifty-two (58%) of the patients *volunteered* that they were fatigued and 39 (43%) were experiencing weakness. The authors noted the high prevalence of asthenia, based on the presence of both these symptoms.

Asthenia is not a term that is widely used by clinicians and is not a term that we use with patients. Fatigue, weakness, and tiredness are the terms that patients more commonly use in reporting their symptoms, as evidenced by the report of Coyle et al.[5] Although these terms are used interchangeably by many, it can be very difficult to successfully distinguish between the terms asthenia and fatigue. What does the term *asthenia* offer that the use of the term *fatigue* does not? To answer this question it is necessary to consider the definitions of fatigue and weakness and the differentiation between these and asthenia.

Fatigue is encountered by most people as a feeling that exists somewhere between tiredness and exhaustion.[6] The prevalence of these symptoms in the cancer population has been studied to a limited extent. Of all symptoms assessed in more than 1000 patients at the Cleveland Clinic,[7] weakness and easy fatigue were ranked numbers 2 and 3 in both severity and prevalence ratings. Pain was the top-ranked symptom in both categories. The authors admit that the terms "easy fatigue," "weakness," and "lack of energy" (collected in patient interviews) may overlap, but "asthenia" was not used. Coyle et al.[5] followed the prevalence of fatigue and weakness prior to the death of patients at the MSKCC. In this select group of patients, there was a decrease (58% to 52%) in the prevalence of fatigue in the 4 weeks prior to death, whereas the prevalence of weakness increased (43% to 49%). In other studies, patients undergoing different modes of antitumor treatment have been studied. Fifty-seven of 91 (63%) patients treated with radiotherapy, chemotherapy, or bone marrow transplant reported that they "felt sluggish." This was the only symptom of the Oncology Treatment Toxicity Tool that could be incorporated into the definition of asthenia.[8]

In common-day usage, fatigue has been defined as a tiredness after physical exercise or mental effort, or as the condition of not arriving at any useful activities or lacking motivation.[9] It has also been defined as a mood state characterized by deactivation or low-action preparedness. From a nursing perspective, Piper and colleagues defined fatigue as the subjective feeling of tiredness that is influenced by circadian rhythm.[10] When acute, it serves a protective function, but when it is unusual, excessive, or constant, it may lead to aversion to activity and the desire to escape. They also classified fatigue as subjective feelings such as weariness, weakness, exhaustion, and lack of energy that result from exertion or stress. Fatigue may lead to discomfort and decreased efficiency, and it causes deterioration of both mental and physical activities. Aistars and co-workers[11] defined fatigue as a condition characterized by subjective feelings of generalized weariness, weakness, exhaustion, and lack of energy resulting from prolonged stress that is directly or indirectly attributable to the disease process. The outcome is an impaired functional status, which ultimately has an impact on a patient's quality of life.

Psychologists consider fatigue as a condition affecting the whole organism, which includes decreased motivation as well as deterioration of mental and physical activities.[6] This diversity yields at least two definitions of fatigue. Fatigue can be described as a subjective sense of weariness or tiredness resulting from exertion and stress. It can also be described as a condition of impaired efficiency resulting from prolonged mental and/or physical activity or from an attitude of boredom or from disgust with monotonous work.

There are also contrasting definitions of fatigue. Fatigue has been defined as a condition characterized by subjective feelings of increased discomfort and decreased functional status related to decreased energy.[12] Factors involved may be physical, mental, emotional, environmental, physiological, and pathological, but importantly, it was stated that there is a voluntary component in fatigue. This concept encompasses the concept of tiredness but contrasts with the concept of weakness, which is a symptom produced by neurological impairment and which does *not* have a voluntary aspect in the performance of the activities. Nail and King[13] defined fatigue "as a human response to the experience of having cancer and to undergoing the treatment of cancer." It is a self-recognized phenomenon involving how the individual feels and how this feeling influences the activities in which one chooses to engage." The authors also state that there is a voluntary component to fatigue, in direct contrast to the symptom of weakness; weakness is produced by neurologic syndromes and does not incorporate a voluntary component in performance of activities.

Asthenia is used interchangeably by some clinicians with the cancer cachexia syndrome which is defined as profound nutritional depletion. Whereas asthenia may by part of that syndrome together with weight loss, anorexia, and anemia, cachexia is not an essential component of asthenia.[14] These conditions may combine to produce the effect of "wasting away," a picture that can present in cancer patients, many elderly patients, and patients with other chronic diseases.[15]

Use of the definition of asthenia as outlined by Theologides[2] and Bruera and MacDonald[4] would suggest that more than fatigue needs to be present for the symptom of asthenia to be present. However, the broader definition of fatigue would allow fatigue and asthenia to be used interchangeably. Given the limited published data on asthenia, fatigue and asthenia will be used interchangeably in this discussion, especially given that this is a symptom to which patients must be able to assign a name. However, some instruments of fatigue confuse it with weakness or with potential responses to fatigue such as decreased activity and depression. The tools for measuring these symptoms need to be evaluated.

How Do We Measure Asthenia?

The measurement of fatigue and weakness has not been a priority within cancer medicine. The Common Toxicity Criteria of the National Cancer Institute do not list asthenia or fatigue in its assessment of treatment-induced symptoms. Weakness is assessed under the heading of "neuro-motor" and the criteria range from no change to paralysis. It is important that self-rating tools be used by patients, as clinicians have assessed fatigue badly when compared with patients' self-assessment.[16]

Only one direct attempt has been made to measure asthenia itself. Bruera and colleagues[17] studied asthenia using four self assessment tests: a visual analog scale in which patients assessed their level of energy, a 27-item questionnaire to rate activity level, 6 visual analog scales (0–100) to rate a patient's ability to perform different activities, and a 7-item questionnaire assessing a patient's ability to complete certain tasks. These scores were averaged and compared with age- and sex-matched controls from the community. Asthenia was considered to be present in those whose score was less than the 10th percentile of the community control group. Forty-one percent of the patients fell below the 10th percentile of the community controls and were considered to have asthenia.

More work has been conducted on the measurement of fatigue, and Irvine and colleagues[18] have published an excellent review of these instruments. Initially, fatigue was measured using tools developed by industry in the late 1960s, both in the U.S. and Japan, to assess the activity level of healthy persons in the work place; these tools were not suitable in a cancer setting.[19] The Symptom Distress Scale (SDS), developed in 1978 by McCorkle and Young,[20] used patient self-report to assess 13 symptoms that commonly result from anticancer treatment. Patients rated the severity of these symptoms, including fatigue and concentration, on a 1–5 scale with verbal descriptors. This scale has been extensively used in patients with cancer and other diseases.[20,21] and has also been validated with adolescents receiving anticancer treatment.[22]

Other scales that specifically assess fatigue have also been developed. The Fatigue Symptom Checklist measures physical and mental fatigue and specific physical symptoms.[23] The Rhoten Scale[24] was developed in 1982 for postoperative patients and is essentially a self-report, 0–10 measure of fatigue. The latter scale correlates with an observation checklist completed by staff but has had limited use in cancer patients. The Piper Fatigue Self-Report Scale,[25] which was developed to measure the temporal, intensity, affective, and sensory dimensions of fatigue, has been tested in radiotherapy patients.

These multidimensional fatigue scales have often been difficult to complete because of their length or they have also assessed other somatic symptoms that might contaminate the assessment of fatigue. To overcome these problems, Smets and colleagues[26] developed the Multidimensional Fatigue Index, initially in Dutch but also available in English and other languages. The dimensions addressed in this index include general, physical, and mental fatigue, as well as motivation and activity level. The tool, which consists of 20 questions, each with a seven-point scale, has been validated in both cancer and noncancer groups. The significance of fatigue measured by this index and the extent to which its presence interferes with a patient's daily activities have not been addressed.

Other tools that have been used in the general assessment of cancer patients undergoing treatment have incorporated an assessment of fatigue. The Profile of Mood States (POMS) includes a fatigue subscale that has been used to assess the effect of psychiatric interventions on the well-being of cancer patients.[27] As quality of life (QOL) has gained prominence in the management of cancer, different QOL measures have incorporated an assessment of fatigue. For example, the European Organization for Research and Treatment of Cancer (EORTC)-Quality of Life Questionnaire, which has been validated cross culturally in lung cancer patients,[28] includes a fatigue subscale. Assessment of fatigue is made from three questions: "Did you need to rest?" "Have you felt weak?" and "Were you tired?" No significant changes from pretreatment to on-treatment assessments for fatigue were found except for those who had a worsening of performance status. The authors claim that this was related to the heterogeneity of the cancer patients and the multiple causes of fatigue.

The Functional Assessment of Cancer Therapy (FACT) has recently been used in the measurement of fatigue and other anemia-related symptoms in 48 cancer patients one month post cancer therapy.[28a] The Brief Fatigue Inventory, modeled on the Brief Pain Inventory, is being developed at the University of Wisconsin Comprehensive Cancer Center and the MD Anderson Cancer Center in Texas.

What Are the Causes of Asthenia in Cancer Patients?

Cancer itself

The prevalence of fatigue is high in many disease states[20] and the specific association between major aspects of the asthenia syndrome and cancer remain unclear. Certainly those patients close to death experience fatigue and could be considered as having fatigue directly as a result of their cancer.[5,7,21,29] Pickard-Holley found a correlation between CA_{125} levels and fatigue in ovarian cancer patients and suggested that increasing tumor burden, reflected by the CA_{125} levels, resulted in more fatigue.[12] In 81 patients treated for breast or lung cancer, there was a significant correlation between the duration of illness and the fatigue.[30] It is important to realize that many of the studies that assess asthenia or fatigue have been performed in small uncontrolled patient groups. It has been difficult to conclude whether disease itself, treatment intervention, or the agent used contributes to the development of asthenia in cancer patients (Table 10.1).

Table 10.1. Causes of asthenia in cancer patients

Cancer	Depression
Malnutrition	Infection
Anemia	Insomnia
Cancer treatment	Pain
Chemotherapy	Metabolic abnormalities
Radiotherapy	Exercise
Opioids	Neurological syndromes
Biological factors	
Steroids	

Malnutrition

The association between asthenia and malnutrition has been clearly established in patients with malignant disease.[3,31] Theologides[2] suggested that variation in enzyme function, lactic acid accumulation, and wasting of type II muscle fibers may be mechanisms in the etiology of asthenia. Some of the mediators of cachexia, such as tumor necrosis factor, cause significant asthenia when administered to animals and to humans.[16]

However, the association of asthenia and malnutrition is not universal for all cancers. Bruera and colleagues assessed the relationship of the nutritional status to asthenia in 64 breast cancer patients.[17] Nutritional status was determined by the measurement of triceps skinfold thickness, arm circumference, actual/usual weight index, and serum albumin, and each was expressed as a percentage of the standard value for each test. Lean body mass was also determined and, on this basis, the study population was assessed as being mildly obese. There was no significant correlation with asthenia score, nutritional status, and lean body mass in this group of breast cancer patients. This may reflect the disease chosen, as cachexia is not a prominent symptom in breast cancer.

Anemia

Anemia is probably overdiagnosed as a cause of fatigue and there is no clear picture of its role in fatigue in cancer patients.[32] The treatment of anemia may be associated more with improvement in exertional dyspnea than fatigue.[33] However, these two symptoms may be inseparable to patients. Although many patients report an increase in energy levels with the correction of anemia, Bruera et al. found no correlation between anemia (Hb < 12gm%) and the asthenia score in 64 breast cancer patients.[17] The authors suggested that asthenia may only be a symptom of anemia when hemoglobin levels are below 7 g/dl.

The FACT subscale for fatigue was used to differentiate between those patients with hemoglobins of greater than 13 g/dl and less than 11.0 g/dl. However, it was not possible to use fatigue symptoms to differentiate hemoglobin levels of less than 13 g/dl.[28a]

Cancer treatment

Anticancer therapy impacts on the energy levels of patients. Fatigue was the most prevalent symptom present in 208 cancer patients treated at six Michigan cancer centers (Table 10.2); the prevalence was 80%.[21] The presence and severity of treatment-induced fatigue depend on the treatment modality.

Chemotherapy

Many chemotherapy agents have been found to cause fatigue. With the development of new drugs with unique modes of action, the incidence of fatigue may be increasing. This increase may also reflect measurement bias; fatigue is now being sought as a symptom of chemotherapy treatment. Fatigue occurred in early studies of busulfan[34] and was commonly associated with the development of pulmonary fibrosis. Gallium nitrate therapy caused fatigue and asthenia in over 70% of patients treated with this agent.[35] Eight percent of colon cancer patients receiving oral levamisole alone in a large comparative phase III trial[36] experienced fatigue or weakness, which disappeared with cessation of therapy. Asthenic symptoms were observed in 11% of those treated with the combination of oral levamisole plus intravenous weekly 5-fluorouracil. Two-thirds of 43 head and neck patients administered docetaxel (100 mg/m² every 3 weeks) in a phase 2 study experienced fatigue and 23% experienced grade 3 or 4 toxicity.[37] In a phase 1 study of a new protein synthesis inhibitor, the dose-limiting toxicities were delayed hypotension and severe asthenia; asthenia was experienced by 9 of 12 patients at all dose levels and its severity was dose related and lasted from 1 to 21 days (median 3 days).[38] Gemcitabine, which has been shown to improve the

Table 10.2. Incidence of fatigue in patients treated with chemotherapy in relation to survival and to age

	No. of patients	% with fatigue	Average severity
Survivor group			
≥ 12 months	111	78.4	1.71
6–12 months	35	77.1	2.12
≤ 6 months	62	83.9	1.83
Age group			
20–49 yr	38	71.4	1.4
50–64 yr	87	91.7	1.82
≤65 yr	83	81.3	1.87

Adapted from data from Kurtz et al.[21]

quality of life of patients with pancreatic cancer, causes fatigue or lethargy, occurring either alone or in conjunction with other flu-like symptoms.[39,40] In a phase 1 study completed at the University of Wisconsin, oral carboxyamidotriazole was administered each morning to cancer patients.[41] Fatigue was a predominant symptom for these patients but nighttime administration of the drug helped 5 of the 6 patients who were switched from morning dosing. However, 6 of 6 patients initially commenced on nighttime administration were also found to have mild to moderate fatigue.

The administration of combination chemotherapy also contributes to the development of fatigue. In one survey, 46 of 56 patients administered normal chemotherapy regimens reported tiredness and 29 reported weakness.[42] Jamar and colleagues[43] measured fatigue (with the Byers Pearson tool) in 16 women with ovarian cancer (stages I–IV) who were receiving chemotherapy (cisplatin and cyclophosphamide) administered every 4 weeks. Twelve of these women (75%) reported that fatigue was worse the first week following chemotherapy but that it lessened during the subsequent 3 weeks of the cycle. Twelve of the 16 patients reported that they had to give up or change activities, including social activities, because of fatigue, and 11 reported a change in sleep pattern. Nine patients had below-normal hemoglobin and hematocrit levels, but there was no association of these with the level of fatigue. Pickard-Holley and colleagues confirmed this peaking of fatigue levels within 7 days of therapy and the subsequent gradual decline back toward baseline before the next course.[12] Twelve ovarian cancer patients with a high performance status and who were at different stages of their cyclophosphamide and cisplatin treatment self-rated fatigue with the Rhoten Fatigue Scale. No correlation was found between the cycle of treatment and fatigue, suggesting that there was no cumulative effect of chemotherapy on fatigue. Other chemotherapy regimens (ranging from 5-fluorouracil alone to platinum, doxorubicin and carmustine treatment) caused fatigue, as measured on a 0–5 scale with verbal descriptors, in another small group of adult cancer patients.[44] Fatigue was the predominant toxicity, with 7 of 9 patients having this symptom at day 2 (mean severity, 3.23 out of 5).

The type of chemotherapy may not be important in the development of asthenic symptoms. In 64 patients with breast cancer, there was no difference in the asthenia scores following the administration of anticancer regimens that included cyclophosphamide, methotrexate and fluorouracil ($n = 19$); cyclophosphamide, fluorouracil, methotrexate, vincristine and prednisolone ($n = 18$); adriamycin and vinblastine ($n = 12$); tamoxifen ($n = 10$); and medroxyprogesterone acetate ($n = 5$).[17] In particular, there was no difference between the chemotherapy group and the hormone treatment groups, and in those treated with chemotherapy, there was no difference in fatigue between the patients administered adriamycin-based chemotherapy and those receiving regimens without adriamycin. The authors concluded that cancer treatment, as used in breast cancer, had no major effect on the incidence of asthenia. It is of interest to note that none of these chemotherapy regimens contained cisplatin, which was present in the regimens used in the ovarian cancer populations.

It is possible that drugs used to control nausea and vomiting following chemo-therapy administration contribute to fatigue, but little work has been performed to address this issue. No correlation for fatigue and the use of antiemetic therapy in the previous 24 hours was found by Blesch and colleagues in 77 patients with breast and lung cancer undergoing chemotherapy treatment.[30] Simms, Rhodes, and Madsen found that the addition of lorazepam in the treatment of chemother-apy-induced emesis significantly reduced fatigue when compared with prochlo-perazine alone.[45]

Radiotherapy

Haylock and colleagues were among the first to systematically document the incidence of fatigue in 30 patients receiving localized radiotherapy.[23] Fatigue was measured using the Pearson Byers Feeling Checklist and the 30-item Fatigue Symptom Checklist of the Japanese Association of Industrial Health, both tools not specifically designed for the cancer setting. Patients were treated each week-day over a 4- to 6-week period and there was an increase in fatigue (15%) during the weekdays of treatment, which accumulated over the treatment period. Im-portantly, there was a decrease in fatigue scores on weekends but not back to the pretreatment levels. The effect of the daily radiotherapy administration time on fatigue was not addressed in this study. The fatigue-sparing effect of weekends was confirmed by Kobashi-Schoot et al., but only in patients with lymphoma and uterine cancer and not in patients with breast or bladder cancer.[46]

In general, radiotherapy-associated fatigue is reversible. Some investigators, however, have suggested that this is not always the case. Fatigue was still present in many patients 3 months after the completion of treatment in patients who were receiving radiotherapy to different regions of the body (Table 10.3).[47] In another study, the physical well-being of 403 survivors of Hodgkin's disease was assessed at Stanford University.[48] Energy levels had been affected adversely by treatment in 90% of patients and had not returned to normal in 37%, despite a median follow-up time of 9 years (range 1–21 years). Patients older than 34 years took much longer to recover from the fatigue associated with Hodgkin's disease.

Opioids

Opioids are known to cause sedation in normal clinical practice but it is difficult from the available literature to assess whether they cause asthenia. Opioids may contribute to the occurrence of daytime drowsiness, which may be perceived as fatigue by these patients. The relief of pain in many patients may allow them to sleep and consequently recover from pain-induced sleep deprivation. Opioids can also impair concentration and may therefore contribute to mental fatigue. Blesh and colleagues found no significant correlation between fatigue and the dose of opioids administered during the previous 24 hours in breast or lung cancer patients, although there was a significant correlation between fatigue and pain intensity.[30] The duration of opioid treatment may be significant, as patients often develop tolerance to the opioid-induced drowsiness.

Table 10.3 Characteristics of fatigue following radiotherapy treatment to different areas of the body in 96 patients with cancer

Site of radiotherapy	n	Incidence week 1 (%)	Max incidence (%)	Week of max. incidence	Post RT incidence 3 months (%)
Thorax	15	60	93	3	46
Head and neck	25	35	68	4	39
Pelvis (Female)	30	52	76	3	32
Pelvis (male)	26	35	65	5	14

Adapted from the data of King et al.[47]

Biological therapy

Perhaps the best known iatrogenic cause of fatigue in cancer medicine are the biotherapy agents.[49] It has been postulated that asthenia caused by these agents is the result of a diffuse encephalopathy.[50] Although a relationship with dose has been suggested,[51] Robinson and colleagues found no significant correlation between the degree or duration of fatigue and the dose of biological response modifier administered.[16] In the latter study, 50% found that treatment caused moderate to severe fatigue and nine of these patients stated that fatigue caused significant changes in their lifestyle, e.g., reduced hours of employment. Although the interferons are most commonly associated with asthenia, growth factors may also cause these symptoms. This is illustrated by the case report of a 47-year-old woman with extensive liver metastases from squamous cell carcinoma of the uterine cervix.[52] Prolonged leukopenia developed after cycle 2 of cisplatin and recombinant human granulocyte-colony stimulating factor (rh G-CSF) was added for the third cycle. Fatigue and asthenia developed on day 4 of the third cycle and the patient became bedridden with severe asthenia. Her symptoms recovered but recurred with cycle 4 in which half the dose of rh G-CSF was administered. rh G-CSF was omitted for cycle 5 and the patient had no recurrence of symptoms of asthenia.

Fatigue is the most frequent adverse effect of interferon alpha (α-IFN) and is reported by 90% of patients.[53] It is generally heralded by the occurrence of a febrile reaction. Fatigue also appears to be the most important dose-limiting toxic effect of (α-IFN). Fatigue is profound at doses exceeding 20 million units daily in older patients or those with a poor performance status.[54,55] In a series of 2500 patients with a variety of malignancies reported by Gauci,[56] fatigue and anorexia occurred in 90% and 70% of patients, respectively, and frequently limited the dose of α2a-IFN administered. The onset of these effects generally occurred in the first 2 weeks of treatment, were persistent throughout the duration of therapy, and resolved upon withdrawal of the drug. Other related symptoms that may have contributed to the symptoms of fatigue following α-IFN administration were severe weight loss in 18%, a decrease in mental function in 12% of patients, confusion in 8%, and depression in 5%. All of these symptoms resolved upon discontinuation of treatment. Fatigue was the dose-limiting toxicity of a phase 1 study of the combination of interleukin 2 combined with α-IFN.[57]

Steroids

Steroids are commonly used in oncology as antiemetics and anti-inflammatory agents. These drugs have been suggested as a possible treatment for asthenia but, in some cases, they may be involved in producing the symptom. Steroid-induced myopathy was the cause of asthenia in a woman with hepatocellular carcinoma who received a steroid for control of severe nausea and vomiting.[58] Withdrawal from steroids used as part of chemotherapy regimens may also contribute to symptoms of fatigue in so-treated patients.

Depression

Depression can be a difficult symptom to assess in relation to asthenia as depression may be both a cause and a result of asthenia. The incidence of depression tends to be overestimated in cancer patients. Although self-report scales suggest a prevalence as high as 25%,[59] only 6% of cancer patients are estimated to have major depression and 2% to have an anxiety disorder.[60] Of the Stanford Hodgkin's Disease patients, those whose energy levels had not returned to normal were more likely to be depressed than those who had returned to a full level of activity.[48] Bruera and colleagues[17] found a significant association between asthenia and psychological distress as measured by the Symptom Checklist-90. This correlation decreased with multiple regression analysis, suggesting that psychological distress cannot independently explain a significant number of cases of asthenia in cancer patients. No correlation between fatigue and depression was found in 12 women receiving chemotherapy for ovarian cancer.[12] In 77 patients administered chemotherapy and or radiotherapy for the treatment of breast or lung cancer, there was a significant correlation between fatigue and depression.[30] Piper and colleagues[25] also found a significant correlation between total fatigue score and depression as measured by the Piper Fatigue Scale and POMS, respectively. Total mood disturbance, also measured by the POMS, correlated with the total fatigue score.

Infection

Almost all patients who have an infection experience fatigue, most likely resulting from the release of cytokines. Prolonged viral infections with agents such as the Epstein Barr virus may produce long-lasting fatigue as the predominant symptom.[61] Cancer patients are at increased risk of infection because of decreased immunity and white cells. Antibiotics such as ketoconazole may contribute to fatigue.[62]

Insomnia

Although lack of sleep can contribute to fatigue, it is not usually associated with weakness. Disturbed sleep in cancer patients may be caused by pain, depression, drugs (such as steroids), or other factors. Pain interferes with the onset of sleep and with the ability to sleep through the night.[63] Pain may also contribute to fatigue itself and to depression, which may cause early morning wakening. Disturbance of sleep is therefore linked to many factors and may not be an independent variable in the etiology of fatigue.

Pain

There was a strong and highly significant correlation between the intensity of fatigue and pain severity in 81 patients with breast and lung cancer,[30] a finding confirmed separately within each disease group. In contrast, Bruera and colleagues found no association of pain with asthenia and also found no improvement in appetite with the diminution of pain.[17]

Metabolic abnormalities

Asthenia is the cardinal sign of Addison's disease, a primary adrenal syndrome rarely encountered in recent times. Many drugs can cause hypoadrenalism, however, and produce symptoms and signs identical to the primary disorder. Among the agents that cause hypoadrenalism are suramin[64] and ketoconazole therapy for prostatic carcinoma (1200 mg daily).[65] Steroid withdrawal is also associated with a secondary Addison's disease and is probably an under recognized syndrome when one considers the use of steroids in oncology. In this author's experience, many patients administered 5 days of steroids as part of a chemotherapy regimen complain of severe fatigue following the sudden cessation of treatment. This "washed out" feeling may be lessened by tapering the steroid regimen, which in turn may increase the toxicity of the chemotherapy regimen. Although hyperkalemia is part of the syndrome of Addison's disease, hyperkalemia alone can contribute to asthenia, particularly through muscle weakness.

Exercise

Exercise is commonly recommended for patients with cancer and some have found that exercise is beneficial in preventing the development of fatigue.[66] However, appropriate levels of exercise need to be suggested for individual patients. Fatigue may develop as a result of either excessive exercise[67] or too much bed rest.

Neurological syndromes

The classic paraneoplastic association of asthenia and cancer is the Eaton Lambert Syndrome, in which patients have weakness and fatigability of proximal limb and torso muscles with relative sparing of extraocular and bulbar muscles. It is more common for the lower limbs to be involved than the upper limbs, and autonomic manifestations occur in half of patients. Seventy-two percent of males and 32% of females with the syndrome have cancer, of which 80% are small-cell lung cancer. This syndrome can respond to immunosuppressants and plasmapharesis and the small-cell lung cancer is responsive to chemotherapy. Resolution of asthenia is variable following treatment of the associated cancer.[68]

Interventions in the Treatment of Asthenia

It is essential prior to treating asthenia that careful consideration be given to those disease processes that may respond to direct therapy e.g., infection, hyperkalemia, and Addison's disease. It is also essential prior to the commencing diagnostics and treatment of fatigue that the relevance of the symptom in relation to a patient's disease process, expected life span, and quality of life be considered.

Correction of anemia

It has already been suggested that anemia may be overestimated as a cause of fatigue in cancer patients. This relationship may become more evaluable as pharmacological treatment of anemia using synthetic erythropoietin becomes more widespread. Among 118 cancer patients not receiving chemotherapy, erythropoietin resulted in a 2.4% increase in hematocrit, which was significantly greater than the change seen with placebo (-0.1%).[69] There was, however, no statistically significant difference in the absolute hematocrit levels between the two groups. Although pretreatment erythropoietin levels were a significant predictor of response in this group, there was no significant difference in the transfusion requirements of patients receiving placebo or erythropoietin over the 8 weeks of the study. One has to question the role of synthetic erythropoietin administration in this group. For those receiving chemotherapy (with and without cisplatin), there was a significant change in hematocrit with the administration of erythropoietin in the first month, but no significant change in transfusion requirements. Transfusion requirements decreased significantly in the erythropoietin group during the second and third months of treatment but only in those patients receiving cisplatin.

One difficulty with the results of this study is the way that the results are presented. QOL data are only presented in the responders, that is, in those who have had a greater than 6% increase in their hematocrit. Whereas these increases were significantly different from the pooled placebo data, the change in visual analog scores for those treated with erythropoietin compared with the placebo group was only 10 mm (out of 100 mm) for energy level, daily activities, and overall QOL. It is difficult to appreciate how meaningful this 10-mm change would be to patients. A 10% decrease in fatigue scores may have little impact on a patient's QOL if similarities are drawn with the measurement of pain.[70] One would also suspect that the inclusion of nonresponders in these results may result in a nonsignificant finding.

The ability to truly treat fatigue, as opposed to other symptoms of anemia, is questionable. Ludwig and colleagues studied the effect of erythropoietin for cancer-associated anemia. They found an improvement in performance status and quality of life for the 50% of 102 patients who had an increase in hemoglobin of greater than 2 gm/dl. Those who did not achieve an improvement in hemoglobin had no change in performance status and little improvement in quality of life. Whereas selected individuals may benefit, further research is required to define those who will benefit.[70a] Breast cancer patients receiving chemotherapy together with erythropoietin maintained a better hemoglobin level than in those receiving chemotherapy alone. However, there was no difference in psychological distress, including physical activity, between the two groups.[70b]

Nutrition

There is little evidence that aggressive improvement in nutrition increases survival, tumor response, or treatment toxicity among those with advanced cancer. There is no evidence that aggressive nutritional therapy improves the quality of life of these patients.[71] Parenteral feeding of cancer patients has little impact on fatigue.[31]

Drug interventions

The cessation of other drug therapies that cause asthenia is recommended. Difficulties arise when these therapies are used with curative or life-prolonging intent. Steroids may need to be tapered slowly in patients who experience fatigue following longer use of these drugs.

Supplemental steroid therapy can ameliorate fatigue and may be particularly indicated during some anticancer treatments, such as high-dose ketoconazole therapy.[65] Moertel and colleagues[72] found a significant improvement in appetite and strength in patients after 2 weeks of dexamethasone treatment (0.75 and 1.5 mg qid), compared with placebo. However, this improvement disappeared after 4 weeks of treatment. Bruera and colleagues observed that methylprednisolone caused a rapid improvement in activity level in a double-blind setting but this improvement was not sustained over a 3-week period.[73] In another randomized, placebo-controlled, double-blind trial, Bruera et al. found that 1 week of megesterol acetate resulted in an improvement in appetite, caloric intake, nutritional status, and level of energy.[74] This improvement may have been a non-specific steroid effect of megesterol, rather than a specific action on fatigue. Although steroids have been used to treat the symptoms of asthenia, a dilemma arises if steroid-induced myopathy occurs. The treatment options in this setting are reduction of steroid dose, changing to a nonfluorinated steroid, alternate-day dosing, and isometric exercise.[58]

Amphetamines may be useful in patients who have treatment-associated asthenia. Mazindol had little effect on the activity score of cancer patients,[75] but methylphenidate resulted in a significant improvement in the level of activity.[76] In the latter study, patients were taking large doses of opioids and the methylphenidate may have had an indirect effect by improving pain control or opioid-induced sedation.

Exercise

Exercise has been helpful in improving symptoms in women receiving chemotherapy.[66] A structured 10-week exercise program reduced fatigue, stabilized weight, and reduced nausea in state II breast cancer patients treated with chemotherapy. However, caution must be urged to ensure that the exercise level is appropriate for the patient and does not result in the development of fatigue.[67]

Group therapy

The effect of group therapy on the symptoms of asthenia has been studied in a number of settings. Forrester and colleagues[77] examined the effect of group therapy on anorexia, fatigue, and nausea in a randomized study of patients receiving radiotherapy. The authors found that a significant decrease in physical symptoms resulted from group therapy, but the clinical significance of this difference is questionable. There was no difference in scores for anorexia, fatigue, and nausea at completion of treatment but 4 weeks later there was a 1.6 (of a total of 21) difference in scores. The clinical utility of a 7.6% decrease in these three symptoms combined is doubtful. In another psychiatric group intervention, which used the POMS to assess symptoms, there was only a nonsignificant decrease in fatigue 6 months following the intervention.[27]

Self-help activities

In the nursing literature, many articles address the value of patient self-help activities to overcome fatigue. In one study, 49 adult patients used a self-care diary (0–5 scale with verbal descriptors) following the administration of chemotherapy (ranging from 5-FU alone to platinum, doxorubicin, and carmustine treatment) to assess the effect of self-help tools. The predominant toxicity was fatigue, with 81% of patients having this symptom at day 2 (severity, 3.23).[44] Of the self-care activities listed, 85% went to bed earlier or had a nap. The efficacy of these maneuvers was 3.17 and 3.57, respectively, which the authors equated to moderate relief. They concluded that many of the activities recommended to overcome symptoms are not uniformly effective but may work for some patients.

Similar findings were found in a population that received biological modifier therapy and reported a high prevalence of fatigue that was more severe in the afternoon and evening (63%).[16] Fifty percent indicated that rest or sleep improved fatigue and the other 50% described continuing their usual routine or lightly exercising as most beneficial.

The use of an activity diary that also records patient self-assessment of fatigue may be useful.[51] This allows patients to make the most of high-energy times and allows clinicians to schedule dose reduction and/or a break from therapy, if possible, within the goals of treatment.

Fatigue in the caregiver

Fatigue in the family caregiver can be physically induced by the demands of the caregiving experience and psychologically induced by concern regarding the diagnosis, treatment, and prognosis of the cancer patient. In 248 caregivers, no correlation was found between fatigue and age, or the duration of caregiving. However, relationships were found among the total number of hours of care provided, the outside employment of the caregiver, and the impact on the caregivers schedule.[78]

Summary

Asthenia is a prevalent symptom in patients with cancer and it multiple etiologies are still poorly understood. It is important to continue research on asthenia and to consider ways to prevent and treat fatigue and weakness. The directly treatable causes of asthenia are currently few, whereas the number of cancer patients affected by the syndrome are many.

References

1. Rowland LP, Schotland DL. Neoplasms and Muscle Disease. In: Brain WR, Norris FH, eds. The remote effects of cancer on the nervous system. New York: Grune and Stratton; 1965; 83–97.
2. Theologides A. Asthenia in cancer. Am J Med 1982; 73:1–3.
3. Theologides A. Anorexins, asthenins, and cachectins in cancer. Am J Med 1986; 81:696–698.
4. Bruera E, MacDonald RN. Asthenia in patients with advanced cancer. Issues in symptom control. Part 1, J Pain Symptom Manage 1988; 3:9–14. [erratum appears in J Pain Symptom Manage 1988; 3(4):211].
5. Coyle N, Adelhardt J, Foley KM, Portenoy RK. Character of terminal illness in the advanced cancer patient: pain and other symptoms during the last four weeks of life. J Pain Symptom Manage 1990; 5:83–93.
6. Hart LK, Freel MI. Fatigue. In: Norris CM, ed. Concept Clarification in Nursing. Rockville, MD: Aspen Publications; 1982:251–261.
7. Donnelly S, Walsh D, Rybicki L. The symptoms of advanced cancer: identification of clinical and research priorities by assessment of prevalence and severity. J Palliat Care 1995; 11:27–32.
8. Youngblood M, Williams PD, Eyles H, Waring J, Runyon S. A comparison of two methods of assessing cancer therapy-related symptoms. Cancer Nurs 1994; 17:37–44.

9. Frijda NH. *The Emotions. Studies in Emotion and Social Interaction.* Cambridge, England: Cambridge University Press, 1986.

10. Piper BF, Lindsey AM, Dodd MJ. Fatigue mechanisms in cancer patients: developing nursing theory. *Oncol Nurs Forum* 1987; 14:17–23.

11. Aistars J. Fatigue in the cancer patient: a conceptual approach to a clinical problem. *Oncol Nurs Forum* 1987; 14:25–30.

12. Pickard-Holley S. Fatigue in cancer patients. A descriptive study. *Cancer Nurs* 1991; 14:13–9.

13. Nail LM, King KB. Fatigue. *Semin Oncol Nurs* 1987; 3:257–362.

14. Langstein HN, Norton JA. Mechanisms of cancer cahexia. *Hematol Oncol Clin North Am* 1991; 5:103–123.

15. Verdery RB. 'Wasting away' of the old old: can it—and should it—be treated? *Geriatrics* 1990; 45:26–31.

16. Robinson KD, Posner JD. Patterns of self care needs and interventions related to biological response modifier therapy: fatigue as a model. *Semin Oncol Nurs* 1992; 8:17–22.

17. Bruera E, Brenneis C, Michaud M, et al. Association between asthenia and nutritional status, lean body mass, anemia, psychological status, and tumor mass in patients with advanced breast cancer. *J Pain Symptom Manage* 1989; 4:59–63.

18. Irvine DM, Vincent L, Bubela N, Thompson L, Graydon J. A critical appraisal of the research literature investigating fatigue in the individual with cancer. *Cancer Nurs* 1991; 14:188–199.

19. Varricchio CG. Selecting a tool for measuring fatigue. *Oncol Nurs Forum* 1985; 12:122–127.

20. McCorkle R, Young K. Development of a symptom distress scale. *Cancer Nurs* 1978; 1:373–378.

21. Kurtz ME, Given B, Kurtz JC, Given CW. The interaction of age, symptoms and survival status on physical and mental health of patients with cancer and their families. *Cancer* 1994; 74:2071–2078.

22. Hinds PS, Quargnenti AG, Wentz TJ. Measuring symptom distress in adolescents with cancer. *J Pediatr Oncol Nurs* 1992; 9:84–86.

23. Haylock PJ. Fatigue in patients receiving localized radiation. *Cancer Nurs* 1979; 2:461–467.

24. Rhoten D. Fatigue and the postsurgical patient. In: Norris CM, ed. *Concept Clarification in Nursing.* Rockville, MD: Aspen Publishing; 1982:277–300.

25. Piper BF, Lindsey AM, Dodd MJ, Ferkerich S, Paul SM, Weller S. The development of an instrument to measure the subjective dimension of fatigue. In: Funk SG, Tonrnquist EM, Champagne MT, Copp LA, Wiese RA, eds. *Key Aspects of Comfort: Management of Pain, Fatigue and Nausea.* New York: Springer-Verlag; 1989;199–208.

26. Smets EM, Garseen B, Cull A, de Haes JC. Application of the multidimensional fatigue inventory (MFI-20) in cancer patients receiving radiotherapy. *Br J Cancer* 1996; 73:241–245. *Psychosom Res* 1995; 39:315-25.

27. Fawzy FI, Cousins N, Fawzy NW, Kemeny ME, Elashoff R, Morton D. A structured psyhiatric interview for cancer patients. *Arch Gen Psychiatry* 1990; 47:720–725.

28. Aaronson NK, Ahmedzai S, Bergman B, et al. The European Organization for Research and Treatment of Cancer QLQ-C30: A quality-of-life instrument for use in international clinical trials in oncology. *J Natl Cancer Inst* 1993; 85:365–376.

28a. Yellen SB, Cella DF, Webster K, Blendowski C, Kaplan E. Measuring fatigue and other anemia-related symptoms with the Functional Assessment of Cancer Therapy (FACT) measurement system. *J Pain Symptom Manage* 1997; 13:63–74.

29. Bruera E, MacDonald RN. Overwhelming fatigue in advanced cancer. *Am J Nurs* 1988; 88:99–100.

30. Blesch KS, Paice JA, Wickham R, et al. Correlates of fatigue in people with breast or lung cancer. *Oncol Nurs Forum* 1991; 18:81–87.

31. Nelson KA, Walsh D, Sheehan FA. The cancer anorexia–cahexia syndrome. *J Clin Oncol* 1994; 12:213–225.

32. Adams R, Victor M. *Lassitude and Fatigue, Nervousness, Irritability, Anxiety and Depression.* New York: McGraw Hill, 1993.

33. Skillings JR, Sridhar FG, Wong C, et al. The frequency of red cell transfusion for anemia in patients receiving chemotherapy: a retrospective cohort study. *J Clin Oncol* 1993; 16:22–25.

34. Dahlgren S, Holm G, Svanborg N. Clinical and morphological side-effects of busulfan (Myleran). *Acta Med Scand* 1972; 192:129–135.

35. Jabboury K, Frye D, Holmes FA, et al. Phase II evaluation of gallium nitrate by continuous infusion in breast cancer. *Invest New Drugs* 1989; 7:225–229.

36. Moertel CG, Fleming TR, MacDonald JS, et al. Levamisole and fluorouracil for adjuvant therapy of resected colon carcinoma. *N Engl J Med* 1990; 322:352–358.

37. Catimel G, Verweij J, Mattijsseen V, et al. Docetaxel (Taxotere): an active drug for the treatment of patients with advanced squamous cell carcinoma of the head and neck. *Ann Oncol* 1994; 5:533–537.

38. Catimel G, Coquard R, Guastalla JP, et al. Phase 1 study of RP 48532A, a new protein-synthesis inhibitor, in patients with advanced refreactory solid tumors. *Cancer Chemother Pharmacol* 1995; 35:246–248.

39. Christman K, Kelsen D, Saltz L, et al. Phase II trial of gemcitabine in patients with advanced gastric cancer. *Cancer* 1994; 73:5–7.

40. Poplin EA, Corbett T, Flaherty L, et al. Difluorodeoxycytidine (dFdC)-gemcitabine: a phase I study. *Invest New Drugs* 1992; 10:165–170.

41. Berlin JD, Tutsch, KD, Hutson P, et al. Phase 1 clinical and pharmacokinetic study of oral carboxyamidotriazole, a signal transduction inhibitor. *J Clin Oncol* 1996; in press.

42. Cassileth BR, Lusk EJ, Strouse TB, Miller DS, Brown LL, Cross PA. A psychological analysis of cancer patients and their next of kin. *Cancer* 1985; 50:72–76.

43. Jamar S. Fatigue in women receiving chemotherapy for ovarian cancer. In: Funk SG, Tornquist EM, Campagne MT, Archer Gropp L, Wiese RA, eds. *Key Aspects of Comfort: Management of Pain, Fatigue, and Nausea.* New York: Springer-Verlag; 1989:224–228.

44. Nail LM, Jones LS, Greene D, Schipper DL, Jensen R. Use and perceived efficacy of self-care activities in patients receiving chemotherapy. *Oncol Nurs Forum* 1991; 18:883–887.

45. Simms S, Rhodes V, Madsen R. Comparison of prochloperazine and lorazepam antiemetic regiments in the control of post chemotherapy symptoms. *Nurs Res* 1993; 42:234–239.

46. Kobashi-Schoot JA, Hanewald GJ, van Dam FS, Bruning PF. Assessment of malaise in cancer patients treated with radiotherapy. *Cancer Nurs* 1985; 8:306–813.

47. King KB, Nail LM, Kreamer K, Strohl RA, Johnson JE. Patient's descriptions of the experience of receiving radiation therapy. *Oncol Nurs Forum* 1985; 12:55–61.
48. Fobair P, Hoppe RT, Bloom J, Cox R, Varghese A, Spiegel D. Psychological problems among survivors of Hodgkin's disease. *J Clin Oncol* 1986; 4:805–814.
49. Piper BF, Rieger PT, Brophy L, et al. Recent advances in the management of biotherapy-related side effects: fatigue. *Oncol Nurs Forum* 1989; 16(Suppl):27–34.
50. Adams F, Quesada J, Gutterman J. Neuropsychiatric manifestations of human leucocyte interferon therapy in patients with cancer. *JAMA* 1984; 7:938–941.
51. Brophy LR, Sharp EJ. Physical symptoms of combination biotherapy: a quality of life issue. *Oncol Nurs Forum* 1991; (Suppl) 18:25–30.
52. Punt CJA, Kingma BJ. Severe asthenia and fatigue caused by recombinant human granulocyte conony stimulating factor (rh G-CSF). *Ann Oncol* 1994; 5:473–474.
53. Jones GJ, Itri LM. Safety and tolerance of recombinant interferon alfa-2a (Roferon(R)-A) in cancer patients. *Cancer* 1986; 57(Suppl):1709–1715.
54. Gutterman JU, Fine S, Quesada J, et al. Recombinant leukocyte A interferon: pharmacokinetics, single-dose tolerance, and biologic effects in cancer patients. *Ann Intern Med* 1982; 96:549–556.
55. Quesada JR, Talpaz M, Rios A, Kurzrock R, Gutterman JU. Clinical toxicity of interferons in cancer patients: a review. *J Clin Oncol* 1986; 4:234–243.
56. Gauci L. Management of cancer patients receiving interferon alfa-2a. *Int J Cancer* 1987; Suppl 1:21–30.
57. Hirsh M, Lipton A, Harvey H, et al. Phase I study of interleukin-2 and interferon alfa-2a as outpatient therapy for patients with advanced malignancy. *J Clin Oncol* 1990; 8:1657–1663.
58. MacDonald SM, Hagen N, Bruera E. Proximal muscle weakness in a patient with hepatocellular carcinoma. *J Pain Symptom Manage* 1994; 9:346–350.
59. Massie MJ, Gagnon P, Holland JC. Depression and suicide in patients with cancer. *J Pain Symptom Manage* 1994; 9:325–340.
60. Derogatis L, Morrow G, Fetting J, et al. The prevalence of psychiatric disorders among cancer patients. *JAMA* 1983;249:751–757.
61. Schooley RT. Epstein Barr virus infections, including infectious mononucleosis. In: Isselbacher KJ, Braunwald E, Wilson JD, Martin JB, Fauci AS, Kasper DL, eds. *Harrison's Principles of Internal Medicine.* 13th ed. New York: McGraw Hill; 1994:790–793.
62. Ross JB, Levine B, Catanzaro A, et al. Ketoconazole for treatment of chronic pulmonary coccidioidomycosis. *Ann Intern Med* 1982; 96:440–443.
63. Dorrepaal KL, Aaronson NK, van Dam FS. Pain experience and pain management among hospitalized cancer patients. A clinical study. *Cancer* 1989; 63:593–598.
64. Stein CA, Saville W, Yarchoan R, et al. Suramin and function of the adrenal cortex (Letter). *Ann Intern Med* 1986; 104:286–287.
65. White MC, Kendall-Taylor P. Adrenal hypofunction inpatients taking ketoconazole. *Lancet* 1985; i:44–45.
66. MacVicar MG, Winningham ML. Promoting functional capacity of cancer patients. *Cancer Bull* 1986; 38:235–239.
67. St Pierre BA, Kasper CE, Lindsey AM. Fatigue mechanisms in patients with cancer: effects of tumor necrosis factor and exercise on skeletal muscle. *Oncol Nurs Forum* 1992; 19:419–425.

68. Drachman DB. Myasthenia gravis. In: Isselbacher KJ, Braunwald E, Wilson JD, Martin JB, Fauci AS, Kasper DL, eds. *Harrison's Principles of Internal Medicine*. 13th ed. New York: McGraw Hill, 1994; 2394.

69. Henry DH, Abels RI. Recombinant human erythropoietin in the treatment of cancer and chemotherapy-induced anemia: results of double-blind and open-label follow-up studies. *Semin Oncol* 1994; 21(Suppl):21–28.

70. Serlin RC, Mendoza TR, Nakamura Y, Edwards KR, Cleeland CS. When is pain mild, moderate or severe? Grading pain severity by its interference with function. *Pain* 1995; 61:277–284.

70a. Ludwig H, Sundal E, Pecherstorfer M, Leitgeb C, Bauernhofer T, Beinhauer A, Samonigg H, Kappeler AW, Fritz E. Recombinant human erythropoietin for the correction of cancer associated anemia with and without concomitant cytotoxic chemotherapy. *Cancer* 1995; 76:2319–2329.

70b. Del Mastro L, Venturini M, Lionetto R, Garrone O, Melioli G, Pasquetti W, Sertoli MR, Bertelli G, Canavese G, Costantini M, Rosso R. Randomized phase III trial evaluating the role of erythropoietin in the prevention of chemotherapy-induced anemia. *J Clin Oncol* 1997; 15:2715–2721.

71. Bruera E, Fainsinger RL. Clinical management of cachexia and anorexia. In: Doyle D, Hanks G, MacDonald N, eds. *Oxford Textbook of Palliative Medicine*. New York: Oxford University Press; 1993; 330–337.

72. Moertel C, Schutt AJ, Reitemeier RJ, Hahn RG. Corticosteroid therapy of preterminal gastrointestinal cancer. *Cancer* 1974; 33:1607–1609.

73. Bruera E, Roca E, Cedaro L, et al. Action of oral methylprednisolone in terminal cancer patients: a prospective randomized double-blind study. *Cancer Treat Rep* 1985; 69:751–754.

74. Bruera E, MacMillan K, Hanson J, Kuehn N, MacDonald RN. A controlled study of megestrol acetate on appetite, caloric intake, nutritional status and other symptoms in patients with advanced cancer. *Cancer* 1990; 66:1279–1282.

75. Bruera E, Carrara S, Roca E, et al. Double-blind evaluation of the effects of mazindol on pain, depression, anxiety, appetite and activity in terminal cancer patient. *Cancer Treat Rep* 1985; 70:295–297.

76. Bruera E, Chadwick S, Brenneis C. Methylphenidate associated with narcotics for the treatment of cancer pain. *Cancer Treat Rep* 1987; 71:120–127.

77. Forester B, Kornfield DS, Fleiss JL, Thompson S. Group psychotherapy during radiotherapy: effects on emotional and physical distress. *Am J Psychiatry* 1993; 150:1700–1706.

78. Jensen S, Given BA. Fatigue affecting family caregivers of cancer patients. *Cancer Nurs* 1991; 14:181–187.

IV

PSYCHOLOGICAL ISSUES IN THE CAREGIVER

Introduction: Defining the Unit of Care: Who Are We Supporting and How?

IRENE J. HIGGINSON

At its outset, hospice and palliative care considered the patient and family as the unit of care.[1] It took care from beyond the narrow attention of patients isolated from their family situation and considered the needs of those close to them and of professionals. An important aspiration of hospices was to create a family-like atmosphere.[1]

But when we talk of family or caregiver, who do we mean? Is it a lay caregiver such as a spouse, daughter, parent, neighbor? Or do we mean a professional caregiver, from one or more of the many professional backgrounds who may be involved? There are also the volunteers, who are trained and supported by professionals and often fall between formal and lay systems of care. The term "caregiver" is generally taken to mean significant-other person(s); these include family, friends, and professional staff and volunteers. But the term can be misleading. Does a caregiver need to be actively giving care to be included in this definition? Clearly not. An important family member or friend may be more severely disabled than the patient—this can occur in instances when a "caregiver" has a chronic health problem. And as our society changes in structure, so, too, do the caregivers, both professional and lay, change. Cartwright has described the increased role of nurses, rather than family doctors, in the care of patients at home.[2] As our society lives to older ages and becomes more mobile, lay care-givers are more commonly sons, daughters, nieces and nephews in their late fifties and sixties. Families are scattered over wide distances. Or the caregiver is a neighbor, friend, or person running supported housing.

Among formal and lay carers, there can be anything between none and several caregivers to consider, such as a spouse, children, siblings, and friends. Each will have different needs. There is a growing body of research which shows that informal and formal caregivers views may differ from the patient's view, and from one another in their assessment of pain, symptoms, quality of service, and information needed.[3-5] The perceptions of carers after the death may be different from the perceptions held during care.[6] These differences affect the way that support and care are needed and provided to both the patient and the caregivers.

Nevertheless, while caring for a dying relative can be a rewarding experience, many carers inevitably find the experience difficult to cope with. It can have major psychosocial and physical effects, including heightened symptoms of depression, anxiety, psychosomatic symptoms, restriction of roles and activities, strain in relationships, and poor physical health. Some studies have reported spouses as experiencing the same level of distress as patients. A longitudinal study suggested that a substantial group of caregivers experience distress 1 year after diagnosis and that mental health status declined for 30% of carers.[7] In a recent study, 32% of carers were rated as having severe anxiety at referral to a home care team; anxiety remained severe for 26% of carers in the last week of life.[8]

These problems may not only increase the health care needs of the carer but also affect the patient. Interventions that address the needs of carers and develop effective coping skills (such as communication) may indirectly affect the well-being of the patient.[9] Problems for carers in advanced cancer predispose them to a poor outcome at bereavement, and interventions during the terminal phase may prove preventative and also avoid demands on bereavement services.[10] Bereavement has long been recognized as causing increased morbidity and mortality.[11]

Therefore, carers need support during the illness and during bereavement to prevent these problems. But what form should this take? Comparative studies of the effectiveness of different interventions are rare. Interventions vary from service to service.[12] Although validation of different bereavement risk stratification has been undertaken, the use of such measurements is varied.[13] In the United States in a randomized controlled trial, Toseland et al. evaluated a 6-week carer support group, in 80 spouses of cancer patients.[9] Fear of the spouse dying was the most common pressing problem reported. The study found improvements in physical aspects, role, and social functioning in the intervention group, compared with the control group, when those carers with the most distress were considered. Coping strategies in the form of support, information, and coping skills were the most effective. However, there was a low uptake (27%) for the study. Such a study would need to be replicated in places where reactions to groups and psychosocial needs may differ. The transactional model of stress and coping postulates that appraisal of events is individual and carers will differ in the extent to which they find coping methods useful.[14] Therefore, interventions that take an eclectic approach may prove the most useful in a group setting.

Professional caregivers also have important needs. Although there is debate about whether palliative care is more stressful than other areas of health and social care, this question is difficult to answer, because staff with different backgrounds, experiences, and personalities choose different specialties. A more important question is how to develop mechanisms of support for professional caregivers, and to reduce unnecessary stresses. This applies to those individuals already working in hospices and specialist palliative care units and those who meet and care for patients with advanced illness in general care settings, such as family medicine, district nursing, on general hospital wards, and in nursing homes. Research is needed to determine effective mechanisms of providing support to lay and professional caregivers that have a clear effect on the outcomes and well-being of patients and their families and enhance the quality of care that staff are able to provide in the long term.

References

1. Saunders C, Sykes N. *The Management of Terminal Malignant Disease.* 3rd ed. London: Edward Arnold, 1993.
2. Cartwright A. Changes in life and care in the year before death 1969–1987. *J Public Health Med* 1991; 13(2):81–87.
3. Epstein AM, Hall JA, Tognetti J, Son LH, Conant L. Using proxies to evaluate quality of life. Can they provide valid information about patient's health status and satisfaction with medical care. *Med Care* 1989; 27(3):S91–S98.
4. Higginson I, McCarthy M. Validity of the support team assessment schedule: do staffs' ratings reflect those made by patients or their families? *Palliat Med* 1993; 7:219–28.
5. Field D, Douglas C, Jagger C. Terminal illness: views of patients and their lay carers. *Palliat Med* 1995 9:45–54.
6. Higginson I, Priest P, McCarthy M. Are bereaved family members a valid proxy for a patient's assessment of dying? *Soc Sci Med* 1994; 38(4):553–557.
7. Ell K, Nishimot R Mantell J, Hamovitch M. Longitudinal analysis of psychological adaptation among family members of patients with cancer. *J Psychosom Res* 1988; 32:429.
8. Hodgson CS, Higginson IJ, McDonnell M Butters E. Family anxiety in advanced cancer. *Bri J Cancer* 1997; 6:120–124 in press.
9. Toseland RW, Blanchard CG, McCallion P. A problem solving intervention for caregivers of cancer patients. *Soc Sci Med* 1995; 40:517–552.
10. Mor V, Horney C, Sherwood S. Secondary morbidity among the recently bereaved. *Am J Psychiat* 1986÷3:158–63.
11. Bowling A. Mortality after bereavement: a review of the literature on survival periods and factors affecting survival. *Soc Sci Med* 1987; 24(2):117–24.
12. Bromberg M, Higginson I. Bereavement follow-up: what to support teams do? *J Palliat Care* 1996; 12(1):12–17.
13. Parkes CM. Bereavement. In: Doyle D, Hanks GWC, MacDonald N, eds. *Oxford Textbook of Palliative Medicine.* New York: Oxford University Press; 1993; 14:663–678.
14. Grahn, G. Coping with the cancer experience. I. Developing an education and support programme for cancer patients and their significant other. *Euro Jo Cancer Care* 1996; 5:176–181.

11

Care of the Cancer Patient: Response of Family and Staff

MATTHEW J. LOSCALZO AND JAMES R. ZABORA

The Person, Family, and Social Network

People with a chronic illness are both encircled by and are connected to interacting systems best conceptualized as three concentric circles. The patient, the family, and the social network form three systems that are simultaneously interdependent with fluid and permeable boundaries. These three systems influence and are influenced by each other. The degree of influence is determined by the current situation and normal drive to maintain, a sense of equilibrium. Threats to the survival of any system cause disequilibrium, and as a result, a reflexive effort is initiated to regain homeostasis and stability.

The core source of influence is generally the patient, and more specifically, the physiological status of the patient. The physical state and the perceived amount of threat to the immediate survival of the organism is the screen through which all experiences are filtered. Meaningful attention to the psychological, existential, spiritual, family, financial, and social concerns can only be perceived and processed in the absence of an immediate threat to physical survival. Uncontrolled noxious symptoms are experienced as life depleting, and consequently deprive the individual of the ability to strive for a sense of efficacy and control. Ongoing acute physical distress is inimical to effective cognitive integration and meaningful action.

The family is the primary system of support which defines expectations for the person identified as being at risk from a life-threatening illness. The greater the shared sense of threat and disruption to the integrity of the family system, the more likely patients and families will act in unison toward resolution of identified problems. Families have the resources and capacity to create an environment in which support and problem-solving can occur. However, families may also lack the ability and willingness to act in a concerted and constructive manner to initiate the complex adjustments that are necessary to care for a loved one with a chronic and life-threatening disease. Each family has resources and liabilities that need to be evaluated and, when appropriate, maximized to the best interests of the patient and family.

The third level of experience relates to the nature of the social environment. The health care team, patients, families, and social systems are influenced by idiosyncratic perceptions of problems and expectations for action. The greater the shared perception of the problem and expectations of each family member, the more likely the systems will work in synergy to pursue an identified goal. The health care team is part of the patient's social system but may transiently be integrated into the family system at crisis points. Given the complexity of the interactions of individuals, families, and external social systems, stress, confusion, and conflict are endemic to most situations. In most cases, patients, families, and the social supportive systems work effectively to create an environment in which adequate communication and coordination of effort are achieved. Health care staff are an important force throughout the illness process and wield varying degrees of influence. Therefore, the roles and impact of health care staff as they occur in clinical practice will be interwoven throughout this chapter, for the staff act as both an initiator and recipient of influence, power, and control. In many ways, the health care team as a system has specific attitudes, values, and rules of acceptable behaviors that may vary significantly from not only the patient and family but also from team to team. An objective appreciation for the impact of staff is essential if medical, psychosocial, and spiritual care is to be tailored to meet the minimal requirements of patients and families. Under the best circumstances, the optimal result is an effective therapeutic fit between the patient, family, and health care staff.

Care of patients with a life-threatening illness is limited by the context in which medical and psychosocial care occurs. The present fragmented system of health care is increasingly based on economic considerations and not on medical or psychosocial principles or values. Since there has not been a public debate concerning the underlying inherent values in caring for the physically ill, patients and families are unaware of this reality until they feel the negative impact of it. Consequently, patients experience confusion and a sense of victimization when they are compelled to make decisions concerning medical care that may be inconsistent with family attitudes and beliefs. For example, hospice and palliative care provide a context in which to understand this dilemma. But in the United States, patients and family members are uniformly asked to produce proof of health insurance before medical systems provide reassurance that care will be provided and decide between curative therapies and palliation. These approaches to care are frequently perceived as mutually exclusive rather than complementary. Currently, patients are compelled to sign Do Not Resuscitate (DNR) or Do Not Intubate (DNI) directives in order to satisfy legal requirements so that essential services can be provided at home or in a hospice. Patients and families are also compelled to accept and formally state that the patient will forego curative treatments for palliation, again, as if the two were incompatible. For some patients and families, this symbolizes the surrendering of life rather than a shift in focus to creating a more meaningful end of life. A focus on living and resources which promotes self-integration into a family and social network can be achieved, regardless of the prognosis. The inability to balance medical and psychosocial demands results in irrational decisions which, in part, explains why so few eligible dying patients are referred for hospice care.

This context of the person with life-threatening illness and their family is one in which ongoing loss is inevitable. In a fragmented system of medical care, patients and families are ill prepared but must make difficult choices of great consequence. It is within this setting of complex demands that the psychosocial needs of people with life-threatening disease and those of their families can be best understood. For medical care, psychosocial support and spiritual guidance exist within a system of care that is often at odds with itself and attempts to treat disease while simultaneously monitoring and balancing the costs in response to wider national interests.

Cancer in many ways has provided the template for care of the chronically ill with life-threatening diseases. Cancer patients comprise the overwhelming majority of patients receiving organized programs of palliative care. This has been determined by the natural course of the disease, dramatic scientific advances in treatment and care, the perception of cancer in the consciousness of the public, and the availability of funding sources in the industrialized nations of the world.

In a series of published studies in Britain, Seale and Cartwright[1] found that cancer patients were sicker and had more symptoms than a general population of noncancer patients in the year prior to death. Cancer disrupts all components of social integration—family, work, finances, friendships—as well as patients' psychological health. Patients enter the cancer experience as a vital member of a family system that simultaneously attempts to adjust and respond to the diagnosis and its challenges. Over the extended course of the illness, physical changes and deterioration create multiple and complex demands on the family. These demands, in conjunction with financial assaults, generate a negative synergy that is often ignored in the care of patients with advanced disease.

Frequently, cancer patients' greatest concern is not pain, death, or other physical symptoms, but rather the impact of the disease on their families.[2] According to the World Health Organization,[3] "family" refers to those individuals who are either relatives or other significant people as defined by the patient. Health care professionals must acknowledge the role of the family in order to maximize treatment outcomes. If the family is actively incorporated into the care of the patient, the health care team gains a valuable ally and resource. Families are the primary source of support and also provide the caregiving roles for persons with cancer. It is noteworthy that women comprise the majority of individuals who serve in these caregiving roles.[4,5]

To the patient and family, a discussion concerning a referral to hospice can seem quite sudden and may be experienced as rejection as care is transferred to a new set of strangers. This transfer of care to a new institution occurs within the context of a dying loved one. Relatively few hospitals have developed a continuum of care that identifies palliation as a potential outcome of curative treatment, despite the sobering survival statistics for many cancers. It can be surmised that the situation is worse for other chronic life-threatening diseases. At present, patients and family members enter hospice care, which is the primary deliverer of comprehensive palliative care services, and attempt to accept that prolongation of life is no longer the goal of care. In addition to the shift in the focus from cure to care, the patient and family experience the loss of the health care team with whom trust has been imbued over months and sometimes many years. The loss occurs simultaneously at multiple levels. Only one-third of all cancer patients receive formal hospice care and often only in the final days of life.[6,7] Although palliative care should be a time of refocusing and resolution, the referral process may cause an iatrogenic crisis rather than comfort when this shift in focus is not perceived as a natural part of a continuous care. Health care providers seldom inform and support patients and families at all stages of illness as to the potential outcomes, despite overwhelming data to highly probable results.

The psychological impact of cancer and its treatments is directly influenced by the interaction between the degree of physical disability, internal resources of the patient, the intensity of the treatment, side-effects, adverse reactions, as well as the relationship with the health care team. In addition, two salient timelines or continua related to patient and family adaptation should be considered. The level of *psychological distress* forms the first continuum; the second consists of the *predictable and transitional phases* of the disease process. Patients with a pre-existing level of psychological distress can experience significant difficulty as they attempt to adapt to the multiple stressors associated with a cancer diagnosis. While most patients experience significant distress at the time of their diagnosis, the majority of patients gradually adjust during the following 6 months.[8] However, the demands of advancing disease are especially insidious in that they are often extended over a long period of time, frequently change, and only offer potential outcomes which are shrouded in ambiguity. Figure 11.1 details potential interventions along the distress continuum. In other words, the level of psychological vulnerability falls along a continuum from low to high distress and should guide the selection of interventions. Given the variation in distress, a major concern emerges in terms of the prevalence of the most distressed cancer patients. Prevalence studies demonstrate that one of every three newly diagnosed patients (regardless of prognosis) needs psychosocial or psychiatric intervention.[9–11] As disease advances, a positive relationship exists between the increase in the occurrence and severity of physiological symptoms and the patient's level of emotional distress and overall quality of life. Schulz et al., in a study of 268 cancer patients with recurrent disease, report that patients with higher symptomatology,

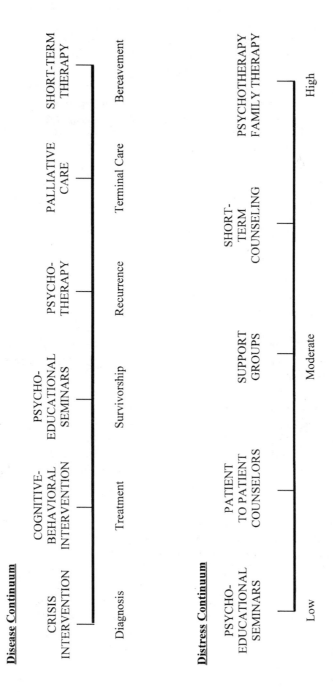

Figure 11.1. Continua of care for cancer patients and their families.

greater financial concerns, and a pessimistic outlook experience higher levels of psychological distress and lower levels of general well-being.[12]

If distress levels can be identified through mechanisms such as psychosocial screening, patients can then be introduced into supportive care systems earlier in the treatment process. Any attempt to identify vulnerable patients and families in a prospective manner is worthwhile. Screening techniques are available through the use of standardized instruments which are able to prospectively identify which patients and families may be more vulnerable to the cancer experience. In many respects, pre-existing psychosocial resources are critical in any predictive or screening process. Weisman and Worden[8] delineated key psychosocial variables in the format of a structured interview accompanied by a self-report measure (see Table 11.1). However, in hospitals, clinics, or community agencies which provide care to a high volume of patients and family members, a structured interview by a psychosocial provider is seldom feasible. Consequently, brief and rapid methods of screening are necessary. Brief screening techniques that examine components of distress such as anxiety or depression can be incorporated into the routine clinical care of the patient. Early psychosocial interventions may be more readily accepted by patients, families, and staff as one component of comprehensive care and be less stigmatizing to the patient.[13] Screening is also a cost-effective technique for case identification, in comparison to an assessment of all new patients.[14]

The second continuum relates to the predictable phases of the disease process. Movements across the disease continuum from the point of diagnosis into cancer therapies and beyond provide patients with experiences, knowledge, and skills that enable them to respond to the demands of their disease. Needs of a newly diagnosed patient with intractable symptoms differ significantly from a patient who has advanced disease and where curative treatments have been terminated. Often, their life perspectives and values are dramatically transformed. Recurrent disease further challenges the adaptive resources of any patient and family. However, as with the newly diagnosed patient, adaptation to

Table 11.1 Variables associated with psychosocial adaptation

Social support	Past history	Current concerns	Other
Marital status	Substance abuse	Health	Education
Living arrangements	Depression	Religion	Employment
Number of family members and relatives in vicinity	Mental health	Work-finance	Physical symptoms
	Major illness	Family	
Church attendance	Past regrets	Friends	
	Optimism vs. pessimism	Existential	
		Self-appraisal	

Adapted from Weisman et al.[16]

recurrent disease does occur. Many of the same variables promote adaptation at this difficult phase on the disease continuum. While the reality of one's mortality confronts virtually every cancer patient, relapse greatly intensifies the focus on terminal care. The potential of dying re-emerges as a distinct reality. In many respects, patients with recurrent disease become chronically and terminally ill. For these patients, the cure of their disease is unrealistic and although they are expected to succumb in the future, a reasonable prediction concerning a time frame is difficult. Their death could occur within 6 months, or the time period could be considerably longer. Consequently, the demands on family caregivers who provide terminal care may be quite demanding and prolonged. In addition, changes in health care personnel on whom the patient and family rely increases a sense of powerlessness and lack of control. Of paramount concern is to maintain the patient and family throughout the illness process and to support the family following the death of the patient. At times, families are overwhelmed by the illness, and as a result, are unable to effectively respond. For some families, a death may represent a loss of the family's identity and may paralyze the family's coping and problem-solving responses. Failure to respond and problem-solve leads to a lack of control and may generate a significant potential for a chronic grief reaction.[15] However, identification of a series of predictable and relevant crisis events and psychosocial challenges that occur as patients and families confront advanced disease can prove helpful to clinicians in anticipating the needs of patients and families (see Table 11.2A,B). Ultimately, even the most challenged families can cope with problems and challenges posed by advancing disease if they are surrounded by health care professionals who support their adaptive efforts by being physically available, provide ongoing expert information, encourage appropriate emotional expression of concerns, and aid in the identification and resolution of problems.

Key Psychosocial Variables and Constructs

Weisman et al.[16] defined the critical variables (which promote effective adaptation) as past history of functioning, social support, and a series of current concerns such as health, work-finance, and family (see Table 11.1). Adjustment to illness is driven by social support and the patient's past history of functioning. Most often, the family is the core of social support.

In Table 11.1, family-related concepts dominate the social support category. Marital status, living arrangements, and number of members in the immediate geographical area represent the availability of the family as a potential source of support. For many patients, the willingness, accessibility, and physical availability of concerned family members is the primary determinant of the quality of care that they will receive as the disease advances. Often, patients are too tired, weak, and confused to advocate for their own needs. One example of this is the prevalence of undertreated pain in cancer patients, even in centers

Table 11.2A. Advancing disease and psychosocial treatment as it relates to patients

Crisis event	Personal meaning/interpretation	Manifestation	Coping tasks	Survivor goals	Professional interventions
Advanced disease	I'm out of control. Will they offer new treatment? What am I doing wrong? Will it be as bad as the last time? Will I go broke?	Depression Anxiety Demoralization Fear Denial Anger Fear of intimacy	Maintain hope and direction Tolerate medical care Enhance coping skills Maintain open communication with family, friends and health care professionals Assess treatment and care options Maintain relationships with medical team	Dignity Direction Role in work, family and community	Support Develop a plan of action Cognitive/behavioral skills training Supportive psychotherapy Physical availability Resource provision/referral Information Education
Terminal	When am I going to die? Does dying hurt? What happens after you die? Why me? Why now? What did I do to deserve this? What will happen to my family? Will I be remembered by my family and friends? What if I start to die and I'm all alone? Can't the doctors do something else, are they holding back on me, have they given up on me?	Depression Fear Anxiety Denial Demoralization Self destructive behavior Loss of control Guilt Anger Fear of abandonment Fear of isolation Increased dependency Acceptance Withdrawal Search for meaning in past as well as present Pain/suffering Need to discuss afterlife	Maintain a meaningful quality of life Adjust to physical deterioration Plan for surviving family members Accept reality of prognosis Mourn actual losses Mourn the death of dreams Get things in order Maintain and end significant relationships Say good-bye to family and friends Accept impending death Confront the relevant existential and spiritual issues Talk about feelings Review one's life	Dignity Family support and bereavement	Physical availability Support Develop a plan of action Cognitive/behavioral skills training Therapeutic rituals Coordination of services Advocacy Information

Recurrence/new primary				
What did I do wrong?	Anger	Re-establish hope	Integrate reality with family	Information
Was it my negative attitude?	Fear	Accept the uncertainty about the future	Functioning	Support
Was I foolish to hope this was over forever?	Depression	Understand information about new situation	Maintain self-worth	Develop a plan of action
God has failed me.	Anxiety	Regain a life focus and time perspective appropriate to the changed prognosis		Education
I beat this last time I will beat it again.	Shock	Communicate new status to others		Cognitive/behavioral skills training
Nothing ever works out good for me.	Loss of hope	Make decisions about the new treatment course		Physical availability
They said I was okay but I'm not.	Denial	Integrate reality of ongoing nature of disease to probable death from cancer		Supportive psychotherapy
Do I have to start all over again?	Guilt	Tolerate changes in routine and roles again		Resource provision/referral
	Loss of trust	Adjust to increased dependency again		
	Feelings of alienation	Reinvest in treatment		
	Increased vulnerability			
	Loss of control			
	Confronting mortality			
	Search for meaning			

Table 11.2.B. Advancing disease and psychosocial treatment as it relates to families

Crisis event for patient	Impact on family	Family survival goals	Professional interventions
Recurrence/new primary	Adjust family roles and tasks again Address growing mistrust of the health care setting Desire to rescue Moderate sense of failure and betrayal	Cope with physical and psychological exhaustion Integrate the experience into everyday life	Information Support Education Physical availability Resource Provision/referral Advocacy Cognitive/behavioral skills training Develop a plan of action
Advanced disease	Disappointment Sense of failure Acceptance of loss Financial concerns	Maintain sense of hope and meaning Maintain open communication Maintain financial solvency Anticipate life without patient	Information Support Physical availability Resource Provision/referral Cognitive/behavioral skills training Develop a plan of action
Terminal	Guilt Focus of resources on patient Delay or cancel life plans Emotional withdrawal from patient Having strangers in home Physical changes to home Time away from work, school, friends	Need to accept impending loss Determine caregiving roles Accept the death of dreams	Information Support Education Physical availability Resource Provision/referral Advocacy Cognitive/behavioral skills training
Bereavement	Anger Intense acute grief Heightened emotional arousal Fears about emotional and financial solvency Confusion Insecurity Longing Sadness	Develop a new relationship with the decreased Permanently reassign family roles, tasks and power structure Re-evaluate financial solvency Integrate the experience into everyday life	Information Support Education Physical availability Resource Provision/referral Cognitive/behavioral skills training Therapeutic rituals

of excellence, throughout the world. A brief clinical example illustrates some of these points.

Camille was the 27-year-old Hispanic daughter of a 67-year-old patient who was sent home to die. The relationship had always been one of distant respect and love. Camille felt increasingly excluded from her father as his disease progressed. She became depressed and withdrew from her family. The patient tried to protect his family from the reality of his progressing disease by maintaining a positive attitude and focusing on hope. Upon return home, the patient quietly complained of severe unrelenting pain. The attending physician was aware of the patient's pain and told the family that there was nothing else that he could do. Camille and her mother felt that it was disrespectful to bother the doctor again despite the patient's now increased verbal complaints, moaning, crying, and begging to die. The family was immobilized and clearly in crisis. The family felt that there was nothing else they could do. The social worker and nurse, through much encouragement and emotional support, information giving (concerning what was realistic pain management), and role-playing (concerning how to best communicate her father's situation), enabled Camille to act. When the physician was unwilling to prescribe additional medications, Camille had been prepared and was able to ask him for a referral to a local hospice. As a result, the patient's pain was quickly controlled and Camille was able to do something meaningful for her father. Communication in the family was enhanced and the patient died at home with family at his side. Camille reported later that caring for her father changed her life forever and made her feel that she too could do things on her own.

A cancer diagnosis stimulates an exploration of the meaning of life and death. Traditional values and belief systems may be questioned and challenged. If a patient and family can find significant meaning in the process of dying and death, a new level of comfort may be attained. Evidence indicates that spiritually decreases psychological distress.[17] Church attendance is one indicator of spirituality as a source of potential support. Quality of life research studies have only recently begun to consider this concept; health care providers frequently ignore the spiritual domain.[18]

Increasingly, health care providers are confronted with patients and family members who do not believe in God and do not have a spiritual system to provide them solace in times of turmoil and crisis. Some agnostics and atheists are "in the foxhole." For some of these patients, their view that there is nothing after this life and that they will never see their loved ones again can be unsettling to the patient and the family, as the unimaginable abstract concepts of "nothing" and "never" can be terrifying and incomprehensible. This unbuffered perception of ultimate loss can lead to significant sadness and confusion, both of which need to be addressed by professionals trained in mental health. For health care staff, spirituality may be quite important or not at all. Staff are confronted with a patient or family member for whom the standard types of support may not be effective or sufficient. Health care staff are left confused by their frustrated attempts to offer solace though verbal encouragement and to send in a chaplain or to support the view that this life is all that there is. Patients and families often perceive the former as unwanted proselytizing and a lack of respect for their belief systems. The latter is defined as a reinforcement and confrontation that they are powerless to ward off an imminent loss for which meaning is elusive. The role of health care providers in this situation is to encourage and support the search for meaning and growth but not to provide it. This dilemma can be a significant challenge to health care professionals who are trained to perform executive functions in times of crisis and discomfort.

Families as a primary source of social support must be assessed on the basis of availability and adequacy. Family composition and size determines the potential for multiple family members to be available to the patient. A common misperception is that large families will be automatically provide an appropriate level of support. However, composition or size cannot be equated with each family's level of capability and willingness to provide necessary support and care. In many respects, each family varies in its ability and willingness to be a consistent source of support.[19]

Family Adaptability and Cohesion

Families are complex and perplexing to health care professionals who are trained to be rational in their approach to problems and obstacles to identified goals. The emotional aspects related to disease and loss are distressing to most people, but they are especially troublesome to health care providers who as a group tend to avoid emotions. One model helpful in deciphering the reactions of families is the Circumplex Model of Family Functioning. This model, developed by Olson et al.,[20] categorizes families by type in order to explain the variation in their behavior. Although not specifically developed for cancer, this model conceptualizes families' responses to stressful events based on two readily understood and salient constructs, i.e., adaptability and cohesion.

Adaptability reflects the capability of a family to reorganize internal roles, rules, and power structure in response to a significant stressor. Given the impact of advancing cancer, families must frequently reassign roles, alter rules for daily living, and revise long-held methods of problem-solving. Families can range on a continuum from low in adaptability (rigidity) to high in adaptability (chaotic). A family characterized as being rigid in their attempts to adapt will reactively persist in the use of specific coping behaviors even when these strategies are clearly ineffective. Families at the opposite or highest end of the adaptability continuum create a chaotic response within the power structure, roles, and rules of the family. Chaotic families lack structure and obvious order in their responses and attempt different coping strategies with every new stressor. Although the majority of families fall in the more functional category of "structured adaptability," 30% of families manifest extreme responses and may be classified as rigid or chaotic. Consequently, these families will experience significant difficulty in their adaptation and as a result, are likely to exhibit problematic behaviors that the health care team will find difficult to manage.[21] See Table 11.3 for specific problematic family behaviors.

Olson's second construct is indicative of the family's ability to provide adequate support. *Cohesion*, or the level of emotional bonding that exists between family members, is also conceptualized on a continuum from low to high. Low cohesion (disengagement) suggests little or no connectedness between family members. A commitment to care for other family members is not evident and as a result, these families are frequently unavailable to the medical staff for support of the patient or the decision-making process. At the other extreme, high cohesion (enmeshment) blurs the boundaries between family members. This results in the perception by health care providers that some family members seem to be just as affected by the diagnosis, treatment, or each symptom as the patient. Enmeshed families possess the ability to demand excessive amounts of time from the health care team and to be incapable of following simple medical directives. These families are not able to objectively receive and comprehend information that may be in the best interest of the patient. Also, these families may assume an overprotective position and may speak for patients even when they could be encouraged to speak for themselves. As a result of social demands, threats to the integrity of the family structure, noxious symptoms, physical deterioration, and disfigurement, patients and families struggle to maintain a meaningful life. Within the context of advancing cancer, the extreme types of family behaviors are likely to occur.

Within the Weisman et al.[16] framework, the patient's past history of functioning also provides a major understanding to how the patient will respond to the demands of the illness and treatments. Previous history of psychiatric illness, substance abuse, or other mental health problems are difficult to separate from

Table 11.3. Problematic family behaviors for the health care staff

Direct interference with the delivery of medical care

Excessive demands of staff time

Alliances with other families against the health care team

Inability to follow guidelines or noncompliance with directives

Encouragement of the patient to be noncompliant

Unrealistic expectations of the health care team

Unavailability to patient or team concerning decision-making or support

Dysfunctional, or potentially destructive, home environment that inhibits
  effective management of the patient outside the hospital

family dynamics. A patient's mental health disturbance is deeply intertwined with the family interactions. Families possess significant power through their ability to encourage, coerce, reinforce, or shame. For example, it is quite difficult for patients to maintain their social isolation without direct or indirect reinforcement by family members. Patients may enter their cancer treatments on the basis of life experiences that breed mistrust and turmoil. Patients emerge from problematic family situations to receive treatment from caring strangers. Although most people experience support as comforting, vulnerable patients may be unable to accept support and families may feel threatened. Men in particular have a tendency to experience dependency and a lack of control as an assault on their integrity which results in shame and social withdrawal. As a result, health care professionals may maintain unrealistic expectations of families even though their ability to function as effective caregivers varies significantly. Patients unconsciously reconstruct their familial relationships with the health care team. Concomitantly, staff may sense rejection from these families and react in an inappropriate or maladaptive manner. When engaging families, it is necessary to gain an appreciation for the rules and regulations of that particular family, for each family has their own rules, regulations, and communication styles. In gaining an understanding of the role of the patient in the family, it is helpful to ask the patient what specific responsibilities they perform in the family, especially during a crisis. Asking for specific experiences and duties of each family member during a crisis is more helpful than generalities. Specificity enables the patient to openly communicate and objectively evaluate their role and importance in the family system and provides a clinical opportunity to assess ongoing progress or deterioration. Generally, most patients and families can tolerate even the worst news and dire prognosis as long as it is framed within a context in which the patient and family know how they are expected to respond and that the health care team will not abandon them.

Psychosocial Screening

Standardized measures such as the Brief Symptom Inventory[22] or the General Health Questionnaire[23] can be employed to prospectively screen and identify patients who may experience significantly elevated levels of distress at the time of their diagnosis. Distress is often directly related to inadequate or a significant lack of social support. Histories of mental health difficulties, substance abuse, or other major illnesses indicate that the patient and family will experience significant difficulty with a cancer diagnosis. For the homebound patient, screening can be administered by the visiting nurse or social worker. If possible, family members should also be screened.

Through use of a standardized measure such as the Brief Symptom Inventory, levels of psychological distress can differentiate patients by a low, moderate, or high degree of vulnerability. Patients with a low level of distress may benefit from a psychoeducational program that enhances their adaptive capabilities and problem-solving skills. High-distress patients possess significant psychosocial needs and as a result, individual psychotherapy or ongoing family therapy may be the most appropriate intervention. For some patients, mental health services are essential, whereas other patients may require assistance only at critical transition points. However, clinical practice suggests that virtually all patients will benefit from some type of supportive interventions, especially at later stages of the illness.

Psychosocial interventions range from educational programs to support groups to cognitive-behavioral techniques to ongoing psychotherapy. Educational programs may enhance the natural adaptive process in patients who possess lower levels of distress, whereas patients with significantly elevated levels of distress require psychotherapy and pharmacology.[24] It should be noted that 15%–18% of newly diagnosed patients may enter their cancer experience with a psychiatric or substance abuse history, severe family dysfunction, or a history of physical or sexual abuse.[25] Given the physical impact of the illness and the rigors of cancer therapies, the coping and problem-solving skills of these patients are significantly compromised. In all probability, these patients experienced significant distress prior to their diagnosis. Now, cancer has significantly compounded their distress and generated a higher level of vulnerability which may inhibit or prevent their adjustment to the diagnosis as well as their ability to effectively resolve the many problems associated with treatment. Regardless of what the patient and family bring to their experience with life-threatening disease and what specific approach is utilized, psychotherapeutic and educational approaches are focused on maximizing problem-solving abilities, independence, and hope.[26]

Psychological Impact of Pain and Other Noxious Symptoms

As is detailed in Part III of this book, asthenia, fatigue, pain, dyspnea, mental confusion, anxiety, depression, vomiting, sleeplessness, etc. are common symptoms associated with advanced disease. The negative impact on quality of life is obvious. Pain and noxious symptoms impair cognition, concentration, and memory[27] and override the underlying mental schema of patients. As a result, patients' perception is confined to only the most immediate and essential elements of their sensory experience. For the person in pain or acute physical distress, there is only a fragmented distant remnant of a past or future. The immediate need and goal is to stop or minimize the noxious experience. Family members of patients with advancing disease are often bewildered and frightened by the dramatic changes they perceive in the person they have known throughout their lives. This is especially true if the person has been a nurturing or powerful figure who provided support and sustenance.

Pain and other untreated symptoms encompass and inevitably absorb the limited psychic energy of the organism. This valuable psychic energy can only be made available to the person if their physical distress is effectively managed. The body is both the interpreter and integrator of the human experience. The psychic life is subservient to and dependent on the bodily experience.

Moderate to severe pain is often present at diagnosis and during the early stages of cancer treatments in 30–45% of patients.[28] Cancer pain is present in nearly 75% of cancer patients with advanced disease and 90% in terminal patients.[28] Pain stands alone in its ability to gain the active attention of others while dramatically demonstrating a sense of being alone and vulnerable. This is especially true of patients with advanced disease and their families. While a patient is experiencing pain, another person only inches away is incapable of truly understanding what is so central and undeniable to the patient. This invisible and almost palpable boundary between the identified person in pain and his or her caregivers has significant implications for the quality and effectiveness of the therapeutic relationship.

It is generally accepted that pain is poorly managed, despite extant technological capabilities. Patients, families, and professional staff share an almost universal reluctance to use narcotic analgesics, even when life expectancy is quite limited. This irrational set of circumstances suggests that a primordial evolutionary process that enables patients to accept suffering also allows the health care team to permit the unnecessary pain to continue. In terms of the immediate survival of the organism, evolutionary benefits of tolerating the pain and harm to others, especially loved ones, are obvious. Evolution has shaped and determined that those who were best able to tolerate the pain and suffering of others, without endangering themselves, are more likely to survive. However, in relation to evolution, pain, and the brain, under some circumstances, it appears that the role of the "primitive" and "emotional" limbic system still maintains a firm grasp over the "evolved" and "rational" cerebral cortex.

Although most cancer patients are psychologically healthy,[29,30] inadequately managed cancer pain, associated symptoms, and side effects are able to produce a wide variety of "pseudopsychiatric" syndromes which are anxiety provoking and confusing to patients, families, and clinicians. Cancer patients with pain are more likely to develop a psychiatric disorder than cancer patients without significant pain.[31] Pain in the short-term provokes anxiety, and over the long-term generates depression and demoralization. At present, the differences between depression and demoralization as clinical constructs have yet to be empirically explored. Although cancer pain is significantly related to higher levels of depression, pain is more likely to play a causal role related to depression.[32] While overall depression rates for cancer patients are 20–25%,[32] the presence of depression in the advanced cancer patient is quite formidable with estimations ranging between 50% and 70%.[31,33] Anecdotal clinical experience consistently demonstrates that once pain and related distressing physical symptoms are relieved, suffering, anxiety, depression, demoralization, and suicidal ideation are ameliorated. The positive impact on the family is equally significant as their sense of powerlessness and guilt subsides.

Depression is of great importance because of its ubiquitous nature in patients with significantly advanced disease. There is a significant correlation between affective disorders and pain,[34] and the negative emotional states pain produces (dysphoria, hopelessness, guilt, suicidal ideation, etc). Depressed patients universally distort reality and grossly minimize their perceived abilities in managing the demands of the illness and its treatment. Furthermore, depressed cancer patients with inadequately controlled pain are at increased risk of suicide.[35] For the depressed patient, acute sensitivity to physical sensations may lead to or exaggerate pre-existing morbid or self-destructive thoughts. The complex and interactive associations between physical feelings (neutral or noxious sensations), mentation (personal meaning given to the sensations), and behaviors (attempts to minimize threat and regain control) are all negatively influenced by depression. The destructive synergy of unrelieved pain and depression may lead to overwhelming suffering in patients and families and to a shared sense of hopelessness and helplessness. Consequently, a patient or family may develop the faulty perception that suicide is their only remaining vestige of control. Within this context, a multimodal approach is essential for combining pharmacology, supportive psychotherapy, and cognitive-behavioral skills training.[36] From a psychological perspective, promotion of compliance with medical regimens, correction of distorted cognitive perceptions, acquisition of coping skills to manage physical tension, stress, and pain, and the effective use of valuable physical energy to maximize engagement of life become the foci of care.

For many patients with advancing disease, physical debilitation may prevent participation or benefit from psychological interventions. Therefore, by necessity, the focus of care becomes the family. This shift in focus enables the family to begin to anticipate the impending separation and loss and to prepare for life without the patient. Health care staff may become frustrated by the hopelessness expressed by the patient and family and may experience this as a commentary on their effectiveness. In some ways, the family's expression of impending loss of the patient anticipates the withdrawal of the health care team from their lives and may simultaneously symbolize fear of abandonment by both the patient and the team. Depression and demoralization is particularly difficult for health care professionals to tolerate. In some cases, health care professionals who choose to care for dying patients are highly motivated "fixers" and "doers" who are confronted by their own limitations, vulnerability, and mortality when they feel powerless.

Sociocultural Influences on Patient and Family Adaptation

Perceptions of illness and death can be conceptualized as experiences with a significant amount of unknown conscious and unconscious associations. Consequently, these experiences generate concerns and fears that are beyond the limits of our objective knowledge. Sociocultural beliefs may sooth anxiety or fear by providing comfort when a vacuum exists because of a lack of experience in a particular area. In addition, sociocultural attitudes exert considerable influence as patients approach the end of their lives.[37,38] Direct observations can be made of how the family cares for the patient, views an afterlife, or uses rituals related to how the corpse is to be managed.

Although there have been efforts to increase sensitivity about the importance of integrating sociocultural influences into an overall assessment of the cancer patient and family, readily accessible tools, methods, and instruments are still virtually absent. In addition, under certain circumstances, culturally sensitive labels have developed into stereotyping by age, gender, race, religion, or economic status. The role of sociocultural influences are complex and not easily put into a formula or compartment. Koenig and Gates-Williams[39] offer a framework to assess cultural responses relevant to the palliative patient that is consistent with a comprehensive psychological assessment: " . . . culture is only meaningful when interpreted in the context of a patient's unique history, family constellation, and socioeconomic status. . . . Dangers exist . . . creating negative stereotypes—in simply supplying clinicians with an atlas or map of 'cultural traits' common among particular ethnic groups" (p. 244).[39]

Each patient and family system ultimately must be accepted on their own terms. Awareness of a specific racial or cultural group is never a substitute for a comprehensive assessment of this particular patient and family at this particular time and place within the context of their unique understanding of the situation.

Finally, patients and their families cannot be adequately understood without knowledge of their sociocultural backgrounds. Patients and families possess different interests, beliefs, values, and attitudes. Often, individuals learn attitudes or values through family interactions, and these patterns influence how patients respond to the health care team. The health care team represents expertise, safety, and authority. They are also an external and foreign force, which only through necessity, has gained influence and power within the family system. It is expected that the health care team will be perceived as supportive and caring but also capable of judging how the family functions. How the health care team role-models communication and support around problems can significantly influence how the family will integrate this outside force. Within the setting of distress, it is assumed that the patient and family will project their own perceptions about themselves onto the health care team. For example, family members may feel angry, frustrated, and exhausted by the demands of caring for a dying loved one. This emotional and distressful experience can easily be projected onto the medical staff. As a result, the health care team may come to be perceived as a representation of this unpleasant experience that is so unacceptable to the family. It is essential that the team be aware of this process and directly correct any distorted and maladaptive perceptions by the patient or family. Table 11.4 defines specific family characteristics that are particularly relevant to cultural influences.[40]

Table 11.4. Family constructs and characteristics relevant to cultural influences

Constructs	Characteristics
Value system	The family's rules and norms for daily living and how family life is structured
Mobility	The concept of "home" may be more than a fixed address. "Home" may connotate relationships, goals, and needs among family members.
Socialization	Implies the level of interaction with the world external to the family. Examples include utilization of community resources, openness to social opportunities, financial means to afford social outlets, etc.
Parent–child interaction	Specific cultural norms may be intimately woven into the frequent interactions between parents and children. An example is the expectation that women devote themselves to the care of their children.
Kin network	Refers to family relationships among in-laws, visiting relatives, and other extended members. In some cultures, families chose to live close to other relatives as an indication of solidarity rather than enmeshment.
Family orientations	Commitments to work is highly valued. Religious orientations often provide a consistent source of moral support and standards.
Parental roles	Roles within the family and in relation to children are clearly demarcated. Mutuality and shared tasks may be preferred.

Although cultural constructs are important, these influences are diminished over time as families are assimilated into the predominant culture. Second-generation families are more similar to the host country than the country of origin. However, immigrants may possess Old-World attitudes and values about authority and illness, whereas the perspectives of their offspring may be more consistent with those of the health care team. In this case, everyone may experience estrangement.

Principles of Effective Patient and Family Management

The family as defined by the patient is virtually always the primary supportive structure for the patient. The family serves as a supportive environment that provides instrumental assistance, psychological support, and consistent encouragement so that the patient seeks the best available medical care. Early in the diagnostic and treatment planning phases, a family's primary functions are to instill hope and facilitate communication. For the palliative patient, caregiving becomes the primary focus for the family, which requires many complex and instrumental tasks. Families must prepare psychologically and financially for the experience of life without the patient, for which they may have little or no practice. Cancer and its treatments are always a crisis and an assault on the family system. As an uninvited intruder, cancer challenges the viability of the family structure to tolerate and integrate a harsh and threatening reality that cannot be overcome by force, denial, or under certain circumstances, even joint action. Joint action requires a clear definition of a goal as well as the ongoing plan that promotes the optimal opportunity for successful goal attainment. The health care team guides the family to develop and organize a problem-solving approach to the demands of the illness. The plan must be clearly communicated because it delineates each individual's responsibility, so that the potential for goal attainment is maximized. For many families with a history of effective functioning, the cancer experience represents the first time that their joint action may not overcome an external threat. Families may never have experienced anything as serious as this before. Consequently, the cancer experience must be reframed into more realistic terms so that the threat can be perceived as manageable rather than destructive. If this is not achieved, the family can manifest anger, avoidance, displacement, or other forms of regressive behavior. For the family with a history of multiple defeats and failures, the cancer experience may be perceived by a family as another event in which they are incapable of managing the demands of an overwhelming and hostile world. The cancer experience temporarily alters the family structure, but it also has the potential to produce permanent change. The health care team can significantly influence how these changes are interpreted and integrated into the family life.

Patients uniformly identify the negative impact of cancer and its repercussions as most upsetting as it relates to their families.[2] Therefore, any effective intervention must include the patient, their family, and other social supportive networks. Guilt, shame, anger, frustration, and fear of abandonment are common reactions of patients in relation to their families. For family members, emotional responses such as anger, fear, powerlessness, survivor guilt, and confusion emerge as they attempt to care for the patient. Displacement as a defense mechanism enables families to transfer emotion from one person or situation to another. Utilization of displacement is quite common when families experience significant stress. Although the defense mechanism of denial (unconscious repudiation of all or one aspect of reality) is quite rare, distancing (conscious postponing, focusing on all or one aspect of reality) as a coping mechanism is very common.[41] As a result, family responses appear confusing to health care professionals, which in turn creates tension between family members and health care providers at a time when clarity and effective interactions are essential. As the role and presence of the family changes, other supportive networks also play a significant function. Often, supportive resources such as religious groups, social clubs, and occupationally oriented groups are frequently overlooked.

With little exception, assessment of the primary members in the family system is a rather straightforward process. However, the attitude and ability to demonstrate open and frank communication is more important in the long run than the actual questions addressed. When possible, family meeting should include all of the relevant family members. Families want detailed knowledge concerning the patient's present status and life expectancy.[42] The patient can be asked the following questions directly. "Who do you rely on most to assist you in relation to the practical needs of your illness (e.g., transportation, insurance company negotiations)? When you get scared or confused, with whom in your family are you most able to talk? Who in your family most concerns you? Is anyone in your family overwhelmed with your ongoing medical and practical needs? Who in your family is coping least well with your illness? Is anyone in your family openly angry with you because of your illness? Are you particularly worried about how a specific person in your family is coping? Are you ever concerned that the demands of your illness will be too much for your family? Who is most dependent on you in your family? For what do they depend on you? What would happen to your family if you were unable to maintain your present level of functioning?"

The answers to these questions communicate to the patient and family that it is appropriate and necessary to gauge the impact that cancer and its treatment has on their lives, and they also provide the groundwork for the coordination of patient and family functions. In addition, role-modeling of open communication provides an environment of emotional support, flexibility in roles, and the implied and spoken promise never to abandon each other. This cannot be achieved unless the patient and family accept that some treatment effects and life events are beyond their control and there are limits to what is possible. The medical team has the responsibility to manage the physical aspects of the disease while the patient and family actively strive to integrate change, maintain normalcy, and accept the reality of the illness. During the early phase of care, the illness and its consequences, including death, must be identified as one of the potentially uncontrollable issues so the patient and family can focus on areas that are amenable to their influence and control.

Financial resources are virtually always a major concern of patients and families. When discussions of money and resources occur within the family system, shame and guilt are a natural consequence and are frequently alluded to, but not openly discussed. This can be a barrier to open communication as financial limitations are a reality of life. This is especially true for patients with advancing disease. When not addressed, the patient is left alone with fears and fantasies of abandonment. Simultaneously, the family may have concerns about life goals after the patient's acute need is past or death occurs. The expected range of emotional reactions include anger, fear, guilt, anxiety, frustration, powerlessness, and confusion. Cancer confronts people with the reality of limitations.

In addition to the increasing costs of health insurance and home care, there are a wide variety of nonreimbursable illness-related costs that can be financially devastating to patients and families. Transportation, nutritional supplements, temporary housing, child care, and lost work days are but a few examples of costs borne almost totally by patients and families for which there is seldom any form of reimbursement.[43] The direct economic cost of recurrent cancer has been shown to be substantial. Schulz et al.[44] found that respondents spent more than $200.00 per month on health-related expenses and reported significant amounts of leave time from work. Other studies have confirmed the negative financial impact of advanced cancer.[45,46] Money is not always just money.

Money, and its use, is a metaphor for value, control, and power.[47] How patients and family members communicate about money can be an indication of their perceptions of whether treatment is progressing or not. It is a latent communication about the state of affairs over the perceived but unexpressed value of care and its potential outcome. For example, at the beginning of treatment, the patient and family may express that money is not object and all must be done to save the patient. Often by the end of treatment, a much more sober and realistic view concerning valuable and vanishing resources may become evident and a greater discussion of investment and return may ensue. At this point, patients and families may become angry at the hospital and health care team, questioning the utility of their efforts. It should be noted that at this point in time, both patient and family may be actually questioning their ability to persevere. Concerns about money may be an expression of exhaustion, diminishing hope, or anger. It is important that this metaphorical communication be seen as inadequate for open and direct communication. A metaphor is a signal which indicates that an open discussion is necessary. Openness is essential for the patient and family to discuss both their common and increasingly diverging needs. Patients and families need to discuss their physical and spiritual fatigue as well as specific financial concerns related to diminishing resources as a result of their struggle with cancer. The following clinical example illustrates a number of these points.

Mrs. S, a 54-year-old married woman with three adolescent daughters, expressed concern to the team over the ongoing cost of care for her terminally ill husband. The team felt that Mrs. S. was selfish and that it was unethical for them to consider the financial impact on the family in caring for the patient. Mrs. S., sensing their resistance to her plight, felt rejected and became irate. A meeting with the patient, family, and relevant staff was organized by the social worker to openly address her financial concerns. The family had existing financial debts due to past medical treatments, and consequently, had ample reason for their concern related to the additional costs of care. Once this meeting resolved concerns over additional unneeded expenditures, the focus shifted to the much more emotionally laden issues related to the slow deterioration of the patient and the family's intense grief over the impending loss. It became evident that money for the family represented, as the spouse declared, the loss of "everything."

In some cases, the family may begin to perceive the dying patient as already being deceased. Anticipatory grief and premature emotional withdrawal from the dying patient creates confusion and a sense of terror in the patient. As a result, the family experiences guilt and shame because they are prepared for the loss; however, the patient is still alive. The health care team has the challenging task of supporting the family's efforts to continue caring for the patient despite physical and psychological depletion. The health care team may also feel exhausted and frustrated by a lingering dying process as they try to simultaneously protect the patient and support the family. Normalization of these emotional responses and respite is often necessary for both family and staff. Role-modeling by staff concerning limitations and expectations can be a powerful motivator to family members to accept the reality of what they themselves can realistically be expected to accomplish.

Physical exhaustion originates from diverse sources, such as multiple and complex physical demands, emotional distress, poor mental health, inadequate coping skills, social isolation, depression, anxiety, insomnia, powerlessness, helplessness, hopelessness, fear, divided loyalties, financial limitations, etc. These common factors, endemic to chronic illness, assault families and generate long-term demands that they may find overwhelming. Extreme family types will select ineffective coping strategies (e.g., isolation, projection, regression, denial, etc.) in their attempts to resolve these problems. However, the strategies they select will simply not solve these problems. Substance abuse, mental illness, history of poor relationships, dependency, poverty, isolation, few family members in the geographical area, and previous medical or psychiatric history may act in synergy to exhaust and immobilize families. A supportive environment within the palliative model can reframe an overwhelming situation into an effective response that provides comfort and the potential for psychological growth.

Specific Problematic Patient and Family Behaviors with Staff

Primary family supportive functions include assistance with instrumental tasks, assistance in medical decision-making, reduction of stress, initiation of effective problem-solving, and provision of physical and emotional comfort to the patient. If the family cannot provide these functions or is unavailable to the patient and staff, the staff may need to assume and fulfill these roles. Staff may become resentful when families are unavailable or withdraw from active participation as the burden to care for these patients is dramatically increased. Within the context of the family milieu, conflicts with staff are inevitable. As a result, vulnerable families struggle through the cancer experience without direction or the ability to effectively problem-solve. Conflicts may result from a family's inability to follow simple unit guidelines or problems, such as their intolerance for any physical discomfort that the patient may experience. It is the management of these conflicts that will determine the quality of the relationship between the patient, family, and professional staff. However, families who are critical of staff frequently are held to a different standard of behavior. Given the structure of medical delivery systems, it is expected that entitled or ungrateful families will irritate and alienate staff. Under these circumstances, unit guidelines become laws and the struggle for control results in fear and mistrust. Conversely, patients and families who endear themselves to staff through verbal praise or gifts receive warmth and flexibility and greater attention to their needs. For example, unit guidelines, such as visiting hours or number of visitors, may be relaxed. In the home setting, battles for control are manifested over compliancy with the scheduling of medications, especially narcotic analgesics, and the relative importance of eating. The professional staff must be flexible in their communication styles or they may be perceived as violating family boundaries. This type of interaction can devolve into a battle for power and control. Conflicts that remain at the level of power and control make it virtually impossible to work with the patient and family to develop action-oriented, problem-solving strategies that unite all in a common set of values and goals. Again, a clinical example may be helpful.

    Mr. P. is a 69-year-old retired history professor with metastatic colon cancer. The patient and spouse have an enmeshed relationship. Mr. P. guards his privacy and attempts to maintain independence by ignoring his pain. Requests for medication by him are delayed until the pain becomes intolerable. Any delay in the staff's response to his agitated demands are perceived by him as punishment for being weak. Dependence on staff and delays in dispensing medications dramatically increases within the patient and his wife, which breeds mistrust and creates a barrier between the patient, spouse, and staff. As a result, the staff are not prone to empathic responses. The staff defined the patient's demands as inappropriate. The wife perceived herself as being marginalized, and the patient felt out of control.

This case example is not unusual with advanced cancer patients who, by virtue of the extent of their disease, developed increased dependence on health care providers. General symptom management and effective pain control possesses the potential to engage the patient, family, and staff toward a common goal or to lead to estrangement and abandonment. Open communication can establish clearly defined goals within the context of the family culture which can significantly reduce these strains. However, health care providers must accept that, at times, any approach may be ineffective because the family structure cannot tolerate the influence of external forces. When this occurs, continued attempts at open communication is the only alternative that can achieve some sense of mutual understanding and trust. Families can exhibit a range of other behaviors (see Table 11.3) that the health care team defines as problematic.

    Family members have the capacity to directly interfere with the delivery of medical care. Families can delay or prevent the completion of a procedure, verbally abuse the staff, or triangulate the team. All of these behaviors disrupt the effective delivery of care to the patient. Families may demand excessive amounts of staff time and manifest significant difficulty in their ability to comprehend technical information associated with cancer therapies. As a result, some families will demand repetitious sessions to review the same material. In these circumstances, anxiety and confusion should be understood as an expression of overwhelming nature of this experience for family caregivers who are highly uncertain concerning their ability to manage. Significant anxiety will disrupt any attempt for effective communication because family members may be unable to comprehend or retain complex or technical information. In addition, these families may also compare the response of one staff member with that of another as families search for inconsistencies. Unwittingly, staff may contradict each other on relatively minor points, that the family manipulate to gain power in the system. The normal competitiveness among staff is elevated to "turf struggles" in which all concerned lose as the system is undermined. The family is able to make the staff experience first-hand the way they have been feeling. Disruption by families is a communication, a disguised and confused plea for help, which is best handled by attending to the underlying concerns of the family and not the distractions, such as imperfections of the staff. The staff can effectively use the situation as presented by the family to role model appropriate team problem-solving techniques. Again, a brief clinical example to illustrate these points follows.

Ms. B. is a 63-year-old married, disabled high school teacher diagnosed with liver cancer. She has a history of alcohol abuse, which she minimizes; "I have only one or two drinks a night, no big deal. Who am I hurting anyway?". Her husband, a member of the clergy, has informed the staff that his wife continues to have a significant drinking problem that very recently resulted in a serious car accident involving another vehicle. According to Ms. B., some staff have told her that one or two drinks would not hurt anyone. In fact, there were some staff who acknowledged saying this to the patient without knowing her history. The patient has the uncanny ability to consistently identify staff who contradict each other, often over inconsequential details. Mr. B. is livid with the staff and makes written complaints to the administrative staff, always on his professional stationary. He perceives the staff as inconsistent and weak and not willing to control his wife's drinking behavior.

In other situations, families may not follow unit guidelines or may encourage the patient not to follow a medical recommendation or directive. Family members may consistently arrive well before visiting hours or persistently delay their departure from the hospital at the end of the day. At times, families may speak for the patient and encourage the patient to withdraw and regress. Families may also possess unrealistic expectations of staff. Family members may perceive the staff as their own personal medical providers and may seek personal care from the team. Problematic families may also find each other in waiting rooms, family groups, or at other events. These families may form alliances with one another against the staff. Through their perceptions, families may identify inconsistencies in medical care, availability of staff, and access to information. Consequently, instead of one family, the staff may be confronted by a number of agitated and indignant families, who together approach the staff with a diffuse list of complaints focusing on how they feel maltreated. The staff in turn feel under siege and exasperated and maltreated.

Special Patient and Family Issues

Children in the home

Often, children of adult cancer patients are an unseen and forgotten population. In acute clinical settings, children are not observed because of the patient's daytime appointments or policies that prohibit visits to inpatient units. Within the palliative setting, children and grandchildren are often present and may play an active role in the caregiving process. Salient developmental differences exist between children of different ages. Generally, young children (3 years or older) are able to verbally communicate their concerns so that an ongoing dialogue can occur. Highly sensitive to emotional and physical changes, regardless of age and maturity, children benefit most from an environment in which they are continually given measured amounts of information in a manner that they can understand and then encouraged to ask questions. Adults should be prepared for questions to be rather concrete and egocentric, centered around the immediate needs of the child and any potential change in the family. Children are specifically concerned about the continued presence of parents and their own safety. Questions from children usually come one or two at a time. Children often need time to interpret and integrate the adult responses before returning for additional information that may occur days or even weeks later.

Consequently, methods to deliver medical information or relieve distress within children must vary according to each child's developmental stage. A child who is 5 years old possesses fantasies related to a parent's illness in terms of its etiology, meaning, and duration. Most often, a cancer diagnosis does not result in immediate physical deterioration. If cancer therapy is unsuccessful, the patient experiences a gradual debilitating course over a 6- to 18-month period of time. Young children need consistent and ongoing information, whether they request it or not, concerning this chronic course of care so that they can anticipate changes and incorporate an understanding of these medical events into their world. Children cannot fully appreciate the concept of permanence. The permanence of death or abstract terms such as "forever" are beyond their ability to integrate these concepts. Children need consistent support, measured doses of information, and an environment that can respond to their questions. In particular, this is true when a parent has a protracted illness or is dying.

Adolescents are also vulnerable to a prolonged course of medical care as their parent, sibling, or grandparent move from a treatment phase into supportive or terminal care. Developmentally, adolescence is the time for testing the limits of independence and dependence as well as a quickened pace to individuation from the family. The natural course is toward increasing participation outside of the family structure as social integration deepens and psychological and emotional growth accelerates. These processes can be delayed because of the family's focus on a loved one who is slowly deteriorating and dying. Competitiveness, sexuality, aggression, and peer relationships may compound and confuse attempts to cope with a loss and the end of a significant relationship. Familial roles can be disrupted or confused, and as a result, adolescents may be forced to prematurely assume adult responsibilities. There is a danger in treating an adolescent as an adult. The demands of adolescence under normal circumstances generate numerous stressors for the family. Chronic illness at this point in the life cycle can significantly exacerbate the family's level of premorbid distress. Of particular concern is that adolescents may be parentified. Often, physical maturity is erroneously equated with the emotional, intellectual, and spiritual development of an adult. Adolescents can easily be overwhelmed with guilt and shame when their normal sense of power and grandiosity cannot control symptoms or death. This may have a long-term negative effect on the ability to tolerate emotional relationships and dependency later in life. If the death of a parent or grandparent is to occur in the home, children must be carefully assessed and appropriate interventions and support should be offered. Health care professionals are in the unique position to protect adolescents from assuming that they are now responsible for the dying parent's role within the family. Given the emotional and stressful environment around the time of death, statements reinforcing or conveying the assumption of the parent's role can have significant connotations for the developing adolescent and should be perceived as having the power of hypnotic suggestions with life-long implications. Adolescents are incapable of replacing the functions of the dying parent, they should not be expected to do so, and they should be told so directly.

Psychiatric illness

Histories of psychiatric disorders present further challenges in the effective management of patients and families as they experience supportive and terminal care. Symptoms such as severe depression may dramatically influence a patient's perception of pain and other noxious symptoms and the ability of the health care team to control it. Psychiatric symptoms must be assessed and appropriately managed if the patient is to truly benefit from supportive care interventions. Furthermore, psychiatric symptoms of a family member can also cause a significant concern, given the health care team's expectations concerning caregiving in the home by family members. The demands of caring for a dying person in the home can produce significant levels of distress, resulting in exacerbation of neurotic and psychiatric symptoms in high-risk individuals. Early intervention and added levels of emotional and instrumental support is especially essential to this population. Frequently, expectations of family members as caregivers are relatively uniform, despite the significant variation that exists in each family's level of functioning. Families must be assessed not only for their availability but also for their ability to provide adequate supportive care.

Finally, patients and families who enter the cancer experience with a history of physical or sexual abuse may exhibit significant difficulty in their ability to develop a trusting relationship with the health care team and may require ongoing psychiatric management. Families with a history of abuse possess the need to protect information related to the abuse and any attempt to assess the patient or family may be perceived as an unwanted intrusion. Trust can only be developed over time, as the health care team demonstrates their concern for patient and family, as well as their availability for support and effective intervention. Families with severe dysfunction isolate and protect themselves from the outside world with a rigid outer boundary. Health care providers define a family as truly problematic when initial offers of assistance are refused. Health care professionals tend to have a need for approval and acceptance and are likely to perceive any variation as a rejection. As a result, the health care team experiences frustration and confusion and withdraws, which is inevitably communicated directly to the patient and family. Consequently, the family is lost as an ally and resource and as a result, their isolation is increased. Helping families with rigid boundaries is a difficult task, and frontal assaults only confirm in the families mind the need to protect themselves from the strangers on whom they are suddenly dependent. Although few in number, timely psychosocial referrals for these patients and family members are essential.

Addictions

History of substance abuse or an active addiction within the patient or the family creates a sense of alarm within the health care team. For example, if the patient possesses a history of narcotic addiction, health care providers may simply not trust the patient's account of past events or may define the patient's behavior as automatically manipulative. This may be true even if the history of abuse is in the distant past. In this circumstance, the patient quickly learns not to trust the staff with sensitive information. In cases related to pain control, physicians may be unwilling to prescribe higher dosages of narcotics even if the patient is in pain or is terminally ill.

Since cancer does not discriminate, patients with histories of substance abuse will also be diagnosed with cancer. These patients should not needlessly suffer through their terminal illness as a result of their past history of abuse or their current treatment in a methadone clinic. Patients with a history of narcotic addiction who are maintained on methadone can remain drug-free of illicit substances, reduce their criminal activity, and maintain full-time employment in a structured and supervised drug treatment program. Consultation with reputable drug treatment facilities is necessary in terms of effective patient management strategies.

Patients who are actively abusing drugs pose a significant challenge to the health care professional who wants to trust and care for the individual with a life-threatening illness and to protect society from the potential of drug diversion simultaneously. Flight into philosophical discourse over the primary responsibility is an oversimplification of the situation. All patients—including the least favored of society—have the right to humane care. Society also has the right to expect that those whom they give special rights and privileges will not ignore their need for protection from antisocial behavior.

Health care professionals are trained and are used to being in control. Their values and unique set of skills and knowledge, combined with the sanction of society to bear the responsibility to protect human life and to reduce suffering, is often in direct opposition to the lifestyle of the active substance abuser. Caring for these patients is never easy. Caring and consistent confrontation and structure is often the best the health care professional can do. Acceptance of realistic limitations to influence the patient and vigilance in maintaining professional ethical standards comprises the foundation for adequate care. Threats of rejection and abandonment almost never work; they only postpone the care until it is emergent and the health care team is forced to act. Sadly, it may not be until the individual nears the end of life and becomes increasingly debilitated that it becomes possible to make meaningful contact and to provide adequate medical and emotional support.

Finally, family members of an active substance abuser may influence or reinforce the drug-seeking behavior of the patient. Substance abuse families frequently possess a high level of cohesion which can be characterized as enmeshed. Within this type of family, boundaries between family members are nebulous and as a result, may appear to be equally affected by the status of the patient. Their level of care may be sporadic or inconsistent because they may be overwhelmed by the severity of the illness. Careful medical and psychosocial coordination between patient, family, staff, and, when appropriate, drug treatment center, is essential to maximize cooperation and maintain quality care.[48] Despite the level of frustration associated this challenging group of patients, dignified care is possible and attainable when objectivity is used to identify realistic goals tailored to the individual patient and family.

Intimacy and sexuality

Advanced disease always affects sexuality and sexual functioning. Within supportive and terminal care programs, the lack of sexual libido and functioning is frequently overlooked or ignored as a concern of the patient. The reticence and discomfort to discuss sexuality and intimacy is usually a result of an uncomfortable health care professional. The patient and spouse are well aware that there have been significant changes in their sexual life. They simply may not know that it is appropriate to discuss such personal matters. The health care professional can serve as a catalyst to this important form of communication. Both patient and spouse often feel guilt over the changes in the nature of their relationship. The patient may feel guilt that they are not meeting the needs of their spouse and that they are physically repulsive. The spouse may experience guilt over feeling deprived and angry that a loved one is seriously ill. Open discussion of intimacy and sexuality with the team can actually result in enhancement of emotional vitality. In fact, an increase in intimacy can evolve as closeness is redefined and openly discussed. Patients' needs for intimacy and sexual activity must be examined and supported. Intimacy between a couple during supportive or terminal care can restore a sense of normalcy and relief in the midst of a highly traumatic course of unpleasant medical events. It can also remind patients that their body can still produce pleasant sensations. As patients enter the terminal phase, these discussions require a high level of sensitivity since most patients long to be touched and held. It is not uncommon for spouses or children to lie in bed with a dying patient in order to provide comfort and experience closeness or intimacy. Although this may make staff uncomfortable, it may represent a last opportunity for family to feel close to the loved one who is leaving them.

Dying at home

Although many patients and families describe a preference for death to occur in the comfort of their home, this goal is not always attainable. Approximately 76%–80% of patient deaths occur in medical institutions whereas only 10–14% of patients die in hospices and the remaining 5%–10% in nursing homes or in patients' homes.[49-51] The return to home, nursing homes, or hospices as the chosen places of death continues to increase in relation to hospitals. The primary impetus for this shift is a direct result of the Medicare Hospice Benefit.[52] A number of key psychosocial variables (which were previously defined in Table 11.1) may inhibit or prevent the occurrence of death in the home even with the highest level of supportive care or hospice services. Families must be assessed carefully and prepared for the death event. Preparations including advance directives, wills, and Do Not Resuscitate orders should begin as early as possible to resolve all questions and informational needs that the family may possess. Often, hospice services are only in the home for a fraction of each day. Consequently, in all probability, the patient's death may occur when the family is alone.

   Key family members can be specifically questioned concerning their level of comfort or tolerance of stressful events within the home. Responses can be quite varied. A family may wish to maintain a dying member at home despite complex needs. Suddenly, they may then request that the patient die in the hospital. Reasons for rapid changes may be obvious and practical or may be irrational and unconscious. Either way, the resources and limitations of the family must be assessed and supported. At times of great stress and crisis, family strengths must be the focus while family deficits can be ignored. If terminal caregiving is prolonged, the family may reach a point when they are unable to sustain the care plan and they may advocate for an admission to an inpatient unit. The family should be helped to see that dying in the hospital is not a failure even if it was against the patient's last wish. Since many terminally ill patients possess acute care needs (e.g., pain control, mental status changes, etc.), an inpatient admission may be warranted to better manage complex symptoms and to provide brief respite for the family or to actually manage the death event.

When the patient dies

Although the final hours of life are usually uneventful, these moments possess significant meaning for the family and offer an opportunity for closure. The ritualistic need to be present at the exact moment of death can be very powerful for family members. At times, the effect on families may be irrational. The desire to be present for the death event is common, and for family members who are absent, significant regrets may result.[53] Unexpected deaths occur in about 30% of patients, so consequently, attempts to notify the family of the impending event is possible in 70% of cases.[54]

While the death occurs, family members require objective information concerning the cause of death especially if the death was unexpected. In other words, despite the terminal prognosis, families still need to understand why the patient died at that time. Information will meditate the high level of distress and address any irrational concerns and fears associated with the death event as it is happening. Verbal interactions that occur immediately following the death can have a long-term effect. Emotional reactions of family members are expected, and crying, sobbing, and wailing are common. The therapeutic demands associated with the provision of terminal care challenges the health care professional to communicate with empathy while facilitating the initiation of essential tasks, such as removal of the body and funeral arrangements. Families vary in their ability to receive information and emotional support. The ongoing relationship between the family and the health care team influences how much of these preparations can be made prior to the death event and what level of professional intervention the family requires and can tolerate. Generally, families elect a spokesperson to provide and receive information, but care must be taken to assess other members of the family. A follow-up meeting with the family by a social worker or nurse in the home can be very helpful to identify any family member who may be at risk for an abnormal grief response.

Bereavement

Bereavement represents the end of the care cycle. At diagnosis, the primary focus is to save the patient from the immediate threat of disease. As disease progresses, the focus of care increasingly shifts to the complex physical needs of patients and emotional support of families. As death approaches, attention is focused on the family and their efforts to cope with the demands of advanced disease. Generally, social workers, nurses, and chaplains are responsible for the provision of emotional support and bereavement counseling. Anecdotal reports, in conjunction with well-designed research studies, have established an increased risk for morbidity and mortality among bereaved spouses.[55]

Social support and tolerance for a grieving family is brief and intense. Following a significant level of attention and care, family members find themselves in an emotional turmoil after the loss. Once the funeral and burial rituals are completed, the full and true impact of the loss is experienced. First, the central issue—caring for the patient—is now gone and little can replace this demanding, meaningful, and intense experience. This void is filled with a longing for the patient, periodic or sustained loneliness, and ambivalence associated with an uncertain future. Many families experience a sense of abandonment by the health care team following the death of the patient. Families may also experience the termination of their relationship with the health care team as an additional significant loss. For the health care team, involvement with supportive and loving families of patients may create a sense of loss and longing, pointing to a lack of intimacy and closeness in their own families. Given the professional demands made on health care professionals and the intensity of the emotional relationships with patients and families, periods of sadness following the death of a favored patient are predictable.

Although most families cope and adapt to the loss, an integral role exists for health care professionals. Periodic and regularly scheduled telephone contact provides an excellent mechanism to provide support and to assess the family's reintegration. The family can be actively encouraged to contact members of the team with specific concerns or unanswered questions. However, the focus on these interactions should guide the family to a return to optimal social functioning and resumption of a future-oriented life. It is not unusual for family members (especially spouses and parents) to believe that they see the deceased in a crowd, hear their voice, smell them, or sense their presence. Vivid nocturnal dreams, nightmares, insomnia, intense sorrow, and social withdrawal are components of the grief process. Many family members and close friends find it helpful to talk to a social worker, psychologist, or a psychiatrist to gain support, learn how to express and manage emotions, and develop plans for action during this period. Family members need to understand that the intensity of their emotional reactions will subside following an acute phase of 3–6 months. For some families, a sense of fear is present which is related to their belief that the absence of sadness disconnects them from memories of the deceased. Families must be assured that once the acute phase of the loss passes, they will still be connected with the deceased since nothing can remove their memories and the life they shared together. Families will also need to be prepared for and supported in openly expressing and working through any ambivalence toward the deceased. If intense ambivalence persistently interferes with daily functioning, a referral to a psychotherapist outside of the medical system should be made in a timely fashion.

Anniversaries and other significant dates act as triggers in remembering and reflecting, and for some, reliving the family's loss. Frequently, family members possess the need to contact those professionals who cared for the deceased. This healthy response represents a time to emotionally connect with the deceased and to make contact with the caring support of the living. The following case example illustrates the needs of the bereaved at this point in time.

A 59-year-old book designer cared for her father for 3 years until his death occurred in her home. Motherless since the age of 5, this bereaved daughter perceived her father as a loving and kind source of support throughout her life. Although quite saddened and depressed following his death, she was able to enter weekly counseling until she returned to normal functioning about 4 months later. Upon each anniversary of his death, the daughter has returned to the hospital for the past 8 years to sit quietly in the lobby for 1 hour. This ritual enables her to feel "connected and healed." Although she continues to miss her father, her level of functioning has not diminished and she has been able to form a significant relationship.

Conclusions

All patients and families possess a personal meaning of disease, prolonged illness, and death. These meanings are influenced and developed over time as a result of numerous factors. A clear understanding of how patients and families perceive supportive and terminal care significantly enhances the health care team's ability to provide care and anticipate potential problems. Information and education must be consistently available as the patient and family move across the disease continuum toward the death event.

Comprehensive psychosocial assessments of the palliative patient must move beyond traditional considerations and include intimacy, sexuality, and spirituality, as well as a realistic appraisal of the capabilities and limitations of each family. Health care providers tend to erroneously assume that all patients are capable of withstanding the multiple and complex demands of a prolonged illness. Because of the ongoing trend toward reducing the inpatient length of stay and help in the home simultaneously, families must be carefully assessed to determine if the level of care and support for the patient is adequate. If indications of marginal or inadequate care exist, the patient may require additional supportive services or an inpatient admission may be necessary.

Health care professionals practice in an extremely demanding environment. Although they are prepared to function well within the context of intellectual challenges and multiple technical and instrumental tasks, staff are seldom prepared for the psychological and emotional demands of patients, families, and their own idiosyncratic responses. Dying and death are essentially emotional experiences. While death is essentially a physical event, dying is a social, spiritual, and disarmingly confrontational occurrence for the survivors. For the patient and family, loss is at the center of the experience. For the health care professional with a commitment to palliative care, facilitation of a dignified death for the patient and adequate support for the family can lead to a sense of completion and satisfaction. For staff who perceive death as a failure, they may consequently experience a pervasive sense of emptiness, powerlessness, and hopelessness. In addition, for health care providers who lack a meaningful emotional life outside of the professional context, death can be a confrontation of a life without adequate meaning and gratification. In this case, staff may despair and experience the death as deeply and as profoundly as the loss of a family member.

Care at the end of life offers a different set of rewards than those associated with cure and extending life. For health care professionals committed to palliative care, the rewards involve active support of living and hope in a place where death is soon to be a visitor. Staff experience an emotional connectedness to patients and families in a very special and at times, sacred place, where most others fear to go. Staff share in this struggle to enable patients and families to tolerate sadness and loss and to find a sense of meaningful completion.

References

1. Seale C, Cartwright A. *The Year Before Death.* Brookfield VT: Ashgate Publishing, 1994.
2. Levin, DN, Cleeland CS, Dar R. Public attitudes toward cancer pain. *Cancer* 1985; 56:2337–2339.
3. World Health Organization. Cancer pain and palliative care. Technical Report 804. Geneva, 1990.
4. Zarit SH, Todd PA, Zarit JM. Subjective burdens of husbands and wives as caregivers: a longitudinal study. *Gerontologist* 1986; 26:260–266.
5. Brody EM. Women in the middle and family help to older people. *Gerontologist* 1981; 21:471–480.
6. Gochman DS, Bonham GS. Physicians and the hospice decision: awareness, discussion, reasons and satisfaction. *Hospice J* 1988; 4(1):25–53.
7. Hyman RB, Bulkin W. Physician reported incentives and disincentives for referring patients to hospice. *Hospice J* 1990; 6(4):39–64.
8. Weisman AD, Worden JW. The existential plight in cancer: significance of the first 100 days. *Int J Psychiatry Med* 1976–1977; 7:1–9.
9. Derogatis LR, Morrow GR, Fetting J. The prevalence of psychiatric disorders among cancer patients. *JAMA* 1983; 249(6):751–757.
10. Farber JM, Weinerman BH, Kuypers JA. Psychosocial distress in oncology outpatients. *J Psychosoc Oncol* 1984; 2:109–118.

11. Stefanek M, Derogatis L, Shaw A. Psychological distress among oncology outpatients. *Psychosomatics* 1987; 28:537–539.

12. Schulz R, Williamson GM, Knapp JE, Bookwala J, et al. The psychological, social, and economic impact of illness among patients with recurrent cancer. *J Psychosoc Oncol* 1995; 13(3):21–45.

13. Fawzy, FI, Fawzy NW, Arndt LA, Pasnau RO. Critical review of psychosocial interventions in cancer care. *Arch Gen Psychiatry* 1995; 52:100–113.

14. Zabora JR, Smith-Wilson R, Fetting JH, et al. An efficient method for the psychosocial screening of cancer patients. *Psychosomatics* 1990; 31(2):192–196.

15. BrintzenhofeSzoc KM. Family functioning and psychosocial distress as related to spousal grief reaction following the death of a cancer patient (Abstract). *Abstract Book—Annual Conference of the Association of Oncology Social Work.* Tucson, AZ: 1996.

16. Weisman AD, Worden JW, Sobel HJ. Psychosocial screening and interventions with cancer patients: a research report. Boston: Harvard Medical School and Massachusetts Hospital, 1980.

17. Smith ED, Stefanek ME, Joseph MV, et al. Spiritual awareness, personal perspective on death, and psychosocial distress among cancer patients. *J Psychosoc Oncol* 1993; 11(3):89–103.

18. Donovan K, Sanson-Fisher RW, Redman S. Measuring quality of life in cancer patients. *J Clin Oncol* 1989; 7(7):959–968.

19. Zabora JR, Smith ED. Family dysfunction and the cancer patient: early recognition and intervention. *Oncology* 1992; 5(2):31–35.

20. Olson DH, McCubbin HI, Barnes HL, et al. *Families: What Makes Them Work.* London: Sage, 1989.

21. Zabora JR, Fetting JH, Shaley VB, et al. Predicting conflict with staff among families of cancer patients during prolonged hospitalizations. *J Psychosoc Oncol* 1989; 7(3):103–111.

22. Derogatis LR, Melisaratos N. The Brief Symptom Inventory: an introductory report. *Psychol Med* 1983; 13:595–605.

23. McDowell I, Newell C. *Measuring Health: A Guide to Rating Scales and Questionnaires.* New York: Oxford University Press, 1987.

24. Zabora JR, Loscalzo MJ. Comprehensive psychosocial programs: a prospective model of care. *Oncol Iss* 1996; 11(1):14–18.

25. Seddon CF, Zabora JR. Psychotherapy needs of cancer patients and their families (Abstract). *Abstract Book of the Association of Oncology Social Work,* San Antonio, TX: May 1995.

26. Houts PS, Nezu AM, Maguth Nezu C, Bucher JA. The prepared family caregiver: a problem-solving approach to family caregiver education. *Patient Ed Counsel* 1996; 27:63–73.

27. Jamison RN, Sbrocco T, Parris W. The influence of problems in concentration and memory on emotional distress and daily activities in chronic pain patients. *Int J Psychiatry Med* 1988; 18:183–.

28. Daut RL, Cleeland CS. The prevalence and severity of pain in cancer. *Cancer* 1982; 50(9):1913–1918.

29. Bond MR, Pearson IB. Psychological aspects of pain in women with advanced cancer of the cervix. *J Psychosom Res* 1969; 13:13–19

30. Cleeland CS. The impact of pain on the patient with cancer. *Cancer* 1984; 54:2635–2641

31. Derogatis LR, Morrow GR, Fetting J, et al. The prevalence of psychiatric disorders among cancer patients. *JAMA* 1983; 249(6):751–757.

32. Spiegel D, Sands SS, Koopman C. Pain and depression in patients with cancer. *Cancer* 1994; 74:2570–2578

33. Razavi D, Delvaux N, Farvacques C, et al. Screening for adjustment idsorders and major depressive disorders in cancer inpatients. *Br J Psychiatry* 1990; 156:79–83.

34. Shacham S, Reinhart LC, Raubertas RF, Cleeland CS. Emotional states and pain: intraindividual and interindividual measures of association. *J Behav Med* 1983; 6:405–419.

35. Bolund C. Suicide and cancer II: medical and care factors in suicide by cancer patients in Sweden, 1973–1976. *J Psychosoc Oncol* 1985: 3:17–30.

36. Massie MJ, Holland JC. Depression and the cancer patient. *J Clin Psychiatry* 1990; 51 (Supp.):12–19.

37. Kagawa-Singer M. Diverse cultural beliefs and practices about death and dying in the elderly. In: Wieland? ed. *Cultural Diversity and Geriatric Care*. New York; 1994:101–?.

38. Hellman C. *Culture, Health and Illness*. 3rd ed. Newton, MA: Butterworth & Heinemann; 1995.

39. Koenig BA, Gates-Williams J. Understanding cultural difference in caring for dying patients, In: *Caring for Patients at the End of Life* (special issue). *West J Med* 1995; 163(3):244–249.

40. Power PW, Dell Orto AE. Understanding the family. In: Power PW, Dell Orto AE, eds. *Role of the Family in the Rehabilitation of the Physically Disabled*. Baltimore: University Park Press; 1980: xxx–xxx.

41. Dunkell-Schetter C, Feinstein LG, Taylor SE, Folks RL. Patterns of coping with cancer. *Health Psychol* 1992; 11(2):79–87.

42. Miller RD, Krech R, Walsh TD. The role of a palliative care service family conference in the management of the patient with advanced cancer. *Palliat Med* 1991; 5:34–39.

43. Lansky SB, Cairns N, Lowman J, et al. Childhood cancer: non-medical costs of the illness. *Cancer* 1979; 43(1):403–408.

44. Schultz R, Williamson GM, Knapp JE, Bookwala MS, Lave J, Fello M. The psychological, social, and economic impact of illness among patients with recurrent cancer. *J Psychoso Oncol* 1995; 13(3):21–45.

45. Houts PS, Lipton A, Harvey HA, Martin B, Simmonds MA, Dixon R, et al. Nonmedical costs to patients and their families associated with outpatient chemotherapy. *Cancer* 1984; 53:2388–2392.

46. Mor V, Guadagnoli E, Wool M. An examination of the concrete of the concrete service needs of advanced cancer patients. *J Psychosoc Oncol* 1987; 5:1–12.

47. Farkas C, Loscalzo M. Death without indignity. In: Kutscher AH, Carr AC, Kutscher LG, eds. *Principles of Thanatology*. New York: Columbia University Press; 1987:133–152.

48. Loscalzo M, Amendola J. Psychosocial and behavioral management of cancer pain: The social work contribution. In: Foley KM, Bonica JJ, Ventafridda V, eds. Advances in Pain Research and Therapy. Vol. 16. New York: Raven Press; 1990:429–442.

49. McCusker J. Where cancer patients die: an epidemiological study. *Public Health Rep* 1983; 98:170–176.
50. Merill D, Mor V. Pathways to hospital death among the oldest old. *J Aging Health* 1993; 516-535.
51. Sager M, Easterling D, Kindig D, Anderson O. Changes in the location of death after passage of Medicare's prospective payment system. *N Engl J Med* 1989; 320:433–439.
52. McMullan A, Mentnech R, Lubitz J, McBean AM, Russell D. Trends and patterns in place of death for Medicare enrollees. *Health Care Fin Rev* 1990; 12:107.
53. Tolle SW, Bascom PB, Hickam DA, Benson JA. Communication between physicians and surviving spouses following patient death. *J Gen Intern Med* 1986; 1:309–314.
54. Tolle SW, Girard DW. The physician's role in the events surrounding patient death. *Arch Intern Med* 1982; 143:1447–1449.
55. Helsing KJ, Szklo M. Mortality after bereavement. *Epidemiol Rev* 1981; 114:41–52.

12

Staff Burnout: Sources, Diagnosis, Management, and Prevention

MARY L. S. VACHON

Providing supportive care confronts caregivers with multiple challenges that are different from those of traditional palliative care. Supportive care in oncology has been defined as "the provision of the necessary services for those living with or affected by cancer to meet their physical, psychosocial, informational and spiritual needs during the diagnostic, treatment, follow-up phases, encompassing issues of survivorship, palliation and bereavement."[1]

Supportive care can be provided by caregivers working in their normal roles throughout the continuum of care in oncology or other specialities. Included in this definition of supportive care are: family physicians, professionals and volunteers in the acute care setting, community care providers, as well as caregivers in hospice and palliative care settings. Alternatively, specialized supportive care may be provided by a team of professionals with particular skills in symptom relief and/or psychosocial assessment, support, and treatment. Such supportive care teams most often target high-risk patients/families and/or those with difficult to control symptoms. While some supportive care teams target their interventions primarily to physical symptoms, this chapter will assume that the physical care of patients with life-threatening illness is not separable from the psychosocial and spiritual needs of patients and their families. We will assume that caregivers in supportive care are involved with patients at various stages of the illness continuum and that there is a tendency to have longer-term relationships with patients and families than has been the traditional role of caregivers in palliative care.

In the mid-1990s, there is a trend for palliative care specialists to see their role as broader and extending throughout the illness continuum. In the United Kingdom, Australia, and New Zealand, palliative care is a postgraduate specialty that involves work with patients/families at an earlier point in time than was usually the case.[2] In the United States and Canada, the specialty of palliative care is still in the process of negotiation. In the United States, palliative care may develop as a subdiscipline within medical oncology.[3] While palliative care as a specialty has yet to be fully accepted in Canada, the Canadian Palliative Care Association has recently published a definition of palliative care that "allows for the variable need and role of primary, secondary and tertiary palliative care along a patient's illness trajectory":

> Palliative care, as a philosophy of care, is the combination of active and compassionate therapies intended to comfort and support individuals and families who are living with a life-threatening illness. During periods of illness and bereavement, palliative care strives to meet physical, psychological, social and spiritual expectations and needs, while remaining sensitive to personal, cultural and religious values, beliefs and practices. Palliative care may be combined with therapies aimed at reducing or curing the illness, or it may be the total focus of care. Palliative care is planned and delivered through the collaborative efforts of an interdisciplinary team including the individual, family, caregivers and service providers. It should be available to the individual and his/her family at any time during the illness trajectory and bereavement."[4] (p. 12)

This chapter recognizes the evolving role of palliative care but will focus attention on the research into the diagnosis, management, and prevention of stress and burnout in caregivers working across the continuum of care. The research on the stress of palliative caregivers has recently been reviewed.[2,5,6] The conclusions drawn are that stress and burnout in palliative care are less than that experienced by professionals in many other settings. However, studies have noted problems of concern, including suicidal ideation, increased alcohol and drug usage, anxiety, depression, and difficulty dealing with issues of death and dying. It was hypothesized that part of the reason that stress was lower than might have been expected in palliative care was because of the early recognition of the potential stress inherent in this field and the development of appropriate organizational and personal coping strategies to deal with identified stressors.[5]

A recent review of the literature of stress and burnout in oncology concluded that stress and burnout in oncology care may be no higher than that experienced by professionals in other specialties but is greater than that reported in palliative care. Stress is associated with empathic relationships with patients and families, particularly those approaching death. However, the greatest difference in stress and burnout in oncology as compared with palliative care is the greater workload of those in oncology. In addition, there is not the same recognition that exists in palliative care settings that personal and organizational support systems are required in order to enable caregivers to care effectively for patients and their families without totally depleting themselves.[7]

This chapter will review the literature on the stress experienced by professionals working in the continuum of supportive care. The primary focus will be on supportive care in oncology and on studies comparing oncology professionals with caregivers in other specialties, but the research studies to be reviewed will also include other nursing and medical groups. Table 12.1 contains a review of many of the relevant studies of the last decade on which this chapter is based.[8-26]

The work of supportive care can be described as being emotional labor which is "the labour involved in dealing with other people's feelings, a core component of which is the regulation of emotions."[27] The nature of the work is such that it is often difficult to define the skills vital to work because they involve emotion, intuition, and instinct—all vague and unscientific terms. "Emotional labour is hard work and can be sorrowful and difficult. It demands that the labourer gives personal attention which means that they must give something of themselves, not just a formulaic response."[27] Such work also involves the regulation of emotion between the carer and the person being cared for, which is one of the sometimes tremendous but rewarding challenges of supportive care.

Burnout[7]

The concept of burnout is generally credited to Freudenberger.[28] Burnout has been characterized as "the progressive loss of idealism, energy and purpose experienced by people in the helping professions as a result of the conditions of their work."[29] Burnout has also been described as a *syndrome* of responses involving increased feelings of emotional exhaustion, negative attitudes towards the recipients of one's service (depersonalization), a tendency to evaluate oneself negatively with regard to one's work, and a feeling of dissatisfaction with accomplishments on the job.[22,30]

Burnout is generally seen as resulting from the interaction between the needs of people to sacrifice themselves for a job and a job situation that places inordinate demands on an individual. The person prone to burnout is apt to have unrealistically high personal expectations for satisfaction in a given area of life. The phenomenon can occur not only in an individual but also within a system.[29,31]

Pines[32] proposed a social-psychological model of burnout positing certain characteristics of the work environment as contributing to burnout. According to her model, professionals with a high level of motivation can either achieve peak performance if working within a positive environment, or develop burnout symptoms if the individual continues to confront a stressful, discouraging environment. Individual differences determine how soon an individual develops burnout and how extreme the experience may be.

The most commonly used instrument to measure burnout is the Maslach Burnout Inventory [MBI],[33] which measures emotional exhaustion, depersonalization, and a lack of personal accomplishment on two dimensions: *frequency* (how often a feeling occurs) and *intensity* (the strength of that feeling). The MBI has been used in numerous studies in oncology.[19,22,24-26,34] Other burnout instruments used in studies of oncology professionals include: the Staff Burnout Scale for Health Professionals,[11,35] and author-constructed burnout questionnaires.[15,16]

Table 12.1. Selected studies of stress in oncology/supportive care

Authors	Description of study	Personal variables	Stressors	Manifestations	Coping/intervention
• Vachon[8,9]	• 81 semi-structured interviews involving an international convenience sample of 110 caregivers in oncology: 38 MDs, 33 RNs, 18 SWs, clergy, psychologists, 21 others. • Part of a larger study of 581 caregivers from a variety of professions and practice settings.	• Younger caregivers had more stressors, more manifestations of stress, and fewer coping strategies. • Social support system served both as a source of stress and a stressor	• More likely to report equal stressors from work environment, occupational role and patient/families. • More likely to report problems with patients and families with coping and and/or personality problems; communication problems with patients/families; role overload; identification with patients and families; unrealistic expectations, and lack of control.	• Depression, grief and guilt • Anger, frustration • Job/home interaction • Helplessness, inadequacy, insecurity • Avoidance of patient	• Sense of competence, control and pleasure in one's work • Develop multiple roles • Personal philosophy • Team philosophy, support, team building • Leave work situation
• Schmale et al[10]	• 147/470 (31% response rate) physician members of American Society of Clinical Oncology. • Average age 43, 83% male, 79% in private practice, in practice an average of 12 years, for 86% more than 50% of		• Dissatisfactions included pressures of practice, negative relationships with patients/families, dealing with dying patients, ineffective treatments, emotional support to patients and families, negative relations with other professionals,	• 61.9% found working in oncology stressful	• 80% somewhat or very satisfied with working in oncology • Satisfactions included effective treatment, the challenge of oncology, positive relations with patients and families, personal satisfactions, symptom man-

Study	Sample/Method	Findings	Implications
	• and impact on personal life.	• agement, positive professional interactions, and emotional support to patients and families. • Activities outside of practice; support systems; personal satisfaction; self-protective behaviors helped to deal with stressful aspects of practice • Coped with stress through recognition of sources of stress, support services to patients and families, and emotional support for oncologist	
• Bram and Katz[11]	• 57 nurses employed full-time in three oncology units and six hospices in urban area of Pennsylvania; convenience sample • Both groups worked with similar proportions of terminally ill patients with cancer and both experienced similar numbers of patient deaths over past month. Similar in their practice was oncology. • Author-constructed mailout questionnaire.	• Burnout for older, married, more experienced and more educated hospice nurses was related to congruence between professional ideals and the goals, philosophy, and environment of hospice. • For younger, single, less educated hospital nurses the perception of dissonance between values and work envi- • Hospital oncology setting more stressful and less reinforcing for nurses caring for terminally ill patients than was hospice • Oncology nurses perceived less opportunity to talk about work-related feelings and discuss problems in the workplace, had slightly more dissonance between their real and • Compared with previous studies using the same instrument, oncology nurses were in the mid-range and hospice nurses had lowest burnout scores • Burnout in both groups associated with perception of less support in the workplace • Oncology nurses had significantly higher	• Staffing practices should take into account that for younger and/or oncology nurses, the number of patients assigned and amount of direct contact with patients/families are associated with stress and burnout. • For older or hospice nurses, the importance of congruence between professional ide-

(continued)

Table 12.1. Selected studies of stress in oncology/supportive care

Authors	Description of study	Personal variables	Stressors	Manifestations	Coping/intervention
• Bram and Katz[11] (continued)	number of hours worked per week and number of night shifts • Staff Burnout Scale for Health Professionals, Corwin's Nursing Role Conception Scale, work-related scale developed by one of authors	ronment did not have a significant relationship to burnout.	ideal work situations, and spent more hours in direct contact with patients/families which was associated with higher burnout scores. • They were less likely to consider communication with administration and quality of supervision as being excellent, had less sense of control over decision-making and practice, but perceived more job mobility. • The more patients for whom the oncology nurse was responsible, the greater was her burnout score.	burnout scores than hospice nurses • Burnout scores interacted significantly with role overload factors. • Caregivers' role in hospital seen as less reinforcing and more stressful than hospice environment	als and philosophy of health care setting is implied; this should be emphasized in hiring practices.
• Cooper et al.[12]	• 1,817 U.K. general practitioners selected at random by 20 family practitioner committees in England • Questionnaires distributed by family practice	• Women general practitioners had job satisfaction and showed positive signs of mental well-being in contrast	• Multivarate analysis showed four job stressors predictive of high levels of job dissatisfaction and lack of mental well-being; demands of the job and patient ex-	• Males were more emotionally anxious but did not reflect this in psychosomatic complaints • Four job stressors and age, sex and type A behavior were	• Highest levels of satisfaction, reported from amount of responsibility given, amount of freedom in choosing working methods, and

committees, returned anonymously to researchers • 48.2% response rate • Warr-Cook-Wall job satisfaction scale, shortened Crown-Crisp experiential index, alcohol and cigarette consumption, personal and job demographic variables, adapted version of Bortner type A questionnaire, job stress questionnaire	with other normative groups. • Male doctors had significantly higher anxiety scores than norms, had less job satisfaction, and drank more alcohol than female counterparts. • Physicians who had qualified in the U.K. had significantly more job satisfaction than those who qualified overseas. • For males, most significant predictors of job and stress were demands of job and patients' expectations; and for women, work/home interface and social life. • General practitioners most at risk of four job stress factors were older, male, and type A.	pectations; interference with family life; constant interruptions at work and home; and practice administration.	significantly predictive of high levels of mental ill health or lack of well-being. • For women the stress of job interfering with family life was the most important factor contributing to negative mental well-being. • For males the work–home interface was least important predictor; most important predictors were interruptions, practice administration, and demands of job and patient expectations. • Dealing with death and dying was prevalent in alcohol drinking behavior analysis, especially for women.	amount of variety in the job • Counseling service for general practitioners and other health care workers who suffer psychological pressure from their work • Training in social and managerial skills, including time management, people management, and work organization skill development
• Cooper and Mitchell[13] • 117/250 (47% usable questionnaire response rate) U.K. nurses from	• Depression was associated with older age and lower status for hospital nurses; for hos-	• Hospital and hospice nurses reported less stress than nurse managers on two "work-	• Hospital nurses dealing with the critically ill were significantly more dissatisfied with	• Hospital nurses need systematic training on dealing with patients and relatives as well as (continued)

Table 12.1. Selected studies of stress in oncology/supportive care

Authors	Description of study	Personal variables	Stressors	Manifestations	Coping/ intervention
• Cooper and Mitchell[13] (*continued*)	oncology, CCU, ICU and hospice • Mailout questionnaire • Nurse Stress Index, Job Satisfaction Scale, Crown-Crisp Experiential Index	pice nurses it was associated with less time since registration and lower status. • Young, inexperienced hospice nurses have more difficulty with death and dying and dealing with relatives and patients.	load" scales, and organizational support and involvement scales • Both groups had difficulty with dealing with relatives and managing the home–work interface. • Hospital nurses were significantly more stressed with a number of issues related to death and dying.	their job than were hospice nurses. Low job satisfaction was predicted by expected reaction of superiors to home–work conflict, lower nurse status, few post-basic qualifications, and lack of support at work. • Hospice nurses' low job satisfaction was related more to lack of staff support and involvement in decision-making and home affecting the work environment. • Hospice nurses were significantly more anxious and showed signs of psychosomatic complaints. • Poor mental health in hospital nurses was predicted by work affecting the home and dealing with relatives and patients; in hos-	outlets to deal with feelings when death occurs • Back-up stress counsellors for hospital nurses to deal with feelings about death and dying • Better management training for hospice administrators; strongest predictors of poor mental health linked to lack of support from senior staff and organizational issues. • Staff support and involvement in decision-making important to both groups but of greater consequence to hospice nurses. • To decrease work–home conflict greater provision for childcare, more flexible work hours, and job sharing needed.

• Ullrich and FitzGerald[14]	• 91 (51% response rate) nurses and 57 physicians (68% response rate) from 13 institutions in Bavaria, half worked only with cancer patients and half worked on units where 25–76% of patients had cancer • Author-constructed questionnaire describing many conflict situations, background information, institutional variables, and checklist of (psycho)somatic symptoms	• Nurses were more likely to have physical symptoms if outside life failed to relieve stress generated on the job. • Gender, not profession affected tendency to cry. • With age, stress decreased. • Young doctors were very tired.	• Nurses had vulnerability to stress involving the empathic component of their relationship with patients. • Physicians had stress associated with decision-making and communicating the diagnosis. Less stress with interpersonal difficulties, symptoms more strongly correlated with space, dealing with patients, and workday. • Working with trainees was a stress for both groups. • In small hospitals nurses had more stress

pice nurses, by staff support, involvement in decision-making and high workload.
• Dealing with critically ill or dying patients has more adverse affects in the home life (and vice versa) of hospital than in that of hospice nurses.

• Nurses showed greater stress levels—primarily interpersonal stress that related to physical distress.
• Overcommitment and identification with patients' suffering led to tiredness. Nurses suffered from exertion-related complaints.
• Physicians' stress was in part from lack of confidence when faced with limited ability to alter course of disease.
• Identification led to almost a physical rejection of patient.

• Intervention into particular problem areas: interpersonal difficulties for nurses and job dissatisfaction for doctors

(continued)

Table 12.1. Selected studies of stress in oncology/supportive care

Authors	Description of study	Personal variables	Stressors	Manifestations	Coping/ intervention
• Ullrich and FitzGerald[14] (*continued*)			• through identification with patients, doctors found such hospitals to be cramped. • Irregular working hours related to both total level of stress and total symptom level. • Caring for the ill and dying is a major stressor		
• Olkinuora et al.[15]	• 2671/3,496 Finnish physicians (76% response rate) • Stress Symptoms Score, Burnout Index, Suicidal Tendency Index	• Stress symptoms in male physicians were similar to those in male managers; female physicians showed slightly less stress than female white collar workers. • Male, but not female oncologists more likely to report burnout. • Those with university position or private practice were less likely to report burnout.		• Suicidal intent was higher in physicians than in the general population and more common among female (26% vs. 22%) physicians. • Oncologists were not among physicians with high suicidal ideation. • Higher burnout was experienced in specialties dealing with chronically ill, incurable, or dying patients. • It is hypothesized that hope, or lack of it	

		• Nonspecialists and those in municipal health centers and other outpatient settings had the highest burnout scores.	significantly influenced burnout. • General practice and occupational health medicine were high burnout specialties with heavy workloads, hectic working tempos and problems of professional identity	
• Whippen and Canellos[16]	• 598 physician subscribers to *Clinical Oncology* (60% response rate) • Mailout, author-constructed questionnaire	• There was no significant relationship between incidence of burnout and specialty within oncology, year medical training ended, or practice location. • Institution or university-based oncologists reported lower incidence of burnout.	• Administering palliative or terminal care, reimbursement issues, and a heavy workload were identified as contributing factors to burnout. • 80% said career had met their expectations from training.	• Frustration or sense of failure (56%) was the most frequent description of burnout. • Insufficient personal and/or vacation time (57%) was the most frequent reason to explain burnout. • The percentage of positive responses to burnout was proportional to total percentage of time spent in patient care.	• The majority (69%) indicated the need for more vacation or personal time to alleviate burnout. • Oncologists need better appreciation of positive contribution in palliative care. • Training programs need to provide more realistic expectations of reality of clinical practice involving total care of cancer patient. • Practicing medical oncologists would benefit from reduced work week with more personal and family time.

(continued)

Table 12.1. Selected studies of stress in oncology/supportive care

Authors	Description of study	Personal variables	Stressors	Manifestations	Coping/intervention
• Herschbach[17]	• 299 MDs and 592 nurses (52% response rate) from 54 hospitals and clinics in Germany • Oncology, cardiac, intensive care, surgery • Author-constructed questionnaire: 64 potentially stressful situations regarding degree of emotional or physical stress caused by each situation	• There may be "premorbid" personality characteristics that predispose staff to work in oncology, which could explain the difference in the experience of stress. • Continual confrontation with cancer patient's suffering and emotional involvement bound up with it influenced staff's values and their sense of the place and worth of their own work.	• Major stressors for nurses and physicians in oncology: disappointment in the power of medicine, patients remind one of one's own relatives, patients' unrealistic expectations of recovery, thinking of incurable children of incurable patients; for oncologists: less stress associated with institutional conditions and difficult patients • Institutional sources of stress move into the background when compared with stress associated with personal, emotional involvement with patients.	• Although oncology and comparison groups experienced the same overall degree of work-related stress and physical complaints, the oncology group suffered more from feelings of emotional involvement and self-doubt. • The oncology staff had more severe stress associated with emotional involvement with patients and had less difficulty with work and private life. They suffered less from stress connected with institutional factors than the comparison group, despite few objective differences in the respective situations.	• Oncology staff had better working conditions with fewer night and weekend shifts; this may be part of the reason they had less stress. They may also come to accept levels of stress in their own lives they would otherwise judge as being unacceptable. • Improving only the practical aspects of working conditions would not be sufficient to decrease stress. • Support groups to reflect on "personal hygiene" need to be established.
• Beck-Friis et al.[18]	• Swedish multidisciplinary staff of hospital-	• Hospital staff were younger and had a	• Hospital staff had less freedom to make their	• Hospital staff had higher levels of stress	• Both groups had high job satisfaction and

based home care unit (HBHC) (N = 35 [100% response rate]) and three hospital wards (N = 113 [94.2% response rate]); all staff worked regularly with severely ill cancer patients
• Self-administered author constructed questionnaire

shorter period of time working with the terminally ill; they were less likely to be registered nurses.
• HBHC staff were older, married, had children and had worked longer within the program—all factors identified as being associated with better coping.
• As staff work with terminally ill over a longer period of time they develop their own coping mechanisms for providing comfort, responding to anger, enhancing the quality of life during dying, and responding to the family.

own decisions, less cooperation between day and night staff, heavier workload, more communication problems with patients, and needed to train new staff more frequently because of turnover.
• Heavier workload of hospital staff attending to physical needs meant less time available for education and led to emotional problems.
• Overall correspondence between formal education and work was better in HBHC.
• Patients in the hospital may be upset with progression of the disease, despite ongoing treatment, and they are suffering the side effects of treatment, thus leading staff to question their roles and quality of care more.
• HBHC patients have accepted terminal stage of disease and

and anxiety, more tension, (groundless) guilt, and sleeping problems.

relatively low levels of stress.
• Continuing education is important. Hospital staff need education regarding problems with patient food intake and nausea/vomiting. HBHC staff probably had fewer problems because of ongoing education.
• Education on death and dying is important and should focus on specific behaviors rather than on anxiety about death.
• HBHC resources to staff on 24 hr basis provided staff with tools needed to perform high-quality palliative care and led to increased job satisfaction.
• HBHC stimulated staff's own initiative but was also capable of supporting staff when necessary and provided a more flexible environment.

(continued)

Table 12.1. Selected studies of stress in oncology/supportive care

Authors	Description of study	Personal variables	Stressors	Manifestations	Coping/ intervention
• Beck-Friis et al.[18] (*continued*)			focus on symptom relief. They and their family choose to go home and are probably more motivated and families have more positive expectations than patients admitted to hospital care.		• HBHC staff received more ongoing praise from relatives, in part because patient/family asked for and wanted home care. • HBHC staff had the opportunity to work with chronically ill patients as well as those terminally ill, thus they possibly decreased their vulnerability to burnout through shifting tasks.
• Van Servellen and Leake (19)	• 237 nurses from 7 hospitals in California • Convenience sample: response rate: 56–82% overall rate: 70% • Maslach Burnout Inventory to study burnout in AIDS and special care units (SCUs), oncology special care units, medical ICUs, and general medical	• Being white was associated with greater feelings of accomplishment. • Male nurses were more likely to report higher levels of depersonalization. • Older nurses and those with more years of practice on the unit scored lower on the	• Medical ICU work continued to show a negative impact on accomplishment when race and other important covariates were controlled. • Working in an ICU environment had a negative impact on feelings of accomplishment independent of cultural or racial effects.	• No significant difference in burnout scores across settings except that medical ICU nurses scored significantly lower on the personal accomplishment scale of the MBI. • Job tension was a key predictor of emotional exhaustion.	• Greater job influence had a significant protective effect on emotional exhaustion and enhanced personal accomplishment. • Methods to decrease job tension and improve nursing staff's sense of influence over work environment was important.

units to measure extent to which delivery method, patient diagnosis and other key personal and work-related variables were related to level of distress

• Primarily nongovernmental, small- to moderate-size hospitals where stress may already be under control

Emotional Exhaustion subscale.

• Those with more years of experience in hospital nursing and on the unit were more likely to have lower personal accomplishment scores.

• Although practice experience may guard against emotional exhaustion, it doesn't enhance one's sense of personal accomplishment as measured by MBI. This suggests a blunting of work effects; a protected group of seasoned practitioners neither suffers from exhaustion nor experiences high levels of personal accomplishment.

• AIDS SCU staff were more emotionally drained, but job tension was still the most important predictor of emotional exhaustion. Job influence and older age had independent protective effects.

• A recent change in shift was associated with higher levels of emotional exhaustion.

• Sources of tension to enhance individual input at unit level and implement changes need to be continuously evaluated where possible.

• Role clarity and congruency about job expectations were important; when these were absent, job tension and dissatisfaction developed.

• Role ambiguity can be detrimental to individuals and management of a unit as a whole. Nurses need a clear sense of direction and influence over decisions about assignments and case loads but should not be promised decision-making power when results of deliberations will not be implemented.

• Nurses who felt they had more influence over their job situation reported higher levels of accomplishment.

(continued)

Table 12.1. Selected studies of stress in oncology/supportive care

Authors	Description of study	Personal variables	Stressors	Manifestations	Coping/ intervention
• Copp and Dunn[20]	• 167 UK nurses from three practice settings—community, hospice, and acute care—were asked to identify the five most common problems when caring for dying and the five most difficult problems to manage. • Community nurses were palliative care Macmillan nurses. • Open-ended, written questionnaire, convenience sample	• 30% had 5 years or less postregistration experience; 21% had less than 1 year experience with dying patients; 49% had 2–5 years of experience.	• Across 3 settings the most common problems were physical, but these were less often seen as difficult to manage. • Nutrition and pain were the most frequently reported symptoms. • In acute care, work-related problems and nurse-related problems were most common. • Pain was the most difficult to manage physical problem. • Team relationship problems were the most common work-related issue; these were sometimes related to difficulties advising medical colleagues to use effective medication for pain and other symptoms	• Feelings of rejection and frustration were experienced when nurses felt their roles and knowledge were not valued. • They also felt feelings of inadequacy about providing support to colleagues.	• Education on pain management may be needed for acute care staff. Alternatively, problem of pain control may be more complex in acute care where patients/relatives are reluctant to use opioids. • Difficulties involved in team work need to be recognized so that conflicts are managed constructively, so staff morale and common goal of patient care are maintained and not eroded. • Improved physical environment in acute care settings needed to allow for privacy. • Improve gap in nursing knowledge about how best to handle conflicts involved in coming to terms with

(in acute care and community settings)

- Providing support to colleagues and needing personal support were the most difficult problems for nurses to manage.
- In hospice and community settings physical problems were reported twice as often.
- Weakness and confusion were the most difficult to manage.
- It was questionable whether higher frequency of pain-related problems was due to greater sensitivity to the physical aspects of care or to more patients presenting with complex pain and symptom management issues.
- The frequency of death- related and emotional problems were fairly uniform across settings.
- Difficulty in management was also reported.

dying, i.e., treatment decisions and palliative care decisions.

- Acute care staff need support in dealing with the intensity of nurse-patient relationships, watching patients die, and fears of loosing emotional control when caring for dying patients.
- Staff also need educational preparation to deal with emotional responses and identification that occur when dealing with dying patients. This includes reflective practice involving self-awareness and acknowledging feelings. These require additional support from educators, mentors, and managers.
- Awareness that more esoteric, less familiar problems, such as spiritual problems may not be identified, need research.

(continued)

Table 12.1. Selected studies of stress in oncology/supportive care

Authors	Description of study	Personal variables	Stressors	Manifestations	Coping/intervention
• Copp and Dunn[20] (continued)			• Patients coming to terms with dying was the main death-related problem.		
• Wilkinson[21]	• 65 U.K. cancer nurses (98% response rate) studied to identify general proneness to stress and characteristics of nurses who experience the most stress • Nurses from 6 wards in 2 hospitals identified 2 most stressful incidents over last 3 months and completed Spielberger State–Trait Anxiety Inventory	• Newly qualified nurses were more anxious than sisters and enrolled nurses, perhaps because they lacked security in their role. • Nurses who attended church weekly had the lowest anxiety levels. • Nurses who had not taken a post-basic course in cancer nursing had more stressors related to nursing advanced cancer patients. • Nurses experienced high job satisfaction perhaps because they had self-selected to nurse cancer patients and had already established that they could cope with cancer nursing.		• Nurses prone to anxiety had the same values as working females • Anxiety and job satisfaction differed across wards. • Low level of stress	• Most nurses reported high levels of job satisfaction. • Preceptorship program for newly qualified nurses may help them to feel less anxious. • There is some indication that religious faith may be helpful in coping with cancer nursing but this finding requires more research. • Ward managers need to create an environment in which open discussion of difficulties and stressors is encouraged. Otherwise, nurses will experience higher levels of stress and lower job satisfaction.

• Papadatou et al.[22]	• 217 Greek oncology nurses and 226 general hospital nurses (82% response rate) in Athens area • Study to determine burnout levels of oncology nurses compared with those in general hospitals and to identify personal and environmental factors that contribute to burnout • Maslach Burnout Inventory, Hardiness Scale, Ways of Coping Scale, Life Style Scale, Type A Behavior Scale, Job Stress Questionnaire, General Information Questionnaire	• Personality characteristics predicted greater percentage of variability in burnout score than occupational and demographic variables. • Hardy personality and sense of control over what happens in life and work environment protected nurses from emotional exhaustion, depersonalization and lack of personal accomplishment. • Nurses who had high initial expectations of career were more likely to have high burnout and low job satisfaction. • Nurses more vulnerable to burnout tended to overestimate their abilities and/or embellish reality. They were more easily discouraged when the situation did not correspond to their ideals.	• Oncology nurses had more free time on the job and fewer night shifts. • Heavy workload was the only job stressor associated with burnout and emotional exhaustion in particular.	• No statistical differences in burnout were experienced by both groups. • Oncology nurses had lower emotional exhaustion. • Oncology nurses had lower levels of stress due to workload and shortage of personnel. • Stress was associated with lack of support from senior colleagues and difficulty balancing demands of work and home life. • Nurses who experienced a higher degree of burnout reported a sense of lack of control over external events. sense of personal control protected nurses from burnout	• Oncology nurses may change their philosophy toward life, become more realistic and re-evaluate their priorities. • They may discover the richness of oncology nursing, and find meaning and get satisfaction from caring for patients in this specialty. • The challenge may counterbalance stress. • Prevention and management of burnout should address individual needs and reduce frequency and intensity of job stressors. • Adequate staffing, flexible scheduling, promotion of support among co-workers, effective leadership, and career enrichment opportunities are needed. • Programs are needed to explore nurses' perceptions, feelings, and attitudes towards their role, as well as toward

(continued)

Table 12.1. Selected studies of stress in oncology/supportive care

Authors	Description of study	Personal variables	Stressors	Manifestations	Coping/intervention
• Papadatou et al.[22] (continued)					health, illness, pain, and death and to enhance coping skills when dealing with stressful job situations. • Educational programs, support groups, interprofessional consultation, and careful staff selection are needed.
• McAbee[23]	• 663 U.S. employed women: 200 oncology nurses (30.4% response rate), 215 nononcology nurses (28.3% response rate), 232 university employees, primarily clerical staff and educators (29% response rate) • Investigated specificity of coping strategies and organizational social supports of oncology nurses • Author constructed, self-administered questionnaire				• The top four coping strategies reported for all groups were exercise, talk, take a break, and relaxation. • Oncology nurses averaged 9.98 people with whom they could discuss their problems. This was nonsignificantly higher than in the other 2 groups. • Organizational support took the form of scheduled support groups, scheduled "rap sessions," and critical inci-

			dent debriefing. Informal support came through an atmosphere for discussion and supportive supervisors and co-workers. • Exercise was the most common strategy reported by all 3 groups. Formal and informal unscheduled facilities need to be available on a flexible basis. • Talking it out was the second most common strategy both at work and at home. An informal lounge was helpful. • Oncology nurses were more likely to report using counseling and EAP programs.
• Ramirez et al.[24]	• 393 U.K. senior oncologists and palliative care specialists' national survey • Mailout questionnaire with 83% response rate • Assessed prevalence and causes of burnout and psychiatric disorder	• Younger age (55 or under) was associated with burnout. • Occupational factors have a causal role in distress experienced by cancer clinicians; they precipitate burnout and psychiatric disorder in those who are	• The stressors of being overloaded and its effect on home life, dealing with patients' suffering and being involved with treatment toxicity and errors were similar to those from junior doctors, general practi-	• The estimated prevalence of psychiatric disorder was 28%, which was similar to that of British junior house officers. • Levels of emotional exhaustion and low personal accomplishment were similar to those
			• Dealing well with patients and relatives was the most important source of job satisfaction. • Increased resources to lessen overload. • Communication skills training reduced stress and enhanced satisfac-

(continued)

Table 12.1. Selected studies of stress in oncology/supportive care

Authors	Description of study	Personal variables	Stressors	Manifestations	Coping/ intervention
• Ramirez et al.[24] (*continued*)	• Maslach Burnout Inventory, 12-item General Health Questionnaire, author-constructed questionnaire on job stress and satisfaction	• psychologically vulnerable. • Family psychiatric history, childhood experience of illness, death and emotional neglect and particular personality traits have previously been described as placing physicians at risk.	tioners, doctors generally and cancer health professionals of all disciplines. • Having organizational responsibilities and conflicts was the second and most important cause of stress for cancer clinicians. This was not previously documented and may reflect ongoing changes in health delivery in the U.K. It did not increase the risk of burnout or psychiatric disorder.	found in American doctors and nurses but lower levels of depersonalization were found. • Burnout was more common among clinical oncologists than among medical oncologists and palliative care specialists. • Psychiatric disorder was independently associated with feeling overloaded, dealing with treatment toxicity and errors and deriving little satisfaction from professional status and esteem. • Burnout was related to the above factors and to high stress and low satisfaction in dealing with patients and to low satisfaction from having inadequate resources.	tion of dealing with patients, reducing stress of dealing with treatment toxicity and errors and enhancing professional esteem. • Training in management skills reduced stress of overload and increased professional esteem. • Changing the criteria for selection to exclude those who are vulnerable to the stress of cancer and burnout might reduce burnout and psychiatric disorder but might also exclude those who are more empathic and self-critical and have an important contribution to make to medicine, albeit at a personal cost. • Overload issue needs to be addressed.

• Ramirez et al.[25]	• 882 U.K. consultants in gastroenterology, surgery, radiology, and oncology • Mailout questionnaire with 78% response rate • Relationship between consultants' mental health and job stress and satisfaction, job and demographic characteristics • Maslach Burnout Inventory, 12-item General Health Questionnaire, author-constructed questionnaire on job stress and satisfaction	• Being 55 or less and being single were independent risk factors for burnout. • There was a higher prevalence of psychiatric morbidity in females but this was not related to gender differences in job stress and satisfaction. It may reflect generally higher rates of psychiatric illness in women.	• The estimated prevalence of psychiatric disturbance was 27%; there was no significant difference across specialties. These results are similar to those of a recent study of 500 Scottish consultants who showed a prevalence rate of 21%. • Feeling overloaded and its effect on home life, feeling poorly managed and resourced, and dealing with patients' suffering were associated with both burnout and psychiatric distress.
		• Those who felt insufficiently trained in communication and management skills had significantly higher levels of distress. • Palliative care doctors had the lowest levels of stress and highest job satisfaction.	• Job satisfaction significantly protected mental health against the adverse effects of job stress. • Consultants may be able to tolerate stresses of medical practice that arise primarily from overload, provided that their sources of job satisfaction are protected. • Having professional status and esteem, feeling well managed and resourced, and having autonomy are all concerned with having effective control over work, which is an im-

(continued)

Table 12.1. Selected studies of stress in oncology/supportive care

Authors	Description of study	Personal variables	Stressors	Manifestations	Coping/ intervention
• Ramirez et al.[25] *(continued)*				• Burnout was also associated with deriving low satisfaction from relationships with patients, relatives, and staff. • Low satisfaction was related to professional status and esteem and to low satisfaction from intellectual stimulation • Burnout was more common amongst consultants who felt insufficiently trained in communication and management skills. • Stress and satisfaction were only weakly related to each other but both influenced burnout and psychiatric morbidity. • Surgeons had the highest scores for stress and satisfaction; radiologists had the lowest scores on stress factors and the lowest scores on satisfaction factors.	portant determinant of mental health. • The high demands of medicine may become intolerable if control over work and autonomy in decision-making is removed. • Mental health may be protected by maintaining or enhancing job satisfaction through autonomy and variety in work as well as by effective training in communication and management skills.

| • Graham et al.[26] | • 126 U.K. palliative care specialists (82% response rate) and 882 consultants in surgery, gastroenterology, radiology, and oncology
• Mailout qeustionnaire
• Instruments as above | • For palliative physicians feeling overloaded and its effect on home life made the greatest contribution to job stress. 35% of palliative care physicians felt inadequately trained in communication skills and 81% felt inadequately trained in management skills.
• Palliative care physicians reported less stress from dealing with distressed relatives, breaking bad news, and dealing with fatal illness and death than other consultants.
• Palliative physicians had more difficulty in relationships with nurses.
• The roles of consultant and nurse should be clarified.
• Physicians working in acute care hospitals who aim to cure disease and prolong life may experience failure when they feel they have nothing left to offer patients. | • Palliative physicians reported less stress from overload, and less stress and more satisfaction with the way they were managed and resourced.
• Hospital-based palliative care physicians experienced more stress and less satisfaction from management and had less resources than those working in hospices.
• Burnout was more prevalent among those who felt insufficiently trained in communication and management skills. | • Palliative physicians reported having good relationships with patients and relatives, and staff made the greatest contribution to job satisfaction.
• Effective training in communication and, management skills would help.
• At least current levels of resourcing and management practices in palliative care should be maintained.
• Health professionals with better mental health may choose to work in palliative care or, alternatively, the culture or approach of palliative care may protect staff from levels of distress experienced by those in other areas.
• Role ambiguity needs to be addressed to decrease burnout. |

Studies assessing the stress of caregivers in supportive care often focus on the concept of burnout, but other symptoms of distress are also important. This chapter will therefore review papers related to stress in supportive care and will not focus exclusively on burnout.

Personal Variables

Demographic variables

Age

Younger staff have often been found to report more stressors, manifestations of stress, and fewer coping strategies than older caregivers (45 and over).[8] Younger, inexperienced hospice nurses had more difficulty dealing with death and dying and dealing with relatives and patients,[13] and nurses who had not taken a post-basic course in cancer nursing had more stressors related to nursing more advanced canver patients.[21] Newly qualified nurses were more anxious than more experienced colleagues.[21] However, younger, less educated caregivers were not as vulnerable to burnout if there was dissonance between their values and the work environment as were older colleagues.[11]

Generally, older caregivers report less stress.[14,18] Palliative care specialists and consultants in oncology, surgery, gastroenterology, and radiology over age 55 were found to be less likely to have burnout than their younger colleagues.[24-26] Older nurses and those with more years of practice scored lower on the Emotional Exhaustion scale of the MBI, although those with more years of experience of hospital nursing and on the same unit on which they were currently working had lower personal accomplishment scores on the MBI.[19]

Other studies however, have found that general practitioners at the highest risk for job distress were older, male, and had type A personalities.[12] Older hospital nurses and those with less status were at greater risk of depression.[13]

Marital status and gender

Being married has been found to be associated with better coping[18] and being single and under 55 were independent risk factors for burnout.[25] The data on gender is inconclusive. In a study of almost 2000 British family practitioners, female general practitioners had greater job satisfaction and showed greater well-being than matched controls. Male physicians had higher anxiety scores than the norms, had less job satisfaction, and drank more alcohol than their female counterparts. Dealing with death and dying was not a major source of stress: however, it was associated with excess alcohol use—particularly for women physicians.[12]

Male physicians did not report as much difficulty with job/home interaction. For males, the demands of the job and patients' expectations were associated with job dissatisfaction.[12] Male oncologists have been found to be more likely to report burnout[15] and male nurses have higher levels of depersonalization on the MBI.[19]

In a recent study of United Kingdom specialists, there was a higher prevalence of psychiatric morbidity among females. This was not due to gender differences in job stress and satisfaction and was hypothesized to reflect the generally higher rates of psychiatric illness among women.[25] In a large Finnish study of physicians, although female physicians had slightly less stress than female white-collar workers, they were more likely than their male colleagues to have either attempted suicide or to have thought about doing so.[15]

Personality and spirituality[7]

Personality factors were found to predict a greater percentage of variability in burnout scores in oncology nurses than did occupational or demographic variables.[22] It has been hypothesized that "premorbid" personality characteristics that predispose staff to work in oncology could explain some of the differences in stress experienced by those in oncology compared with those in cardiac, intensive care, and surgical units.[17] It has also been suggested that health professionals with better mental health may choose to work in palliative care, or alternatively, the culture, or approach of palliative care may protect staff from levels of distress experienced by those in other areas.[26]

Research on the personality of oncology nurses using the Personal Style Inventory,[36] which is based on the 1923 work of Jung,[37] showed that the most common personality type for oncology nurses was ISFJ: feeling is introverted and perception is practical so that helping others is both a responsibility and a pleasure. Caregivers with these personality characteristics value interpersonal interactions and they have a great ability to empathize. The strengths of this personality type include independence, ability to work alone, diligence, and attention to detail. Traits that could be a hindrance include the proclivity to work alone and the tendency to act on internal reasoning without consulting others.[38]

Theories that emphasize the role of the individual in the development of burnout assert that the degree of burnout depends on personal characteristics, such as the individual's cognitive appraisal and coping strategies under stressful circumstances, motivation for entering the health field, expectations of self and others, and a failure to live up to one's ideals.[22]

The Hardy Personality has been found to be effective in combatting work stress and avoiding burnout.[39,40] The Hardy Personality involves a sense of commitment (as opposed to alienation) to oneself and the various areas in one's life, including work, which reflects the hardy person's curiosity about and a sense of meaningfulness of life; control (as opposed to powerlessness), reflecting the belief that one has the power to influence the course of events; and challenge (as opposed to threat), epitomizing the expectation that it is normal for life to change and for development to be stimulated. Hardiness is associated with fewer mental and physical symptoms of stress. "Hardiness is said to lead to a perception, interpretation, and handling of stressful events that prevents excessive activation of arousal and therefore results in fewer symptoms of stress."[41]

Hardiness was inversely related to burnout and physical illness in house officers at Memorial Sloan-Kettering Cancer Center.[34] A Hardy Personality and sense of control over what happens in life and the work environment was found to protect oncology nurses from emotional exhaustion, depersonalization, and a lack of personal accomplishment. Nurses who experienced higher degrees of burnout reported a lack of a sense of control over external events.[22]

Nurses who had high initial expectations of their career were more likely to have high burnout and low job satisfaction. Those who were more vulnerable to burnout tended to overestimate their abilities and/or to embellish reality. They were more easily discouraged when situations did not correspond to their ideals.

Religious beliefs were associated with decreased burnout in oncology house officers.[34] Nurses who attended church weekly had lower anxiety levels. It was felt that there was some indication that religious faith may be helpful in coping with cancer nursing but the finding requires more research.[21]

Occupational Stressors

When 581 professionals from all major disciplines and specialty areas working with the critically ill and dying were compared, the stressors of those in oncology differed from those in other settings in that they reported equal numbers of stressors in the areas of *patients and families* (patients and families with coping or personality problems, patients and families with whom they had communication problems, and identification with patient and family); *occupational role* (role over-load, role ambiguity, role conflict, lack of control); and *environmental stressors* (team communication problems, inadequate resources, communication problems with others in the system and unrealistic expectations of the organization.[8,9] The other specialty areas were far more likely to report the major stressors as coming from their work environment. Mount[42] delineated the stressors of oncologists as including exposure to death as an existential fact, emphasizing the finite nature of life; the cumulative grief associated with repeated unresolved losses; the pressures of a medical care system fueled by the medical information system; the inability to achieve the idealistic goals embraced by holistic medical care; and the stressors inherent in working as a team and the issues involved in treatment failure.

Patients and families

A number of issues related to patients and families were found to be associated with increased stress or burnout. These included communication problems with patients and families,[8–10,13] patient expectations,[12] identification with patients[8,9,14,17] dealing with critical illness, death and dying,[12–15,20] and administering palliative or terminal care.[16] It has been suggested that oncology nurses may be particularly susceptible to the more chronic situational stressors associated with the nature of their responsibilities and patient/family needs associated with deteriorating illness.[43] Compared with physicians in oncology, nurses reported greater stress associated with the empathic component of their relationship with patients, whereas physicians had less stress associated with interpersonal difficulties. Physicians' symptoms were more strongly associated with space, dealing with patients, and workday.[14] Nurses and doctors in oncology had more severe stress associated with patients than did colleagues in cardiology, intensive care and surgery.[17] When compared with those in palliative care, those in acute care settings were found to have more difficulty dealing with patients and their families.[8,11,13,24,26]

One of the major issues that may confront caregivers in supportive care is the difficulty that patients and families may experience when it becomes clear that continued active treatment aimed at the prolongation of life may no longer be appropriate. Patients coming to terms with dying was the main death-related concern of nurses working in acute care, hospice, and community settings in the United Kingdom.[20] The stress experienced by staff in the acute care setting was contrasted with that of staff in a hospital-based home care (HBHC) unit in Sweden. Patients in the hospital may be upset with the progression of their disease, despite ongoing treatment. These patients may be suffering the side effects of treatment, thus leading staff to question the quality of their care more. Patients and families in the HBHC have accepted the terminal nature of their disease and focus on symptom relief. They and their families have chosen to go home and are probably more motivated, and families have more positive expectations than those who stay in the hospital. The staff in the hospital experienced more stress, anxiety, tension, (groundless) guilt, and sleeping problems connected with their work.[18]

Medical consultants, other than those in palliative care, had difficulty dealing with patients' suffering and being involved with treatment toxicity.[24-26] Burnout and psychiatric distress were associated with these issues.[25] Burnout was far more common among clinical oncologists (formerly known as radiotherapists) and psychiatric disorder was in part related to dealing with treatment toxicity and errors and feeling insufficiently trained in communication skills.[24] Palliative care physicians reported less stress associated with dealing with distressed relatives, breaking bad news, and dealing with fatal illness than did other specialists.[26]

In supportive care it is important that when chemotherapy or radiation is being prescribed primarily for symptom control, then it is imperative that the treatment team communicate clearly with both the patient and family regarding the specific purpose of the therapy—e.g., for symptom control, not for prolongation of life. "The ideal informing process becomes one of shared learning. Patients learn about the medical facts, and the potential benefits and burdens of treatment, in the context of a realistic appraisal of their overall medical condition. Physicians, in turn, must learn of their patient's personal experiences and perceptions about the diagnosis, their current quality of life, and the amount of suffering they are willing to tolerate."[44]

These conversations are difficult. Caregivers must be prepared to give this information in a caring and sensitive manner, being ready to deal with the difficulty patients and families have in accepting this information. Caregivers must also be aware that patients and families may sometimes deny the reality of what is being said. Conversations to clarify the purposes of palliative therapies may have to take place periodically over the course of treatment.[45]

The process of adjusting to terminal illness is not easy. In Hinton's study of patients referred to the St. Christopher's Hospice Home Care Service, awareness of dying and coping attitudes of these patients at their first visit by the home care team were better predictors of which patients were likely to die at home than the symptoms they presented at that time.[46] Patients who stayed at home for death showed more awareness of dying than those who later became inpatients. Only 2 of the 22 patients (out of 77) who died at home initially denied or partly suppressed their prognosis, compared with 30 of the 55 patients subsequently admitted to the hospice for death. "At first the inpatient death group were more optimistic and declared stronger intention to fight the illness, although they later came closer to the home death patients in attitude."[46]

Occupational role

Reviewing studies from the past decade, Wilkinson noted that the stressors in oncology nursing have changed and are now work overload, lack of resources, and staff shortages. Conflicts with other healthcare workers (doctors in particular) seem to have decreased, possibly because of changes in pain and symptom control management. Nurses continue to be concerned about patient deterioration and death.[47]

The pressures of practice and work overload were associated with stress and burnout in many studies,[8–10,16,24–26] as were problems managing the home–work interface.[8–10,12–14,16,22,24–26] The more patients for whom the oncology nurse was responsible, the greater was her burnout score,[11] and heavy workload was the only job stressor associated with burnout, with emotional exhaustion being a particular stressor in a study of Greek oncology nurses.[22]

The experience of senior oncologists and palliative care physicians with respect to being overloaded and its effect on home life, dealing with patients' suffering, and being involved with treatment toxicity and errors, was similar to comparable results from junior doctors, general practitioners, doctors in general, and cancer health professionals of all disciplines.[24] Physicians working in acute care hospitals who aim to cure disease and prolong life may experience failure when they feel that they have nothing left to offer patients.[26] Although palliative care physicians found that feeling overloaded and its effect on their home life made the greatest contribution to their job stress, they had less stress from overload than did colleagues in surgery, gastroenterology, radiology, and oncology.[25]

Having organizational responsibilities and conflicts was the second most important cause of stress for cancer clinicians in the United Kingdom. Ramirez et al. note that this has not previously been documented and may reflect the ongoing changes in health delivery in the U.K. This variable did not increase the risk of burnout or psychiatric disorder in these clinicians.[24]

Caregivers sometimes felt inadequately prepared to carry out their jobs. Physicians who felt inadequately trained in communication and management skills had increased distress as measured on the General Health Questionnaire[24] as well as increased burnout on the Maslach Burnout Inventory.[25] Hospital nurses' heavy workload and attending to the physical needs of patients kept them from being able to attend continuing education courses to learn how to deal with the problems they were experiencing. They had difficulty dealing with the physical symptoms concerned with food intake, nausea, and vomiting as well as the emotional problems of patients and families.[18] Nurses caring for cancer patients in acute care, hospice, and community settings were compared. Hospice and community nurses reported physical problems twice as often as their colleagues in acute care. In the hospice and community settings, weakness and confusion were the most difficult to manage physical problems. Nurses in acute care found pain the most difficult to manage physical problem. Copp and Dunn questioned whether the higher frequency of pain-related problems in their study was due to the greater sensitivity of hospice and community nurses to pain or whether their patients presented with more complex pain and symptom management issues.[20]

Oncology nurses experience difficulty with "excessive demands, negative expectations from patients/families, unexpected crises, poor staffing/overwork/inadequate time, patient deaths, and balancing work and personal life"[38] (p. 484, quoting ref 48). Physicians had stress associated with decision-making and communicating diagnoses.[14] For both nurses and doctors in oncology one of the major stressors was disappointment in the power of medicine,[17] leading them to question their roles and the quality of care.[18] Similar problems were found in studies of oncologists[10,16] and other physicians.[15]

Work environment

Caregivers with university positions report less burnout.[15,16] Hospital-based palliative care physicians had more stress and less satisfaction from their management and resources than those working in hospices.[26] Hospital oncology nurses had less opportunity to talk about work-related feelings and problems than hospice nurses, were less likely to perceive communication with administration and quality of supervision to be excellent, and had less sense of control over decision-making.[11] Compared with hospice nurses, hospital nurses experienced more dissonance between their real and ideal work situation and had more hours spent in direct contact with patients, which was associated with higher burnout scores.[11] Hospital staff had less freedom to make their own decisions, less cooperation between day and night staff, heavier workload, more communication problems with patients, and a more frequent need to train new staff because of turnover.[18] Work-related problems were most common in acute care as were nurse-related problems.[20] The hospital oncology setting was more stressful and less reinforcing for nurses caring for oncology patients than was hospice.[11]

Team stress has consistently been identified as a major stressor in palliative care[5] but is also a problem in supportive care. Communication with other colleagues was a problem for oncologists.[10] Work-related and nurse-related problems were major stressors in acute oncology care in the United Kingdom. Providing support to colleagues and needing personal support were key concerns within the nurse-related categories and were ranked as the most difficult to manage problem.[20] Team relationship problems, which were sometimes related to advising doctors to use effective medication for pain and other symptoms, were problems in both acute care and community settings.[20] Interestingly, whereas nurses in palliative care in the United Kingdom did not report team communication problems with physicians and these problems were speculated to have decreased in oncology settings,[47] palliative care physicians in the United Kingdom reported more difficulty in their relationships with nurses than did their colleagues in other specialties. It was hypothesized that this finding was due to the lack of clarity of roles in the two disciplines.[26]

Manifestations

Physical

Few studies have investigated the physical problems associated with job stress. Elrich and FitzGerald reported that the stress–complaints relationship for physicians and nurses was quite different. For nurses, it was primarily interpersonal stress that related to physical distress. Nurses were more likely to have physical symptoms if their outside life failed to relieve the stress generated on their job. Overcommitment and identification led to tiredness and nurses suffered from exertion-related complaints.[14]

Physicians had much less stress associated with interpersonal difficulties. Their symptoms were much more strongly correlated with space, dealing with patients, and workday. Physicians' dissatisfactions with the job and working conditions, including space problems involving the work environment and dealing with patients, related to a general malaise.[14] The authors described a subpattern of symptoms that "linked stress to loss of control, in the form of irregular heartbeat, diarrhoea, discomfort in the throat, dizziness and breathlessness. The doctors' stress may derive in part from lack of confidence when faced with their limited ability to alter the course of the illness. Identification with the patients' suffering, which was linked to tiredness amongst nurses, had effects amongst doctors which suggest an almost physical rejection of the patient."[14]

Measuring burnout (Table 12.2)

Compared with previous studies using the same instrument, oncology nurses had significantly higher burnout scores than hospice nurses. Oncology nurses were in the mid-range and hospice nurses had the lowest burnout scores. Burnout was associated with less support in the workplace for both groups and interacted significantly with overload factors.[11]

Higher burnout in physicians was associated with specialties dealing with the chronically ill and incurable or dying patients. The authors hypothesized that hope or lack of it significantly influenced burnout.[15] Frustration or sense of failure was the most frequently chosen description of burnout in oncologists. The percentage of positive responses to burnout was proportional to the total percentage of time spent in patient care. Insufficient personal and or vacation time was the most frequent reason chosen to explain the existence of burnout.[16]

In the Ramirez et al. study of U.K. oncologists and palliative care specialists, the percentage of cancer clinicians reporting high levels of exhaustion and low personal accomplishment was similar to that of the normative sample for the Maslach Burnout Inventory.[50] Significantly fewer of the U.K. cancer clinicians reported high levels of depersonalization compared with the American sample (23% vs. 33%, $P < 0.0001$). Demographic factors associated with burnout included being age 55 or younger and being a clinical oncologist, rather than a medical oncologist or palliative care specialist. Job characteristics associated with burnout included being overloaded and its effect on home life, dealing with patients' suffering, low levels of satisfaction from having adequate resources, as well as low levels of satisfaction from dealing well with patients and relatives.

Table 12.2 Signs and symptoms of burnout

Fatigue

Physical and emotional exhaustion

Headaches

Gastrointestinal disturbances

Weight loss

Sleeplessness

Depression

Boredom

Frustration

Low morale

Job turnover

Impaired job performance (decreased empathy, increased absenteeism)[49]

Being a clinical oncologist and working part-time were independent risk factors for depersonalization. "Low personal accomplishment was associated with stress from 'being involved with treatment toxicity and errors' and low levels of satisfaction from 'dealing well with patients and relatives and from 'having professional status and esteem.' " (p. 1268) Feeling overloaded and its effect on home life, feeling poorly managed and resourced, and dealing with patients' suffering were associated with both burnout and psychiatric distress.[25] Burnout was also associated with deriving low satisfaction from relationships with patients, relatives, and staff.[25] Burnout was more common among consultants who felt insufficiently trained in communication and management skills.[25,26]

A study of burnout in oncology clinical nurse specialists showed that although the oncology group had lower burnout scores than other nursing groups previously studied, the best predictors of burnout were dissatisfaction with one's role, high levels of job stress, feelings of apathy and withdrawal, and inadequate psychological support at work.[51] A replication of this study with oncology nurses[52] found similar results, suggesting that oncology nurses experienced moderate amounts of burnout. Those nurses with relatively higher scores indicating burnout reported greater levels of job stress, a greater degree of job dissatisfaction, and lower levels of available perceived support in their work environment. Papadatou et al.[22] caution that both of the previous studies must be viewed with some caution because no control groups were used.

At Memorial Sloan-Kettering Cancer Center, studies found that oncology nurses showed high levels of emotional exhaustion, but relatively lower levels than house staff members of diminished empathy. The author hypothesized that this finding might have a particularly adverse effect on sensitivity and compassion in patient care for the house staff.[43] No significant difference was found in burnout scores for nurses in AIDS, oncology, special care units, medical ICUs and general medical units, except that nurses in medical ICUs scored significantly lower on the personal accomplishment scale of the MBI. Job tension was the key predictor of emotional exhaustion. Job influence and older age had significant protective effects. Recent changes in shifts were associated with higher levels of emotional exhaustion.[19]

Using a control group, Papadatou et al. found no statistically significant difference in burnout scores when comparing Greek oncology nurses with nurses in general hospitals, although oncology nurses had lower emotional exhaustion.[22] Personal characteristics were found to predict a greater percentage of variability in the burnout experience than either occupational or demographic variables. Among the personality dimensions, the existence of the Hardy Personality, especially the perceived control aspect of this personality type, seemed to be significant.[22] A sense of control was found to protect nurses from burnout. Nurses who experienced higher degrees of burnout reported a lack of a sense of control over external events. Among house staff hardiness was found to be negatively related to burnout and physical illness; negative work stressors were positively related to burnout as was supervisor support.[41]

Psychological distress

Almost two-thirds (61.9%) of oncologists found working in oncology stressful.[10] The estimated prevalence of psychiatric disorder for consultants in gastroenterology, surgery, radiology, and oncology was 27%. There was no significant difference across specialties. This finding is similar to that in British house officers and 500 Scottish consultants.[24,25] Low job satisfaction was related to professional status and esteem and low satisfaction from intellectual stimulation.[25] Psychiatric disorder in oncologists and palliative care specialists was independently associated with feeling overloaded, dealing with treatment toxicity and errors, and deriving little satisfaction from professional status and esteem. Oncologists and palliative care specialists who felt insufficiently trained in communication and management skills had significantly higher levels of distress.[24]

For general practitioners, four job stressors—demands of the job and patient expectations, interference with family life, constant interruptions at work and home, and practice administration—and age, sex, and type A behavior were significantly predictive of high levels of mental ill health or lack of well-being and accounted for over 15% of the variance in predicting lack of mental well-being. For women, the stress of the job interfering with family life was the most important factor contributing to negative mental well-being. For men, the work–home interface was the least important predictor, the most important predictors were interruptions, practice administration, demands of the job, and patient expectations. Male general practitioners were more emotionally anxious than females but did not reflect this in psychosomatic complaints.[12]

Oncology nurses reported feelings of rejection and frustration when they felt that their roles and knowledge were not adequately valued. They also felt inadequate when trying to provide emotional support to colleagues.[20] Studies comparing those in oncology with other specialties generally found few consistent differences. Oncology staff were more likely to report feelings of anger and frustration, helplessness, inadequacy, and insecurity.[8,9] Oncology nurses' proneness to general anxiety was no different from the normal values for working females; however, anxiety and job satisfaction differed across wards.[21] Greek oncology nurses had lower levels of stress due to workload and shortage of personnel, but stress was associated with a lack of support from colleagues and difficulty balancing the demands of work and home life.[22] The caregiver's role in the hospital was seen as less reinforcing and more stressful than in a hospice environment.[11] Poor mental health in hospital nurses was predicted by work affecting the home and dealing with relatives and patients, whereas for hospice nurses, poor mental health was predicted by staff support and involvement in decision-making and high workload.[13]

Although oncology, cardiac, intensive care, and surgical specialists suffered the same overall degree of work-related stress and physical complaints, the oncology group suffered more from feelings of emotional involvement and self-doubt. They had more severe stress associated with emotional involvement with patients and less difficulty with work and private life. They had less stress from institutional factors than comparison groups despite few objective differences in their situations.[17]

Behavioral

Work in supportive care can have a significant impact on home life.[8–10,12,13,22] The job of dealing with critically ill or dying patients had more adverse effects on the home life (and vice versa) of hospital nurses[13] and other specialists as compared with palliative care specialists.[26] Low job satisfaction was predicted by the expected reaction of superiors to home–work conflict and lack of support at work.[13]

Behavioral manifestations of stress can also include avoidance of patients[8,9] and inadequate symptom management, which may be due to a lack of education, inadequate assessment, carelessness, or overwork. Studies of pain severity have found that there was no statistically significant correlation between 103 patents with pain from solid tumors, their primary nurse, house officer, or oncology fellow on a visual analogue scale (VAS) rating pain on a 10-cm line. When patients rated their pain from 7 to 10 on the VAS scale, nurses placed the patient's pain in this range only 7% of the time (compared with house officers 20% and oncology fellows 27% of the time).[53] When the management of pain and constipation was assessed in 25 hospice and 19 cancer center patients being treated for pain, it was found that the patients in both settings continued to experience pain (VAS $M =$ 38.6 and 29.7, respectively) in spite of pain management regimens. However, the cancer center patients were given only 38% of the maximum dose of analgesia ordered whereas the hospice patients self-administered 93% of the ordered dose. Patients in the cancer center had daily mean VAS scores as high as 66.7 and in the hospice, as high as 96.7; single scores for cancer patients were as high as 79 and for hospice patients up to the maximum of 100. The study showed a lack of adequate assessment and lack of pain management strategies. For 79% of patients in the cancer center and 72% of patients in the hospice with constipation there was no documentation or in the chart revealing a remarkable lack of concern about this common problem.[54]

Coping

Satisfactions in work

Job satisfaction has been found to protect mental health against the adverse effects of job stress[25] and to have significant protective effects on emotional exhaustion and enhanced personal accomplishment.[19] A sense of competence, control, and pleasure in one's work was the primary coping strategy identified in caregivers across professional disciplines and in multiple specialties.[8,9] Nurses with high job satisfaction preferred a coping mechanism labeled "effort and reasoning," which was similar to a sense of competence and involved a sense of mastery. This group showed little depressive withdrawal compared with a group that did not use this coping mechanism.[55] Nurses who felt they had more influence over their job situation reported higher levels of accomplishment.[19]

The personality types of those in supportive care[17,26,38] may be complementary to the stressors identified in the work setting,[48] leading presumably to increased job satisfaction. In addition, the challenge of working with cancer patients may serve as a reward that counterbalances the stressful aspects of practice.[22] There is some evidence, however, that job satisfaction in oncology nurses is declining.[47]

In a study of 147 physician members of the American Society of Clinical Oncology (ASCO), 80% reported that they were somewhat or very satisfied with working in oncology. Their satisfactions included effective treatment, the challenge of oncology, positive relations with patients and families, personal satisfactions, symptom management, positive professional interactions, and emotional support to patients and families.[10] Similar findings were reported from the British study in which 20 sources of satisfaction items were aggregated into four factors. The four satisfaction items were dealing well with patients and relatives, which contributed most to overall job satisfaction, followed by having professional status and esteem, deriving intellectual stimulation, and having adequate resources. The overall pattern was for clinical oncologists to report the lowest levels of satisfaction for all the factors. Medical oncologists reported higher levels of satisfaction from deriving intellectual stimulation than did either of the other two groups. Palliative care specialists reported the highest levels of satisfaction from dealing well with patients and relatives and having adequate resources. Palliative care physicians had the lowest levels of stress and the highest job satisfaction.[24] They reported that having good relationships with patients, relatives, and staff made the greatest contribution to job satisfaction. In addition, palliative care physicians had more satisfaction with the way they were managed and resources.[26] For general practitioners, the highest levels of satisfaction were reported from the amount of responsibility given, the amount of freedom in choosing working methods, and the amount of variety in the job.[12]

The three most important sources of rewards for oncology nurses were patients, co-workers, and new skills, but each of the sources of rewards could also be a source of difficulty (e.g., relationships with patients were rewarding but emotions could be evoked as nurses watched patients suffer). Critical incidences that showed the essence of oncology nursing were handling emergencies, preventing serious errors, helping with emotional distress, and empathizing with patients.[49] The rewards of oncology nursing were identified as patients getting well and patients' expressions of gratitude for emotional support.[48]

A comparison of the stressors and rewards in oncologists and oncology nurses found that both disciplines received their greatest rewards from helping patients, but physicians more often described satisfaction from curing cancer and learning and advancing research whereas nurses emphasized the rewards of meeting personal goals for patient care.[56]

Personal coping strategies

The top four personal coping mechanisms of oncology nurses, nononcology nurses, and women employed in a university setting were exercise, talk, taking a break, and relaxation. Oncology nurses had nonsignificantly more people with whom they could share their problems than did the other groups.[23] Social support, both on and off the job, is generally considered to be one of the most effective coping mechanisms.[8–10,23,55]

Recognition of the sources of one's stress is also important.[10] Weisman recommends that caregivers learn how to cope better with their own needs and know enough not to get caught in the subtle promises that are often made that "if only you take your treatment the way we prescribe, meditate on your white blood cells knocking out your cancer, and change your lifestyle, all will be fine." He also recommends learning how to share one's concerns with colleagues, and attempting to make a series of small contributions towards a patient's welfare rather than trying to be all things to all people. The ability to maintain realistic goals with the patients with whom one works allows caregivers to continue to experience pleasure even during many years of work in the field.[57]

Caregivers in oncology were the only group to speak of developing multiple roles as a way of coping with job stress. This is interesting in view of the fact that they were the only group to report major problems with work overload.[8,9] This finding is congruent with more recent research stressing the importance of intellectual stimulation to those in oncology.[10,24,25]

Personal philosophy of illness, death and professional role

A personal philosophy of illness, death and one's professional role is an important coping mechanism.[8,9] It was recommended that oncologists need a better appreciation of the positive contribution they can make to palliative care.[16] Oncology nurses were found to change their philosophy to life, become more realistic, and re-evaluate their priorities.[22]

A personal philosophy takes considerable time and thoughtfulness to develop. A philosophy that is helpful has been articulated by Weisman, who said that when he sent young medical students to interview dying patients and they expressed their hesitancy to do so, he told them, "When you go to see these people don't feel guilty that they are dying and you are living. Remember, your time will come, and it may be sooner than you think. As you speak to these people ask yourself, 'What can I do now when it's not my turn that I hope someone else will do tomorrow when it may be.'"[8]

For some, a religious philosophy, centered around a commitment to serve others, may be both helpful and key to deriving a sense of meaning in difficult times. Religion can be a helpful coping mechanism.[21,34,55] However, when caregivers use their own personal religious beliefs to reach out to patients, this may or may not be helpful to patients.[58]

It may also be useful to assume the perspective that "it's not my fault that this person has the disease, but my responsibility is to do what I can to help to lift the burden." Decision-making is thus a shared responsibility. By participating in a collaborative relationship, caregivers can enable patients to heighten their sense of control through increased self-awareness and understanding of the disease process and treatment.[59]

Inherent in a philosophy of practice is the right, and indeed obligation, to mourn for those who have died. Although not all patients will touch caregivers equally, in many situations, patient deaths and the ensuing staff grief deserve recognition. Acknowledging the deaths of individual patients can enable practitioners to avoid the accumulation of grief that comes from repeated, unresolved losses.[42] However, at times, multiple losses can lead to a sense of grief overload that may need to be dealt with in a variety of ways, including memorial services, journaling, staff "wakes," or attending a funeral. In addition, participating in a grief process can enable caregivers to assess what one has gained from this relationship in a manner which may be helpful to future clinical practice.[59,60]

Lifestyle management
While lifestyle management is certainly not a panacea for dealing with work stress, it enables one to have the energy to cope with stressors. It reflects an acknowledgment of an individual's need to learn his or her own body's response to stress to detect signals of significant overload. When one finds oneself experiencing symptoms of stress, such as headaches, gastric disturbances, increased infections, a lack of pleasure in one's professional roles and responsibilities, or feeling overwhelmed by responsibilities, it is often time to take a break, before one develops more serious symptoms. This break may be a few hours away from one's desk to pursue another interest or a longer break of a few days or weeks.[60] Oncologists found it helpful to engage in activities outside of their practice[10] and felt that more vacation or personal time was needed to alleviate burnout.[16]

Effective lifestyle management involves developing a balance between one's personal and professional lives. The emotional health of oncology nurses was predicted more by work affecting the home and dealing with patients and relatives, compared with hospice nurses.[13] Controlling job–home interaction can be very difficult, particularly for those who have developed multiple professional roles, such as clinician, researcher, and writer. One technique for managing such role conflicts can be to use the "ten-year rule." Ask yourself: "Ten years from now, which will matter more, that this article was a few days or weeks late or that I consistently sacrificed myself or members of my personal network for career goals, many of which may have been imposed by others?" Certainly there are times when career demands must take precedence, but if one always bows to career demands at personal and family sacrifice, one may need to look at one's sense of self-esteem.[60] Although lifestyle management and good health habits, including diet, exercise, and rest are all helpful in stress reduction, caregivers often do not mention using these coping strategies.[49]

Additional techniques found to be useful include the development of totally different outside activities, meditation, relaxation, and hobbies. There is some evidence from AIDS caregivers that escapist leisure engagements—those that involve high levels of distraction and allow little capacity for reflection—appear to be ineffective solutions for preventing burnout, particularly the aspect of attentional fatigue that is associated with continued, focused caring. Such escapist leisure activities actually appear to incur negative psychological effects. In contrast, restorative activities—those which engage attention but still provide room for reflection (e.g., walking, gardening) influence functioning in a positive way and provide for restoration and renewal.[61]

Environmental coping mechanisms

Team philosophy, support and team building

Although personal coping mechanisms are important, the work environment also has a role to play in helping caregivers provide effective supportive care. The most important environmental coping strategy identified in an international study of caregivers was a sense of team philosophy, support, and team building.[8,9] Within the work environment, the development of supportive, collaborative relationships may be fundamental to an enhancement of self-efficacy and self-esteem. Improving interprofessional cooperation and team processes and group support in nursing was found to provide the best protective or buffering approach to many health stressors, especially burnout.[55] The perception of social support at work was also correlated with lower burnout.[11] Staff support and involvement in decision-making was important to both acute care and hospice nurses but was of greater consequence to hospice nurses.[13] In a study of social workers, the most important source of social support was their relationships with other staff in the hospital. Specific social work support groups and peer supervision did not provide the support that interaction with those from other disciplines did.[62]

There is a need for recognition of difficulties involved in team work so that conflicts are managed constructively and staff morale and the common goal of patient care are maintained and not eroded.[20] However, caregivers reported difficulty in the areas of developing trust within an interdisciplinary team, communicating information, resolving power struggles, handling conflict, and ensuring team longevity.[8]

Team development always involves tension and conflict.[63] This may be viewed as the result of competition, lack of role definition, or poor leadership, but it can also be viewed as a reflection of contradictory institutional goals. Team members may become entrapped in conflicting relationships through the interaction of limited resources, competing demands, and unrealistic institutional priorities and, as a consequence, come to represent differing value systems within the organization. Team members of different disciplines may become involved in rivalry and "turf wars" in the current tight economic climate in which the roles of many professional groups are being challenged.

An effective team must have clarity of objectives, mission, and priorities that are shared by all team members. Role expectations should be realistic and well defined when they overlap. Effective decision-making and problem-solving processes should be in place to arrive at the best possible solution. Environmental norms should exist that support the tasks of problem solving. There should be a concern for each other's needs and an opportunity for individuals to enlarge their roles and optimize their chances for personal growth.[64]

Counseling

The availability of individual counseling was suggested in numerous studies to deal with the pressures of work,[12] feelings about death and dying,[13] as well as to deal with consultants experiencing stress and burnout.[26] Such services must, of course, be confidential and independent of management.[26] When oncology nurses were compared with nurses from other specialties as well as university women, the oncology nurses were found to be most likely to use employee assistance programs.[23]

Education

Educational programs were suggested for general practitioners. This involved training in social and management skills, including time management, people management, and work organization skill development.[12] Better management training is needed for hospice administrators given that the strongest predictors of mental ill health in nurses were linked to a lack of support from senior staff and organizational issues.[13] Training programs for oncologists need to provide more realistic expectations of the reality of dealing with clinical practice involving the total care of patients.[16] Communication skills training is recommended to reduce stress and enhance satisfaction in dealing with patients, to reduce the stress of dealing with treatment toxicity and errors, and to enhance professional esteem.[13,14,24-26] Education for death and dying is important and should focus on specific behaviours, rather than on anxiety regarding death.[18] Assistance is needed to help staff become more aware of how best to handle conflicts, such as patients and families coming to terms with dying, treatment decisions and palliative care decisions, dealing with the intensity of staff–patient relationships, watching patients die, and fears of loosing control while caring for dying patients.[20] Communication skills training should include role-playing of difficult situations with other health professionals as well as with patients and relatives.[26]

An educational and supportive intervention for house staff at Memorial Sloan-Kettering Cancer Center compared staff rotating to a medical oncology unit with a control unit. Surveys were completed after at least 4 weeks on the unit and 2 months after completing the rotation. The intervention decreased burnout in residents. From the patients' perspective, the house staff on the unit were perceived as being more empathic, sensitive, and compassionate. Hardiness was inversely related to burnout and physical illness, negative work stressors were positively related to burnout, and supervisor support was inversely related to burnout. House staff who had religious beliefs reported less burnout.[34]

Training in management skills to reduce the stress of overload and increase professional esteem is needed.[24,26] Improved education is also needed for the assessment and management of physical symptoms, including appetite disturbances, nausea, and vomiting,[18] and pain, including patient–family education, such as the effective use of opioids.[20,54] Programs are needed to enable nurses to explore their perceptions, feelings, and attitudes towards their role, as well as towards health, illness, pain, and death. Programs also needed to enhance coping skills when dealing with stressful job situations.[22]

Support groups

Support groups are recommended, but caregivers often report finding them to be ineffective.[8] Nurses and university employees reported finding formal scheduled support groups, scheduled "rap sessions," and critical incident debriefing to be helpful.[23] Weekly interdisciplinary "pizza rounds" have been found to be helpful in "enhancing patient care by improving interdisciplinary functioning and by providing staff with the opportunity to exchange ideas, solve problems involving difficult patients and families, develop consistent plans for patient management and ventillate their emotional responses to job-related stress."[69] Private space is needed for these meetings and for staff to take a break either alone or with colleagues.[20,23]

Administrative policies

Changing the criteria for selection to exclude those who might be vulnerable to the stress of cancer and burnout might reduce burnout and psychiatric disorder, but it might also exclude those who are more empathic and self-critical and have important contributions to make to medicine, albeit at a personal cost.[24] The issue of overload needs to be addressed.[24] Practising medical oncologists might benefit from a reduced work week with more personal and family time. This may lead to a reduction in their income unless services are reimbursed at a higher rate.[16] The high demands of medicine may become intolerable if control over work and autonomy in decision-making is removed. Mental health may be protected by maintaining or enhancing job satisfaction through autonomy and variety in work as well as effective training in communication and management skills.[25]

Administrators need to create an environment in which open discussion of difficulties and stressors is encouraged. If it is not encouraged, staff will experience higher levels of stress and lower job satisfaction.[21] The prevention and management of burnout should address individual needs and reduce the frequency and intensity of job stressors. This requires adequate staffing, flexible scheduling, the promotion of support among co-workers, effective leadership, and career enrichment opportunities.[22]

Role ambiguity can be detrimental to individuals and management of a unit as a whole; nurses need a clear sense of direction and influence over decisions regarding assignments and case loads. Administrators must not promise decision-making power when the results of deliberation will not be implemented.[20]

Discussion

Caregivers prone to burnout tend to have unrealistically high expectations for satisfaction in one area of life—often in work.[29,31] They overinvest initially and tend to work harder and harder to meet their own increasingly high expectations of perfection. They tend to have difficulty balancing work with home life and to sacrifice their personal life for work, unconsciously hoping to fill a vacuum that may exist from an earlier point in their life. In the supportive care environment in which work overload from multiple sources is an increasing problem, the needs of patients are immediate, communication skills with patients, family, and colleagues need to be improved, and managerial skills may be lacking, it is easy for caregivers to find themselves sacrificing all aspects of their personal life for work, leaving themselves vulnerable to burnout and psychological and physical distress. Caregivers with a high initial expectation of their career may be particularly vulnerable to burnout.[22] For this reason, caregivers, particularly oncologists, should be taught to appreciate the value of a role at the palliative phase of disease.[16] If caregivers come into supportive care, primarily wishing to cure patients, they will be most vulnerable to the problems involved with treatment toxicity and communicating with patients and families struggling with illness and death. The provision of effective supportive care requires caregivers with a solid knowledge base, access to ongoing educational programs, a clear sense of their value and self-worth as individuals and as professionals, and an ability to maintain an effective balance between work and home life. Caregivers need a work environment that avoids overload, allows for some control enhancing job satisfaction, and has good managerial policies. This balance will enhance job satisfaction and decrease the risk of psychiatric distress and burnout.

References

1. Supportive Care Program Committee. *Providing Supportive Care for Individuals Living with Cancer*. Toronto: Ontario Cancer Treatment and Research Foundation, May, 1994:15.
2. Vachon MLS. The stress of professional caregivers. In: Doyle D, Hanks GW, MacDonald N, eds. *Oxford Textbook of Palliative Medicine*. 2nd ed. Oxford: Oxford University Press; 1998: 919–929.
3. Walsh D. Palliative care: management of the patient with advanced cancer. *Semin Oncol* 1994; 21(4 Suppl 7):100–106.

4. Ferris F, Cummings T. *Palliative Care: Towards a Consensus in Standardized Principles of Practice*. Ottawa: Canadian Palliative Care Association, 1995.

5. Vachon MLS. Staff stress in hospice/palliative care: a review. *Palliat Med* 1995; 9:91–122.

6. Vachon MLS. Burnout and symptoms of stress in staff working in palliative care. In: Chochinov HM, Breitbart W, eds. *Psychiatric Dimensions of Palliative Medicine*. New York: Oxford University Press; in press.

7. Vachon MLS. Stress and burnout in oncology. In: Berger A, Levy MH, Portenoy RK, Weissman DE, eds. *Principles and Practices of Supportive Oncology*. Philadelphia: J.B. Lippincott; in press.

8. Vachon MLS. *Occupational Stress in the Care of the Critically Ill, Dying and Bereaved*. Washington: Hemisphere Publishing, 1987.

9. Vachon MLS. Stress in oncologists. *Can J Oncol* 1993; 3:166–172.

10. Schmale J, Weinberg N, Pieper S. Satisfactions, stresses and coping mechanisms of oncologists in clinical practice. *Am Soc Clin Oncol* 1987; 6:A:1003.

11. Bram PJ, Katz LF. A study of burnout in nurses working in hospice and hospital oncology settings. *Oncol Nurs Forum* 1989; 16:555–560.

12. Cooper GL, Rout U, Faragher B. Mental health, job satisfaction, and job stress among general practitioners. *Br Med J* 1989; 298:366–370.

13. Cooper CL, Mitchell S. Nursing the critically ill and dying. *Hum Relations* 1990; 43:297–311.

14. Ulrich A, FitzGerald P. Stress experienced by physicians and nurses in the cancer ward. *Soc Sci Med* 1990; 31:1013–1022.

15. Olkinuora M, Asp S, Juntunen J, Kauttu K, Strid L, Äärimaa M. Stress symptoms, burnout and suicidal thoughts in Finnish physicians. *Soc Psychiatry Psychitr Epidemiol* 1990;.25:81–86.

16. Whippen DA, Canellos GP. Burnout syndrome in the practice of oncology. *J Clin Oncol* 1991; 9:1916–1921.

17. Herschbach P. Work-related stress specific to physicians and nurses working with cancer patients. *J Psychosoc Oncol* 1992; 10:(2);79–99.

18. Beck-Friis B, Strang P, Sjödén P-O. Caring for severely ill cancer patients: a comparison of working conditions in hospital-based home care and in hospital. *Support Care Cancer* 1993; 1:145–151.

19. Van Servellen G, Leake B. Burn-out in hospital nurses: a comparison of acquired immunodeficiency syndrome, oncology, general medical, and intensive care unit nurse samples. *J Prof Nurs* 1993;9: 169–177.

20. Copp G, Dunn V. Frequent and difficult problems perceived by nurses caring for the dying in community, hospice and acute care settings. *Palliat Med* 1993; 7:19–25.

21. Wilkinson SM. Stress in cancer nursing: does it really exist? *J Adv Nurs* 1994; 20:1079–1084.

22. Papadatou D, Anagnostopoulos F, Monos D. Factors contributing to the development of burnout in oncology nursing. *Br J Med Psychol* 1994; 67:187–199.

23. McAbee R. Job stress and coping strategies among nurses: results of a self report survey. *Am Assoc Occup Health Nurs J* 1994; 42:483–487.

24. Ramirez AJ, Graham J, Richards MA, Cull A, Gregory WM, Leaning MS, Snashall DC, Timothy AR. Burnout and psychiatric disorder among cancer clinicians. *Br J Cancer* 1995; 71:1263–1269.

25. Ramirez AJ, Graham J, Richards MA, Cull A, Gregory WM. Mental health of hospital consultants: the effect of stress and satisfaction at work. *Lancet* 347:724–728. 1996.

26. Graham J, Ramirez AJ, Cull A, Gregory WM, Finlay I, Hoy A, Richards MA. Job stress and satisfaction among palliative physicians: A CRC/ICRF Study. *Palliat Med* 1996; 10:185–194.

27. James N. Emotional labour: skill and work in the social regulation of feelings. *Social Rev* 1989; 37:15–42.

28. Freudenberger HJ. Staff burnout. *J Soc Issues* 1974; 30:159–165.

29. Edelwich J, Brodsky A. *Burn-out: Stages of Disillusionment in the Helping Professions*. New York: Springer-Verlag, 1980.

30. Maslach M. *Burnout—The Cost of Caring*. New York: Prentice Hall Gilmore, 1982.

31. Vachon MLS. Battle fatigue in hospice/palliative care. In Gilmore A, & Gilmore S, eds. *A Safer Death*. New York: Plenum; 1988:149–160.

32. Pines AM. Who is to blame for helper's burnout? Environmental impact. In: Scott CD, Hawk J, eds. *Heal Thyself: The Health of Health Care Professionals*. New York: Brunner/Mazel; 1986:19–43.

33. Maslach C, Jackson SE. *The Maslach Burnout Inventory* (Manual). 2nd ed. Palo Alto: Consulting Psychologists Press, 1986.

34. Kash K, Breitbart W, Holland Jr, Berenson S, Marks E, Lesko L, Ouellette-Kobasa S. A stress-reducing intervention for medical oncology housestaff. *Am Soc Clin Oncol* 1989; 8:A1214.

35. Jones JW. The staff burnout scale: a validity study. Paper presented at the 52nd annual meeting of the Midwestern Psychological Association, St. Louis MO, 1980.

36. Hogan C, Champagne D. Hogan-Champagne reference survey. In: Champagne D, Hogan C, eds. *Supervisory and Management Skills: A Competency-Based Training Program for Middle Managers of Educational Systems*. Pittsburgh: University of Pittsburgh Press: 1979.

37. Jung C. *Psychological Types*. Princeton: Princeton University Press, 1980.

38. Bean CA, Holcombe JK. Personality types of oncology nurses. *Cancer Nurs* 1993; 16:479–485.

39. Kobasa SC. Stressful life events, personality and health: an inquiry into hardiness. *J Pers Soc Psychol* 1979; 37:1–11.

40. Kobasa SC, Maddi SR, Kahn S. Hardiness and health: a prospective inquiry. *J Pers Soc Psychol* 1982; 42:168–177.

41. Kash KM, Holland JC. Special problems of physicians and house staff in oncology. In: Holland JC, Rowland JH, eds. *Handbook of Psychooncology*. New York: Oxford University Press; 1989:647–657.

42. Mount BM. Dealing with our losses. *J Clin Oncol* 1986; 4:1127–1134.

43. Hansell PS. Stress on nurses in oncology. In: Holland JC, Rowland JH, eds. *Handbook of Psychooncology*. New York: Oxford University Press; 1989:658–663.

44. Quill TE. *Death and Dignity: Making Choices and Taking Charge*. New York: W.W. Norton, 1993.

45. Vachon MLS. The emotional problems of the patient in palliative medicine. In: Doyle D, Hanks GW, MacDonald N, eds. *Oxford Textbook of Palliative Medicine*. 2nd ed. Oxford: Oxford University Press; 1998: 882–907.

46. Hinton J. Which patients with terminal cancer are admitted from home care? *Palliat Med* 1994; 8:197–210.

47. Wilkinson SM. The changing pressures for oncology nurses 1986–93. *Eu J Cancer Care* 1995; 4(2):69–74.

48. Cohen M, Sarter B. Love and work: oncology nurses' view of the meaning of their work. *Oncol Nurs Forum* 1992; 19:1481–1486.

49. Cohen MZ, Haberman MR, Steeves R, Deatrick JA. Rewards and difficulties of oncology nursing. *Oncol Nurs Forum* 1994; 21 (Suppl.): 9–17.

50. Maslach C, Jackson SE. Burnout in health professions: a social psychological analysis. In: Sanders GS, Suls J, eds. *Social Psychology of Health and Illness*. London: Erlbaum; 1982:227–251.

51. Yasko JM. Variables which predict burnout experienced by oncology clinical nurse specialties. *Cancer Nurs* 1983; 6:109–116.

52. Jenkins JF, Ostchega Y. Evaluation of burnout in oncology nurses. *Cancer Nurs* 1986; 9:108–116.

53. Grossman SA, Sheidler VR, Swedeen K, Mucenski J, Piantadosis S. Correlation of patient and caregiver ratings of cancer pain. *J Pain Symptom Manage* 1991; 6(2):53–57.

54. McMillan SC, Tittle M. A descriptive study of the management of pain and pain-related side effects in a cancer centre and a hospice. *Hospice J* 1995; 10:89–107.

55. Heim E. Job stressors and coping in health professionals. *Psychother Psychosom* 1991; 55:90–99.

56. Peteet JR, Murray-Ross D, Medeiros C, Walsh-Burke K, Rieker P, Finkelstein D. Job stress and satisfaction among the staff members at a cancer center. *Cancer* 1989; 64:975–982.

57. Weisman AD. Understanding the cancer patient: the syndrome of caregiver plight. *Psychiatry* 1981; 44:161–168.

58. Steeves R, Cohen MZ, Wise CT. An analysis of critical incidents describing the essence of oncology nursing. *Oncol Nurs Forum* 1994: 21(8) (Suppl) 19–26.

59. Vachon MLS Losses and gains: a theoretical model of staff stress in oncology. In: McCorkle R, Hongladarom G. eds. *Issues and Topics in Cancer Nursing*. Norwalk, CT: Appleton-Century-Crofts; 1986:41–59.

60. Vachon MLS, Stylianos SK. Caring for the caregiver: a person-centered framework. In: Baird SB, McCorkle R, Grant M, eds. *Cancer Nursing: A Comprehensive Textbook*. Philadelphia: W.B. Saunders; 1991:1084–1093.

61. Canin LH. Psychological Restoration Among AIDS Caregivers: Maintaining Self-Care. Doctoral dissertation, University of Michigan, 1991.

62. Davidson KW. Social work with cancer patients: stresses and coping patterns. *Soc Work Health Care* 1985; 10 (4): 73–82.

63. Nason F. Team tension as a vital sign. *Gen Hosp Psychiatry* 1981; 3: 32–36.

64. Beckhard R. Organizational implications of team building. In: Wise H, Beckhard R, Rubin I, Kyte Al, eds. Making Health Teams Work. Cambridge: Ballinger; 1974:69–94.

65. Maguire P. Barriers to psychological care of the dying. *Br Med Bull* 1985; 291:1711–1713.

66. Faulkner A, Maguire P. *Talking to Cancer Patients and their Relatives*. Oxford: Oxford University Press, 1994.

67. Faulkner A. *Effective Interaction with Patients.* Edinburgh: Churchill Livingstone, 1992.
68. Faulkner A. *Teaching Interactive Skills in Health Care.* London: Chapman & Hall, 1993.
69. Horowitz SA, Passik SD, Brish M, Breitbart WS. A group intervention for staff on a neuro-oncology service. *Psycho-Oncol* 1994; 3:329–332.

13

The Spectrum of Grief in Palliative Care

LAURENCE KATZ AND HARVEY MAX CHOCHINOV

"No one ever told me that grief felt so like fear. I am not afraid,
but the sensation is like being afraid. The same fluttering in the
stomach, the same restlessness, the yawning. I keep on swallowing."

—*A Grief Observed*, C. S. Lewis

The experience of losing a loved one as a result of death is an inevitable part
of adult life. It has been estimated that for every person who dies, *at least five
close friends, relatives, and loved ones are left behind*.[1] The annual incidence
of bereavement in the population is estimated at between 5% and 9%.[2,3] Because of the nature of progressive medical illness, a substantial portion of the
newly bereaved will have been intimately involved with the deceased during
their medical treatment. It is a salient aspect of grief in this situation that there
is usually a period of anticipatory grieving preceding the death. This presents
an opportunity and an obligation for palliative care teams to combine care and
comfort of the patient with guidance and assessment of the family through the
final phases of terminal illness and death. If this is done with understanding,
concern, and sensitivity, this care can substantially benefit the subsequent grieving process.[4]

To best understand, guide, and, if necessary, treat those experiencing bereavement, it is necessary to be aware of the spectrum of grief and its associated
complications. Familiarity with this spectrum allows for differentiation of normal
from complicated grief and, when appropriate, the diagnosis of bereavement-
related, major depression. Knowing the risk factors for an abnormal grieving
process allows for assessment, monitoring of and early intervention by the treatment team for those most vulnerable. Finally, understanding this spectrum
guides management decisions and directs future research. Although it is often
very difficult to distinguish normal from abnormal bereavement, a review of the

literature can guide assessment and begins to provide a structure for understanding the spectrum of grief reactions.

Definitions

For clarity of discussion here, definitions of the relevant terminology are as follows. *Bereavement* refers to the loss of a person as a result of death.[5] *Grief* describes the feelings and behaviors resulting from loss. The *grieving process* entails the changing feelings and behaviors that occur over time.[6,7] *Mourning* refers to the social expressions in response to loss and grief, including rituals and behaviors specific to each culture and religion.[6] *Anticipatory grief* refers to the psychological and emotional reactions to the anticipation of loss.[5] *Complicated grief* is the failure to return to pre-loss levels of performance or states of emotional well-being.[8]

Normal Grief

To delineate the spectrum of the grieving process, one must begin with a description of "normal" grief. The first systematic study of acute grief was reported in 1944 by Lindemann.[9] Since that time, numerous authors have proposed different models for understanding the nature and stages of grief. However, the manifestations of grief vary greatly from person to person and from moment to moment. Thus, any attempt at staging the grieving process must not be taken too literally. Grief is a fluid process that ebbs and flows over time.[7] Nonetheless, staging provides a useful construct within which the grieving process can be understood. The interpersonal model of grief is based on the work of John Bowlby[10,11] and focuses on the nature of attachment bonds and the psychosocial consequences of breaking them. Parkes[5,12] later revised these phases and created the following structure for conceptualizing the grieving process.

Phase of numbness and blunting

Many people find it hard to take in the full reality of the loss. As a result, they experience varying degrees of disbelief and denial. Frequently, the newly bereaved will make comments such as, "I can't believe it," or, "it's not true." They may also describe themselves as feeling numb or not feeling anything at all. This phase typically lasts from 1 to 14 days.[5,7,13] Mourning rites and the gathering of family and friends can help facilitate passage through this stage. Ideally, a family should be present at the time of death if they wish to be,[14] as this helps make the event real. For many patients receiving palliative care, there has been significant forewarning of the impending death (see Anticipatory Grief). However, if the death is sudden or unexpected, this phase may be magnified or prolonged.

Phase of pining and yearning

Before long, the death is acknowledged both intellectually and emotionally. The sense of unreality and disbelief also diminishes. Episodes of intense feeling states, which occur in waves lasting 20 minutes to 1 hour, were referred to by Lindeman[9] as the "pangs of grief." These "pangs" include sensations of somatic distress (i.e., tightness in the throat, sighing respirations, shortness of breath, and an empty feeling in the abdomen); preoccupation with the image of the deceased; strong feelings of guilt; hostile reactions to attempts at consolation by loved ones; and loss of normal patterns of conduct, including aimless wandering and a lack of organized activity. The hostility may also be directed at the deceased,[15] the bereaved themselves, the physician, the treatment team, the hospital, God, or the world in general. Accompanying the guilt may also be feelings of relief, especially if the illness was prolonged. These pangs are often interspersed with periods of anxiety and tension. The bereaved may experience an intense preoccupation with the memory of the deceased and an intense yearning for their presence.[15,16] Every aspect of the past relationship is recalled and examined in detail. Past grievances, unresolved anger, neglect and guilt are re-examined.[13] There may be bad dreams and transient hallucinatory experiences such as believing they have heard the deceased's voice. These events are often misinterpreted and taken as evidence of illness or madness.[5]

Phase of disorganization and despair

As time passes, the intensity and the frequency of the pangs of grief diminish and a period of social withdrawal and introversion may occur. This phase marks acceptance of both the reality and permanence of the loss.[17] Parkes[5] notes that during this time, the appetites are diminished and people live from day to day, preferring not to look at the future. It is during the transition into this phase that the grieving process can become arrested,[15,18] resulting in constant rumination, self-derogation, and continually unanswered questions. At this time, differentiating normal grief from abnormal grief—especially from clinical depression—is a difficult task. Unlike depression, however, uncomplicated bereavement does not normally present with morbid preoccupation with worthlessness, marked psychomotor retardation, or active suicidal ideation; those who are grieving also generally regard their depressed mood as a normal response.[17] However, it is becoming generally accepted that evidence of major depression extending beyond 2 months after the loss warrants treatment consideration (for further discussion see Bereavement-Related Depression).

Phase of reorganization and recovery

During this phase bereaved individuals break down attachments to the deceased and begin to establish new relationships. They are able to resume old roles, acquire new ones as needed, experience pleasure without guilt, and seek the companionship and love of others.[19] In spite of their grief, they begin to shift attention to the world around them. The bereaved are now able to recall past events with sentimental pleasure, although there may still be occasional pangs of grief, particularly on anniversaries, birthdays, etc. However, these usually diminish in intensity and duration over time.[13,7] As Silverman stated, "You really don't get over it, you get used to it."[20]

This brings us to the question regarding the normal duration of grief. Although many authors have grappled with this question,[6,7,21–23,66,67] its answer remains unclear. Clayton[24] found crying, depressed mood, and sleep disturbance to be cardinal symptoms during the first year of bereavement. Parkes[22] reported that after 13 months of bereavement, only a minority of widows were optimistic and most had the same experience as described by Clayton. Byrne and Raphael[25] found that 76.5% of bereaved elderly men had intrusive memories of their spouses at 13 months; 49% reported feelings of distress; 43% were preoccupied with mental images of their spouse, 41% were still yearning for their spouses, and 25% had looked for their spouse in familiar places. Hays et al. [26] found that bereavement produced a significantly elevated level of distress (i.e., depression, hopelessness/helplessness, anxiety) over a control group at 6 months. They also found that the best prediction of duration and severity of grief was the intensity of initial distress, which correlated closely with distress over the next 2 years. Other studies[23,27] have documented significant distress as much as 2 years into the bereavement course. Thus, it is not possible to clearly demarcate an endpoint for the grieving process. Rather, as Chochinov notes: just as each human relationship is unique, its disruption through death will precipitate a bereavement reaction shaded by the nature and intensity of the severed bond, the life-cycle stages of both the deceased and the bereft, as well as the social and cultural backdrop in the context of which the relationship began, evolved and would ultimately be mourned. Each of these will colour the quality and quantity of a particular bereavement course.[28]

Anticipatory Grief

Anticipatory grief was first described by Lindemann[9] in reference to instances in which a spouse (or parent) becomes so concerned with their adjustment in the face of a potential death that they go through all the phases of grief prior to the actual death. While this reaction was felt to be a safeguard against the impact of a sudden death, it can be problematic when patients follow a more protracted terminal course than originally anticipated. Since Lindemann's first description, there has been significant debate over the nature of anticipatory grief. Some observers feel that the emotional responses of actual bereavement begin in anticipation of loss.[13,28] There has also been evidence that emotional preparation can ease the grief reaction and decrease associated medical, psychological, and social morbidity.[29,20] However, others[4,30] report that true grieving does not begin until the death has occurred. Parkes[30] differentiates the anticipatory grief reaction from grief that follows a death. He believes that anticipatory grief is a reaction of intense separation anxiety or fear. Unlike the separation anxiety seen in postmortem grief, despair and hopelessness are not as prominent. In fact, the attachment is actually transiently enhanced by the threat of loss through death. This may have immediate value for the relationship and later value for the survivor. Finally, Hays et al.[26] recently looked at the course of psychological distress following threatened and actual conjugal bereavement. They found that the premortem psychological symptoms in the weeks and months prior to the death were not reliably distinguishable from the earliest and most intense experiences of postmortem grief. There were nonsignificant differences in mean depression scores and hopelessness/helplessness scores between the prebereaved, those already bereaved, and spouses of critically ill patients who survived. Hays et al. concluded that some dimension of threat or uncertainty is as adverse an experience as an actual loss, according to depressive and hopelessness/helplessness measures. Thus, given the contrasting studies described above, there remains considerable disagreement in the literature regarding the nature of anticipatory grief.

Complicated Grief

Thus far, we have reviewed aspects of the grieving process contained within the "normal" range of the spectrum. However, for reasons that are not entirely clear, a subgroup of bereaved persons develop complications of grief. The relationship between risk factors and outcome is complex (see Assessment), but certain patterns of reaction may be predictable if one considers the emotional circumstances that precede them and the bereaved's previous coping style. General tendencies toward anxiety, depression, and alcohol abuse are predictors of a complicated grief reaction.[5,7] Parkes[5] states that this group represents approximately half of those referred for psychiatric help. The other half represent a large group of individuals (many of whom do not seek psychiatric help) whose complicated grief is a reflection of the nature of the relationship or the type of bereavement that preceded the reaction.

Parkes and Weiss[30] developed a typology to allow for classification of those grief reactions that are unduly influenced by the nature of the relationship or the type of bereavement. Once again, this typology is a fluid structure with frequent overlap among the different types of complicated grief.[31] The *unexpected loss syndrome* may occur with deaths that are sudden and unexpected, associated with multiple losses, mutilation, or situations in which the survivors life was also threatened. It is a pattern of grieving in which attempts to avoid, repress, and delay grief continue for months or years but do not prevent high levels of anxiety and tension.[5,32] These reactions can be viewed as a type of post-traumatic stress disorder.[8,31] This is a dysfunctional syndrome in which recurrent intrusive recollections of the dying (flashbacks and nightmares) and hyperactivity (startle reactions, panic attacks, explosive anger) alternate with emotional numbness, decreased social functioning, and hopelessness regarding the future. This syndrome persists for extended periods of time and interferes with the normal grieving process, as the bereaved often attempts to maintain a fantasy relationship with the deceased who is now seen as ever-present and watching over the living.[5] This syndrome represents a distortion of the "normal" grieving process. Many aspects of "normal" early grief become fixed and magnified, making progress slow or impossible.

The *dependent grief syndrome* results from the end of a relationship in which one member was dependent on the other. Although initially believed to be a syndrome that occurred when the survivor was dependent on the deceased, it is now thought that it can also occur when the deceased was dependent on the survivor.[5] The self-esteem, confidence, and identity of one or both partners was dependent on the relationship; when this system is disrupted, the survivor is left with a gaping wound. Horowitz et al.[33] believe that this results in the reactivation of an image of the self as weak, abandoned, and needy, with intense fear that rescue will never occur. Once the breakdown of the relationship has occurred, severe grief may be perpetuated by the everyday gains associated with this process. Overt mourning allows withdrawal from social and other responsibilities and often dignifies the mourner in the eyes of others.[5] This may provide a needed boost to one's self-esteem and also provides an identity within which to function. This admixture results in a chronic grief syndrome, which is marked by continuous symptoms of grief typical of early phases of loss that continue unchanged as grief fails to resolve.[8,18,30,34]

The final element of the Parkes and Weiss typology is the *conflicted grief syndrome*. The nature of this syndrome is not as clear and its validation and placement on the spectrum of grief reactions has been debated in the literature. This syndrome was first proposed by Freud[35] and Abraham,[36] and was thought to be a product of relationships in which the survivor had ambivalent feelings toward the deceased. The angry component of the ambivalence is turned inward resulting in guilt, self-blame, and self-derogation. Freud and Abraham saw this dynamic as leading to depression. Parkes[5] believes that this dynamic may sometimes result in delayed grief. While an initial reaction may be one of relief, in time, the relationship is reviewed and there is a feeling of unfinished business. The bereaved find themselves having intrusive memories and associated feelings of anger and guilt. Some authors[7,31] do not believe that this construct has held up or been empirically validated; it thus remains a controversial explanation for understanding certain grief reactions.

The nature and specificity of these three syndromes of complicated grief continues to be debated and revised. It is likely, as demonstrated by Prigerson[8] and discussed by Rynearson,[31] that most bereaved persons who present with complications of grief do not present with a single, clean-cut syndrome but rather, with a mixture of these reactions. Nevertheless, an understanding of these three constructs allows for better assessment, understanding, and management of complicated grief.

Bereavement-Related Depression

In continuing our review of the spectrum of grief reactions, we now move to the most frequent and potentially significant complication of bereavement—the presence of depressive symptoms. The Diagnostic and Statistical Manual of Mental Disorders (DSM)-IV[37] lists nine cardinal symptoms of major depression: decreased concentration, fatigue, suicidal ideation, loss of interest, depressed mood, psychomotor retardation, anorexia, social withdrawal, and sleep disturbance. To meet criteria for a major depressive episode, one must have either depressed mood or loss of interest and four of the other symptoms. Prigerson et al.[8] have postulated a bereavement-related depression constellation consisting of hypochondriasis, apathy, insomnia, anxiety, suicidal ideation, guilt, loneliness, depressed mood, psychomotor retardation, hostility, and low self-esteem. This syndrome is associated with significant psychosocial dysfunction.

Depressive symptoms can appear at any point during a bereavement course[27,38] and they raise the clinical question of when these symptoms constitute a disorder requiring treatment. Opinion regarding this distinction has changed over the years as the high prevalence and serious consequences of depression have been delineated. Most investigators have found a significantly higher prevalence of major depression in widows and widowers than in control groups. The rates for major depression peak at approximately 1 month postmortem, reaching nearly 50%,[39] then decline at 2 months to 27%–30%[8,40,41] and continue to drop to 16% at 1 year,[41] after which it stabilizes at this level for up to 2 years.[23,27]

In the past, despite the frequent occurrence of syndromal magnitude depressive symptoms, the diagnosis of major depression was not made in the context of bereavement. It was felt that this reaction was understandable, given the extenuating circumstances. Currently, DSM-IV[39] stipulates that a diagnosis of major depression should only be made when the symptoms are not better accounted for by bereavement, i.e., after the loss of a loved one, the symptoms persist for longer than 2 months or are characterized by marked functional impairment, morbid preoccupation with worthlessness, suicidal ideation, psychotic symptoms or psychomotor retardation. Recent investigators[27,40,42] have found that bereavement-related depressions tend often to be chronic and lead to protracted biopsychosocial dysfunction.

Karam[42] found that bereavement meeting criteria for major depression does not differ from major depression in the community with respect to age of onset, degree of dysfunction, visits to doctors, or taking medication. Zisook and Schuchter[27] found that despite the high prevalence of bereavement-related depression and evidence that is as debilitating as major depression, 83% of bereaved spouses who met criteria for a major depression received no antidepressant medications. This means that a highly disabling and potentially life-threatening illness is either not being diagnosed or not being treated. Zisook thus believes[7,27] that severe major depressive syndromes at any time, and all major depressive syndromes beyond the second month of bereavement, should be carefully evaluated and treated as aggressively as other nonbereavement-related depressions. Major risk factors for major depression 1 year after the death include major depression at 2 months, past and family history of depression, younger age, and poor general medical health.

"Normal" grief is an intense psychological response to a catastrophic event. It is easy to attribute many symptoms and incapacities to the situation and lose sight of the presence of significant illness and disability. The nature of the relationship, the circumstances of the death, the bereaved's personality, coping style, and predisposition to psychiatric illness may cumulatively be predictive of future complicated grief or prominent depressive symptoms. Understanding and awareness of these possibilities allows for appropriate monitoring and more in-depth assessment and intervention when required.

Assessment

As stated previously, palliative care creates an opportunity and presents an obligation for assessment and guidance to help families and loved ones deal with anticipated death as adaptively as possible. This period begins with the delivery of the news of impending death (see Anticipatory Grief) and continues throughout the bereavement period. The death of the patient is not the end of the treatment team's mandate for care but rather, the time at which the focus of care is transferred from the patient to the family and loved ones. Parkes[5] notes that "it is a real paradox that just when the family are most aware of their need for help and most likely to accept it, help is usually withdrawn. Doctors, nurses and others who may have befriended the family while the patient was in hospital say goodbye and the family is left with nothing but a death certificate to take away."

In order to adequately assess imminently bereaved or newly bereaved individuals, it is necessary to be aware of the psychiatric and medical complications of bereavement and their associated risk factors. Some of these psychiatric complications have already been discussed (see Complicated Grief, Bereavement-Related Depression). It has long been widely assumed that bereavement predisposes individuals to exacerbation of pre-existing disease and places them at increased risk of death. Some less severe problems may reflect a disturbance in psychophysiological functioning associated with anxiety and tension. Disturbance of sleep, appetite, concentration, and mood are so common in the first month that they can be regarded as "normal."[5] Reynolds et al.[43] in a controlled study of sleep disturbance during "normal" bereavement, found REM sleep abnormalities in the bereaved compared with non-bereaved controls. It appears that these REM sleep abnormalities were distinct from those found in major depression.

There are several physiological systems thought to be affected by bereavement, including abnormalities in the cardiovascular,[6,21] endocrine,[44] and immunological[45,46,68] systems. These were thought to lead to increased morbidity and mortality from cardiac disease,[6,21] certain cancers,[47] and a nonspecific decline in general medical health.[6] Questions still exist as to the clinical significance of changes in these systems in relation to altering vulnerability to disease.[48,49] Of note, however, is substantial evidence of increased mortality among bereaved individuals,[69] especially older men. Helsing and Szklo[50,51] and recently Schaefer et al.[52] have conducted large, well-controlled longitudinal studies looking at mortality in bereavement. Both studies confirmed that the bereaved had an increased mortality rate, particularly in older men. They also demonstrated that the increased mortality rate persists for years. Helsing and Szklo reported a protective effect of remarriage and an increased mortality rate that was largely nonspecific as to its cause; diseases significantly associated with cause of death included infectious diseases, accidents, and suicide in men, and cirrhosis in women. Li[53] has also found increased rates of suicide in bereaved men over controls. It would thus appear that bereaved elderly men may be particularly vulnerable and require closer monitoring of their bereavement course.

According to Parkes,[5] "the assessment of risk factors in those family members who are most affected by a patient's death should be routine and can be part of the family assessment which is made by a primary care nurse or other care givers whenever it is clear that a patient is entering the terminal phase of care." Psychiatric complications of grief (complicated grief, major depression, anxiety, suicide) can be expected when one or more of the known predictors of poor outcome are present. These include poor social support, prior psychiatric history, unanticipated death (particularly of a young person[5]), other significant stresses or losses, high level of initial distress with depressive symptoms, death of a child, or being an elderly male who has lost a spouse.[4,54–56] Prior dependence on alcohol, drugs (especially tranquillizers), and tobacco predict increased consumption during bereavement.[4] A history of alcoholism increases the suicide risk and likelihood of psychiatric hospitalization shortly after bereavement.[57,58]

Comprehensive care of the dying must thus include assessment of families and loved ones. Understanding the risk factors that predispose to complicated grief and its associated morbidity allows for prevention and early treatment. The palliative care team is in an opportune position to ensure that this is performed adequately or, when required, that referral is made to a more specialized treatment setting.

Management

The assessment and management of bereavement often begins with delivering the news of impending death. Such news is often met with denial and numbness, requiring frequent follow-up discussions and ample opportunity to answer questions. These questions must be answered openly, honestly, and in a caring manner. Open responsiveness to questions and discussion allow the bereaved to understand intellectually the circumstances leading to death and may alleviate misconceptions of personal responsibility (e.g., "if only I had not agreed to that surgery/treatment"). The family will long remember in detail how this information was conveyed and their concerns addressed. Ideally, the news should be delivered by the physician who has taken care of the patient and who knows the surviving relatives/friends well enough to frame the news in a manner that anticipates their likely response. If it is not possible for the responsible physician to be present, then another physician known to the family should convey the information.

People vary in their willingness and ability to deal with the physical unpleasantness of dying. Far from attempting to relieve families of the whole burden of care, some families may see this as their last chance to make restitution with the dying person for any failure or other psychological debt.[7] We do not serve all families best by taking away the whole care of the patient, as this may interrupt the anticipatory grieving and restitution that can occur during this time.

Worden [59] has proposed that mourning can be understood in terms of specific tasks the bereaved individual must accomplish. These include accepting the reality of the loss, experiencing the pain of grief, adjusting to an environment in which the deceased person is missing, and finally, withdrawing emotional energy from the deceased person so it can be reinvested in other relationships.

It is important to recognize that most bereaved individuals recover from their loss without any professional assistance. Facilitating normal bereavement may require nothing more than availability and willingness to listen to the grieving person.[38] Often, adequate support is gleaned from family, friends, and spiritual resources. For many people, however, such support is not available in their immediate social environment. When intervention is attempted, it should be directed toward those who are at known risk for a poor bereavement outcome.

Social workers, psychologists, and psychiatrists have an important role to play in support of front-line palliative care providers.[5] Initially, however, care providers can encourage family members to take care of themselves, eat and sleep well, take any medication they were already on, and visit physicians for routine medical care.[7] This kind of proactive response may ultimately decrease health care costs, as widowers who are not routinely monitored utilize the health care system significantly more than nonwidowers.[60] Similarly, individuals on medication or in psychotherapy should continue in an attempt to prevent pre-existing psychiatric difficulties from being exacerbated by the loss.[7] The nursing staff can provide prebereavement support, assess families for bereavement risk, and support the family at the time of death.[5] Medical staff can provide guidance, meet with the bereaved family to answer questions, discuss the need for an autopsy when necessary, and ensure adequate medical follow-up with general practitioners.[5] It is crucial that the individualized spiritual needs of the family are met through active interaction with the clergy. When added support is needed, mutual support through nonprofessional services and professional interventions (consisting of psychotherapeutic and psychopharmacological approaches) are two beneficial models.

Mutual Support

There is no greater immediate alliance than that which is felt between two individuals who have shared the same stressful experience. The widow-to-widow program[20,30] was developed on the basis of this premise. It offers one-to-one emotional support by an individual who presents a positive model for coping. Fundamental information about practical concerns and bereavement are discussed. Groups promote the personal examination of coping and offer alternative ways that may be more effective. Such programs are available throughout Canada, the United States, and the United Kingdom. The effectiveness of this program in reducing distress has been demonstrated.[61] Mutual support interventions have also been shown to reduce physician visits during bereavement.[60]

Professional Interventions

There are some individuals who experience persistent somatic complaints, prolonged depressive symptoms, drug or alcohol abuse, other health injurious behaviors, breakdown of social relationships, or exacerbation of other medical or psychiatric disorders. Such difficulties sometimes require referral to a more specialized treatment setting. Individuals often respond in six to ten psychotherapeutic visits to assist expression of grief and confrontation with the loss. Individuals at high risk, however, may require much more protracted psychotherapeutic intervention.[31] Sometimes family therapy is the best approach for enhancing communication between surviving family members around residual bereavement issues.

Psychotherapeutic intervention with the bereaved requires that the therapist be familiar with the clinical features of normal and complicated grief. The therapist must be empathic to an individual experiencing great pain. Zisook and Schuchter[62] offer several key tasks in bereavement therapy, including giving permission for expression of feelings and recounting the details of the experience, assessing defenses for dealing with the painful emotions, integrating the continuing relationship with the deceased spouse into the present, encouraging healthy functioning, handling altered relationships, and achieving a new view of the personal world and the self in it, with a willingness to try new experiences. Unfortunately, there are few outcome studies looking at the efficacy of various psychotherapeutic approaches. However, the few controlled trials that targeted patients with high levels of distress showed benefit to both physical and psychological well-being.[63]

Medication may be used either alone or in combination with psychosocial modes of intervention. For individuals who develop insomnia during bereavement, short-term intervention with hypnotic agents may be both helpful and humane.[7] Rather than preventing the ability to face up to grief, this intervention may help facilite the grieving process. The presence of a protracted, significant sleep disorder may herald the onset of a major depressive episode.[43] While the dysfunction associated with bereavement-related depression has been delineated, there are no controlled studies of antidepressant treatment with this population. There are two open studies that support their efficacy.[64,65] This is an area that urgently requires controlled studies.

Areas of Future Research

To ensure that future research brings maximal benefit, it is critical that researchers establish a common terminology. This will allow for broader application and clearer communication of results from longitudinal studies describing the nature and phases of grief, as well as randomized clinical trials. Prospective, descriptive, longitudinal trials looking at the nature and phases of grief are required for validating the current typology or defining another more accurate schema. Further studies delineating the course of bereavement-related depression are also required in an attempt to differentiate this disorder from normal bereavement.

Randomized, prospective, controlled trials assessing the efficacy of mutual support and various types of psychotherapy are required. Randomized, double-blinded, placebo controlled trials of antidepressants should provide a long-overdue answer to the question of the efficacy of pharmacotherapy in bereavement-related depression. The results of such research will no doubt inform our ability to understand the grieving process and, when necessary, intervene effectively.

Summary

Bereavement is a common clinical problem facing palliative care staff. Knowing the nature of "normal" grief and its phases allows for support of grieving families and identification of abnormal reactions. Most individuals will recover from the early phases of grief in 1 to 2 months, and with resolution largely within a year. This usually occurs without professional help. However, some individuals will not progress through the grieving process and will require help. Individuals likely to be at risk include those with a history of emotional problems, maladaptive coping responses, and poor social support; those who have experienced a sudden death of the deceased, are male and elderly, and have other major stressors, high initial distress, or have lost a child. Professional and mutual support are helpful for those at high risk or individuals experiencing unusually intense initial distress. Medications may occasionally facilitate progress through the initial phase of grief and may treat bereavement-related depression. Bereavement-related depression is profoundly underdiagnosed and often goes untreated. Given the substantial general medical and psychiatric morbidity and mortality, it is imperative that palliative care teams make every effort to include assessment and management of bereavement as part of their treatment mandate.

References

1. Cleiren MP. *Adaptation after Bereavement*. Leiden University, Leiden: DSWO Press, 1991.
2. Imboden JB, Canter A, Cliff L. Separation experiences and health records in a group of normal adults. *Psychosom Med* 1963; 25:433–440.
3. Frost NR, Clayton PS. Bereavement and psychiatric hospitalization. *Arch Gen Psychiatry* 1977; 34:1172–1175.
4. Chochinov HM, Holland JC. Bereavement: A special issue in oncology. In: Holland JC, Rowland JH, eds. *Handbook of Psychooncology*. New York: Oxford University Press; 1989:612–627.
5. Parkes CM. Bereavement. In: Doyle D, Hanks GWC, MacDonald N, eds. *Oxford Textbook of Palliative Medicine*. Oxford University Press; 1993:663–678.
6. Osterweis M, Solomon F, Green M. (eds.) *Bereavement: Reactions, Consequences and Care*. Washington, DC: National Academy Press, 1984.
7. Zisook S. Understanding and managing bereavement in palliative care. In: Chochinov HM, Breitbart W, eds. *Psychiatric Dimensions of Palliative Medicine*. New York: Oxford University Press; in press.
8. Prigerson HG, Frand E, Kasl SV, et al. Complicated grief and bereavement-related depression as distinct disorders: preliminary empirical validation in elderly bereaved spouses. *Am J Psychiatry* 1995; 1:22–30.
9. Lindemann E. Symptomatology and management of acute grief. *Am J Psychiatry* 1944; 101:141–148.
10. Bowlby J. The making and breaking of affectional bonds, I: aetiology and psychopathology in the light of attachment theory. *Br J Psychiatry* 1977; 130:201–210.
11. Bowlby J. The making and breaking of affectional bonds, II: some principles of psychotherapy. *Br J Psychiatry* 1977; 130:421–431.
12. Parkes CM. Seeking and finding a lost object: evidence from recent studies of the reaction to bereavement. *Soc Sci Med* 1970; 4:181–201.
13. Brown JT, Stoudemire A. Normal and pathological grief. *JAMA* 1983; 250(3):378–382.
14. Engel GL. Grief and grieving. *Am J Nurs* 1964; 64:93–98.
15. Vargas LA, Loya F, Hodde-Vargas J. Exploring the multidimensional aspects of grief reactions. *Am J Psychiatry* 1989; 146:1484–1488.
16. Bowlby J. Processes of mourning. *Int J Psychoanal* 1961; 42:317–340.
17. Chochinov HM. Management of grief in the cancer setting. In: Breitbart W, Holland JC, eds. *Psychiatric Aspects of Symptom Management in Cancer Patients*. Washington, DC: American Psychiatric Press; 1993:231–241.
18. De Vahl R, Zisook S. Unresolved grief: clinical considerations. *Postgrad Med* 1976; 59:267–271.

19. De Vahl RA, Zisook S, Faschingbauer TR. Clinical aspects of grief and bereavement. *Prim Care* 1979; 6:391–402.

20. Silverman PR. The widow as caregiver in a program of preventative intervention with other widows. In: Killelie CG, ed. *Support Systems and Mutual Help*. New York: Grune and Stratton; 1976:233–243.

21. Engel GL. Is grief a disease? A challenge for medical research. *Psychosom Med* 1961; 23:18–22.

22. Parkes CM. Psychosocial transitions: a field study. *Soc Sci Med* 1971; 5:101–115.

23. Harlow SD, Goldberg EL, Comstock GW. A longitudinal study of the prevalence of depressive symptomatology in elderly widowed and married women. *Arch Gen Psychiatry* 1991; 48:1065–1068.

24. Clayton P. Mourning and depression: their similarities and differences. *Can J Psychiatry* 1974; 1:309–312.

25. Byrne GSA, Raphael B. A longitudinal study of bereavement phenomena in recently widowed elderly men. *Psychol Med* 1994; 24:411–421.

26. Hays JC, Kasl SV, Jacobs SC. The course of psychological distress following threatened and actual conjugal bereavement. *Psycho Med* 1994; 24:917–927.

27. Zisook S, Schuchter SR. Uncomplicated bereavement. *J Clin Psychiatry* 1993; 54:365–372.

28. Chochinov HM. Bereavement: a review for oncology health professionals. *Cancer Invest* 1989; 7:593–600.

29. Bowlby J. *Attachment and Loss. Vol. 3. Loss: Sadness and Depression*. New York: Basic Books, 1980.

30. Parkes CM, Weiss RS. *Recovery from Bereavement*. New York: Basic Books, 1983.

31. Rynearson EK. Psychotherapy of pathologic grief. *Psychiatr Clin North Am* 1987; 10(3):487–499.

32. Lundin T. Morbidity following sudden and unexpected bereavement. *Br J Psychiatry* 1984; 144:84–88.

33. Horowitz M, Wilner N, Marmar C. Pathological grief and the activation of latent self-images. *Am J Psychiatry* 1980; 137:1157–1162.

34. Raphael B, Middleton W. What is pathologic grief? *Psychiatr Ann* 1990; 20:304–307.

35. Freud S. Mourning and melancholia (1917). In: Gaylin W, ed. *The Meaning of Despair*. New York: Jason Aronson; 1968:50–69.

36. Abraham K. Notes on the psychoanalytical investigation and treatment of manic-depressive insanity and allied conditions. In: Gaylin W, ed. *The Meaning of Despair*. New York: Jason Aronson; 1968:26–49.

37. American Psychiatric Association. *Diagnostic and Statistical Manual of Mental Disorders*. 4th ed. Washington, DC: American Psychiatric Association, 1994.

38. Lieberman PB, Jacobs SC. Bereavement and its complications in medical patients: a guide for consultation-liaison psychiatrists. *Int J Psychiatry Med* 1987; 17:23–39.

39. Clayton PJ. Bereavement and depression. *J Clin Psychiatry* 1990; 51:34–38.

40. Zisook S, Shuchter SR. Depression through the first year after the death of a spouse. *Am J Psychiatry* 1991; 148:1346–1352.

41. Zisook S, Shuchter SR, Sledge PA. The spectrum of depressive phenomena after spousal bereavement. *J Clin Psychiatry* 1994; 55(4, Suppl):29–36.

42. Karam EG. The nosological status of bereavement—related depressions. *Br J Psychiatry* 1994; 165:48–52.

43. Reynolds CF, Hoch CC, Buysse DJ, et al. Sleep after spousal bereavement: a study of recovery from stress. *Biol Psychiatry* 1993; 34:791–797.

44. Hofer M, Wolff C, Freedman S, Mason J. A psychoendocrine study of bereavement: parts 1 and 2. *Psychosom Med* 1972; 34:481–507.

45. Bartrop R, Lazarus L, Luckhurst E, Kiloh LG, Penny R. Depressed lymphocyte function after bereavement. *Lancet* 1977; 1:834–836.

46. Irwin M, Daniels M, Weiner H. Immune and neuroendocrine changes during bereavement. *Psychiatr Clin North Am* 1987; 10:449–465.

47. Schmale AHS, Iher HP. The affect of hopelessness and the development of cancer. I. Identification of uterine cervical cancer in women with atypical cytology. *Psychosom Med* 1966; 28:714.

48. Levav I, Friedlander Y, Kark S, Pentz E. An epidemiologic study of mortality among bereaved parents. *N Engl J Med* 1988; 319:457–461.

49. Jones DR, Goldblatt PO, Leon DA. Bereavement and cancer: some data on death of spouses from the longitudinal study of Office of Population Censuses and Surveys. *Br Med J* 1984; 289:461–464.

50. Helsing KJ, Szklo M. Mortality after bereavement. *Am J Epidemiol* 1981; 114:41–52.

51. Helsing KJ, Comstock G, Szklo M. Causes of death in a widowed population. *Am J Epidemiol* 1982; 116:524–532.

52. Schaefer C, Quesenberry CP, Sorra W. Mortality following conjugal bereavement and the effects of a shared environment. *Am J Epidemiol* 1995; 141:1142–1152.

53. Li G. The interaction effect of bereavement and sex on the risk of suicide in the elderly: an historical cohort study. *Soc Sci Med* 1995; 40(6):825–828.

54. Vachon MLS. Predictors and correlates of adaptation in conjugal bereavement. *Am J Psychiatry* 1982; 139:998–1002.

55. Hays JC, Kasl S, Jacobs S. Past personal history of dysphoria, social support and psychological distress following conjugal bereavement. *J Am Geriatr Soc* 1994; 42:712–718.

56. Prigerson HG, Reynolds III CR, Frank E, Kupfer DJ, George CJ, Houck PR. Stressful life events, social rhythms and depressive symptoms among the elderly: an examination of hypothesized causal linkages. *Psychiatry Res* 1994; 51:33–49.

57. Murphy GE, Robins E. Social factors in suicide. *JAMA* 1967; 199:303–308.

58. Robins LN, West PA, Murphy GE. The high rate of suicide in older white men: a study testing ten hypotheses. *Soc Psychiatry* 1977; 12:1–20.

59. Worden W. *Grief Counselling and Grief Therapy: a handbook for the Mental Health Practitioner.* New York: Springer-Verlag 1982.

60. Tudiner F, Permaul-Woods JA, Hilditch J, Harmina J, Saini S. Do widowers use the health care system differently? Does intervention make a difference? *Can Fam Physician* 1995; 41:392–400.

61. Vachon MLS, Sheldon AR, Lancee WJ, et al. A controlled study of self-help: intervention for widows. *Am J Psychiatry* 1980; 137:1380–1384.

62. Zisook S, Schuchter SR. The first four years of widowhood. *Psychiatr Ann* 1985; 16:288–294.

63. Marmar CR, Horowitz MJ, Weiss DS, Wilner NR, Koltreider NB. A controlled trial of brief psychotherapy and mutual-help group treatment of conjugal bereavement. *Am J Psychiatry* 1988; 145:203–209.

64. Jacobs SC, Nelson JC, Zisook S. Treating depressions of bereavement with antidepressants: a pilot study. *Psychiatr Clin North Am* 1987; 10:501–511.

65. Pasternak RE, Reynolds CR, Schlernitzauer M, et al. Acute open-trial nortriptyline therapy of bereavement-related depression in late life. *J Clin Psychiatry* 1991; 52:307–310.
66. Middleton W, Burnett P, Raphael B, Martinek N. The bereavement response: a cluster analysis. *Br J Psychiatry* 1996; 169:167–171.
67. Lichtenstein P, Gatz M, Pederson NL, Berg S, McClearn GE. A Co-twin-control study of response to widowhood. *J Gerontol Ser B Psych Sci Soc Sci* 1996; 51:279–289.
68. Goodkin K, Feaster DJ, Tuttle R, et al. Bereavement is associated with time-dependent decrements in cellular immune function in asymptomatic human immunodeficiency virus type 1 seropositive homosexual men. *Clin Diagn Lab Immunol* 1996; 3:109–118.
69. Martikainen P, Valkonen T. Mortality after the death of a spouse: rates and causes of death in a large Finnish cohort. *Am J Public Health* 1996; 86:1087–1093.

14

Conflict Between Families and Staff: An Approach

CATHERINE JENKINS AND EDUARDO BRUERA

Almost half of the families of palliative patients are dissatisfied with some aspects of the care received[1] and approximately 5% develop a conflict with staff.[2] It is not known how frequently staff perceive families as interfering with care; however, anecdotally, family displeasure is a major stressor for staff. This chapter will examine both the causes and management of family–staff conflict.

Definition

For the purposes of this chapter, "conflict" will be defined as an expressed dissatisfaction by either staff or family about the other's care or concern towards the patient. This will include any situation where either *(a)* the family communicates that the staff are not acting in the best interest of the patient or *(b)* the staff let the family know that they are acting inappropriately. A secondary definition will include any situation in which the family expresses a belief that their needs are not being met.

The reasons for choosing this definition are threefold. First, it avoids focusing only on overt conflict. Although a loud argument at the nurse's desk is a dramatic manifestation of conflict, a family member who silently undermines treatment plans may be more destructive. Second, it reduces assigning blame. Whether family members are being vigorous patient advocates or troublemakers is a matter of perspective. Third, it puts the patient's interests before that of the family or staff. Although harmony between staff and family is important, in some situations, conflict may be preferable to compromising patient care.

Sources of Conflict

Although indices of family satisfaction have been extensively studied,[3-5] little research has been done on factors that cause this dissatisfaction to be manifested as conflict. We have therefore constructed a model for analyzing the sources of conflict (Table 14.1). Although any conflict will usually have multiple etiologies, it is hoped that this model will make the analysis of individual conflicts easier. For purposes of discussion, conflict will be divided into two sections: physiological conflict, or conflict that occurs when both staff and family are motivated by their concerns for the patient; and pathological conflict, when the personal needs of either the family or staff override that of the patient.

Table 14.1 Sources of conflict

Physiological conflict

Difference in opinion about the patient's needs

    Patient unable to express needs

    Patient's expressed needs are not seen as valid

    Patient decides to withhold information from one party

    Cultural differences

Difference in opinion about the feasibility of achieving goals

Pathological conflict

Family

    Stress factors

        Nature of illness

        Trajectory of illness

        Guilt

        External stresses

    Distrust of the health care system

    Maladaptive coping

Staff

    Group

        Fractionated team

        Team style

    Individual

        Personal stress

        Maladaptive coping

Milieu

Physiological Conflict

Studies that have asked family members what they consider important have found that family members place patient comfort and competent medical care first.[3,4] Self-reported information is subject to bias, as few people would admit to placing their needs before that of a dying family member. Nevertheless, the perception that the patient is not receiving adequate care is a major source of conflict. Presuming that the staff are also motivated by concern for the patient, there are two major reasons why conflict can occur in this situation. First, there may be a difference in opinion about the patient's needs. Second, there may be a difference in opinion about the feasibility of fulfilling these needs. Both these issues will be dealt with separately.

Difference in opinion about the patient's needs

There are four potential situations where this can occur.

1. *Patient is unable to express her needs.* This situation has two risk factors for provoking conflict. First, both staff and family must interpret needs in an information vacuum and different interpretations will be common. Second, both parties may feel a heightened responsibility to be advocates. This situation occurs commonly when a patient is delirious, which has been recognized as a major risk factor for staff–family conflict. On a palliative care unit, family–staff conflict was found to be six times more frequent when the patient is delirious, specifically, in 30% of cases compared with 5% overall.[6] Compounding the stress is the fact that delirious behavior is inherently subject to misinterpretation—particularly about the patient's degree of pain.

2. *Patient's expressed needs are not seen as valid.* In this situation, only one party accepts the patient's statements. For example, a depressed patient may express a wish to die. Staff, with a greater understanding of depression, may see this as a temporary manifestation of a treatable disease; the family may feel that the patient's wishes should be honored. Or, a patient who has become too weak to walk may be seen by the family as having given up, whereas the staff interprets these changes as a function of the disease progression. Conflict may develop as the family tries to force the patient to walk while the staff focuses on helping the patient adjust to his weakened state.

3. *The patient decides to share information with only one party.* For example, the patient may decide to use the staff as a buffer to avoid dealing with family conflict or to "protect" family members. At one extreme, the patient may hide the terminal diagnosis from his family. One AIDS patient elected not to tell his family about his underlying diagnosis and

conflict developed when the family could not understand why the doctors could not cure a "simple" pneumonia. More mundane decisions to withhold information can also result in conflict. For example, a patient may request not to see certain relatives. The staff, who are unable to divulge the reason for turning the family away for reasons of patient confidentiality, become targets by default. Patients can also decide to withhold information from staff. An elderly patient who is accustomed to deferring to authority may be reluctant to disagree with a physician outright but may delegate a family member to refuse treatment. The staff, not knowing the background information, then sees the family member as uncooperative.

4. *Cultural differences.* "Ethical" behavior is often culturally determined. For example, in North American aboriginal cultures, direct communication may be viewed as impolite. Staff members who are accustomed to such Western traditions as making direct eye contact will be seen as unnecessarily confrontational.[7] In some Oriental cultures, discussing death with a patient is taboo. And it is acceptable for family members to make decisions and to speak for the patient in a way that would be considered patronizing in Western culture.[8] Staff may perceive this as meddling and feel required to bypass relatives to speak directly to the patient, thus starting a conflict. Because the degree of acculturation to Western values varies, assumptions cannot be made based on heritage. Indeed, severe conflicts may occur when only part of the family retains their traditional beliefs. Not only does the staff have to deal with the conflict between the family's values and their own but they may be required to mediate between family members. This can be exemplified by our experience in the care of an elderly Hindu man with a delirium. One son felt that suffering pain would help the patient redeem his soul and obtain a better reincarnation, whereas the other son opted for optimal pain control.

Difference in opinion about the feasibility of achieving goals

Family members who still believe a cure is possible will see anything short of this outcome as a treatment failure. But physical impossibility is not the only reason goals are not achievable; limited resources may also a factor. Families may, for example, demand more nursing care than funding allows. This is particularly common when the patient changes in acuity and is moved down to a less intensive level of care. Families often assume that the initial level of care should be the norm and do not understand the reason for the change in services. This situation is made even more difficult because in the short term this may be achievable. Staff can either choose to neglect other patients or to work voluntary overtime. Families may see creating conflict as an acceptable tool in this situation, particularly if it results in a short-term improvement in service. For the staff, this cause of conflict can be particularly difficult to deal with because articulating their position sounds unacceptable—how can regular coffee breaks be put before suffering patients? Staff can also demand unreasonable altruism from families. A staff person who believes families should be constantly present—without regard for work schedules or child care duties—will see most families as inadequate.

Pathological Conflict

The next section will examine factors other than concern for the patient which make staff or families more prone to experience conflict.

Family dynamics

Stress factors

It is well recognized that persons under stress are at increased risk of overreacting to everyday disagreements. Within the palliative care setting, certain factors have been postulated as increasing the degree of stress. These include the following.

Nature of the illness. It has been hypothesized that palliative care families are more prone to dissatisfaction because the nature of the disease means that the patient will inevitably worsen and die. Because there is no possibility for a control group in the palliative care population, this hypothesis has not been tested. However, in other settings, patient death has not resulted in increased family dissatisfaction. Indeed, in one study of family assessment of acute stroke care, satisfaction increased when the patient had died.[9] Eighty carers of stroke patients who survived the hospital admission and 34 bereaved carers were interviewed 4 weeks after discharge or death. Of the bereaved carers, 73.5% were very satisfied with the patient's overall hospital stay compared with 45.8% of the caregivers whose family member survived. This was true even though these deaths were unexpected, whereas on a palliative unit, families know the patient will die from the outset. Other aspects of a palliative diagnosis may also increase stress. In particular, poor symptom control has been noted to be a major stressor, especially if the family blames the staff for the poor control. Occasionally, families will try to take over what they perceive to be inadequate care. For example, the family of a delirious patient may interpret the agitation as pain and insist on increasing the opioids. Not only will this make the staff defensive, but the inappropriate treatment, by exacerbating the delirium, may increase the family's stress.

Trajectory of the illness.[1] Illness stage has also been presumed to affect stress levels, particularly the speed of decline. However, the effect of a rapid illness course is subject to debate. It is possible that short time between diagnosis and death will result in poorer coping, as the family has had less time go through the stages of adjustment to the terminal disease.[10] This was not found in one study of family behavior in the intensive care unit (ICU) setting.[11] Twenty-six family members of "long-term" ICU patients (2 or more weeks)

were interviewed and the results compared with those in previous studies involving families of short-stay ICU patients. No significant differences were
found. Two weeks may be an insufficient period of time to expect adjustment,
and this study may not be applicable to a cancer population in which the time
from diagnosis to death can stretch to years. And in the ICU setting, there is
continued uncertainty about the outcome, therefore adjustment is more
difficult, whereas in palliative care the outcome is known from the start. Al-
ternately, it can be argued that stress will increase with the length of the illness
as families exhaust their coping mechanisms and, thus, increase the risk of
conflict. In a survey of satisfaction with nursing home care, 452 families responded to a questionnaire about their perceptions of care.[12] Contrary to the
original hypothesis of the study, satisfaction decreased as the stay lengthened,
and in a multivariate analysis, this factor was found to be statistically significant.
Whether this reflects increasing stress on the part of the family or, as the authors
suggest, that there had been more time in which inadequacies in care could
occur, was beyond the scope of the study. The effect of length of diagnosis
on families of demented patients is also mixed. As part of one study on the
health of family caregivers of demented patients, 86 caregivers were interviewed
at the time of their initial geriatric assessment and 1 year later.[13] Depression
and physical symptoms were used as indices of stress. Equal numbers of family
caregivers (36%) reported either a significant increase or decrease in their depression rating; and 26.7% decreased their number of physical symptoms by
more than one, 34.9% reported an increase in the number of physical symptoms, and 38.4% showed no significant change. Thus, although stress seems to
vary longitudinally for individuals, there was no overall trend as to direction.
It may be that the relative weight of the shock over a recent diagnosis versus
the burnout from a long illness differs with individual families, but to date,
there are no studies focusing on what makes one factor likely to predominate.

   Guilt can also increase the risk of conflict, both because it increases stress
and because family members may create unreasonable demands as a way of
overtly demonstrating their concern. In our experience, family members who
fall short of their own expectations of what they should have been able to
provide are at high risk for conflict. Thus a family who had to abandon their
plans for a home death may be overly critical of the new caregivers. In the
aforementioned study of caregivers of demented patients,[13] families who had
institutionalized their relatives during the year had a higher increase in stress-
related indices. Whether this increase in stress was the cause or result of the
decision to institutionalize was not addressed. Family members who have mixed
feelings about a patient's death—for example, wanting everything to be over
so that their lives can return to normal—may overcompensate by being demanding of staff.

   External stressors. Stressors unrelated to the dying relative can also increase
the risk of conflict. In our experience, unemployment and social isolation are both
risk factors for conflict.

Distrust of the health care system

Families who distrust the health care system will be more prone to question the actions of the palliative care team. This distrust may not be reality based; families can make unrealistic attributions about the responsibilities of health care providers.[14] However, families who have had genuinely bad experiences with the health care system—for example, when the diagnosis was delayed—may see maintaining an oppositional attitude as the best way to prevent future errors. Diseases with a social stigma, such as HIV, may predispose family members to distrust of the health care system, as sufferers and their families define themselves as outsiders.[15]

Maladaptive copers

Difficult persons will continue to be difficult in times of stress. At one extreme, family members may have personality or mood disorders that predispose them to conflict. Persons who have a history of coping chemically will have less well-developed coping mechanisms[16] and will therefore be more prone to initiate conflict. Intrafamilial conflict may also be reflected in increased staff–family conflict if dominating the hospital staff is used to establish authority within the family system.

"Daughter-from-California" syndrome

One situation that combines multiple risk factors for staff–family conflict is the "daughter-from-California" syndrome.[17] This term, which was originally coined as a risk factor for intrafamilial conflict, refers to the return of an absentee relative to the patient in the midst of the disease process. This person may have the following characteristics. First, this person will suddenly have to confront the size of the patient's deterioration. Second, because she has not been present for much of the deliberations about treatment options, she may have unrealistic expectations about what is possible. Third, there may be compounding guilt about being previously absent. Fourth, conflict is one way that this person can reassert her role as an involved caregiver.

Staff characteristics

Patient–staff conflict, as manifested by physical aggression, has been shown to vary widely among care facilities.[18] Although the full reason for this is unknown, differences in environment and staff behaviors are presumed to be major factors. It is a reasonable assumption that staff characteristics will also affect the degree of family–staff conflict, but the particular attributes that predispose staff to conflict have not been studied. Some potential contributory factors follow.

Fractionated team

Teams that convey contradictory information, particularly if members openly criticize each other, will create distrust. A study of malpractice suits found that in 54%

of cases, a medical professional advised suing.[19] However, team unity may be difficult to achieve for several reasons. If the team feels strongly that previous medical advice has been inappropriate, they may need to convey that to the family in order to change the direction of treatment. And the family may interpret changes in the treatment plan as the patient's condition changes as signifying disagreement. The technique of using one family member as a spokesperson and information relater can inadvertently create the impression of discord as the message may be altered during transmission. Teams that are physically separated, for example, when care is being provided in the home, or who have insufficient resources to conference regularly, are in danger of innocently giving contradictory information.

Team style
Involving a health care team means relinquishing some family autonomy. Teams that are too authoritarian may provoke conflict as families rebel against these constraints. Theoretically, teams that are completely flexible could also be a source of conflict. For if families learn that any protest will result in change, this behavior may be re-enforced.

Personal stress/maladaptive behavior
Staff are at risk for many of the dysfunctional behaviors that affect families; they stem from either the particular stresses of working in palliative care or from longstanding coping difficulties. Since these have been discussed in the previous section on the family, these risk factors will not be repeated here.

Milieu

Little is known about how the milieu affects patient–staff conflict. One study did indicate a higher degree of satisfaction with home rather than hospital care; however, this may have been secondary to particular differences in care in those two programs and may not be generalizable.[20] Hospice care has been associated with a high degree of family satisfaction,[21] but this may represent a highly selected group of families. It has not been studied whether other specialized palliative care services have a higher degree of satisfaction than generalized services. Anecdotally, one dissatisfied family can incite other families to complain, and units have been noted to go through fluctuating levels of family satisfaction.

Diagnosis of Conflict

Overt conflict is easy to diagnose. Ideally, however, conflict should be diagnosed before it becomes obvious. Recognizing the risk factors for conflict may help identify which families or situations should be closely monitored. These are summarized in Table 14.2. Behaviors which indicate a distrust of the staff may indicate the start of conflict. For example, families who demand to see the chart

Table 14.2. Risk factors for conflict

Patient characteristics

Agitated delirium

Poor symptom control

History of substance abuse, psychiatric illness

Family characteristics

Family previously heavily involved in care

History of intrafamilial conflict

History of substance abuse, psychiatric illness

Social isolation

Unemployment

Previous conflict with health care giver

are signalling that they do not trust the staff to give accurate information. Non-compliance with medical advice may also be a warning. Splitting the team by complaining about one staff member to another may also presage a conflict against the entire staff.

Management of Conflict

Because staff are presumed to have the greater responsibility to adapt to the family, this section will focus entirely on how staff can manage conflict. Assessment and management are interwoven in practice; they will therefore be dealt with together. Delaying management until assessment is complete allows conflict to fester. And the family's responses to various management strategies can be diagnostic. The algorithm in Figure 14.1 shows how assessment and management are combined. Content and style also cannot be separated in actual practice, but for the sake of clarity, they will be dealt with separately here.

Content

The first point to consider is whether the complaints are valid. Justifiable and remediable complaints can be dealt with simply. Unfortunately, many complaints may be understandable but not remediable. Some problems are outside of the team's control to remedy. For example, the family may wish to have more intensive nursing care than is feasible, given the program's resources. Redirecting the family's complaint to a more appropriate source—in this case, the funding authority—may suffice. Getting the family to provide supplementary care, for example, by hiring private duty nurses, may fill the gap in services. However, this

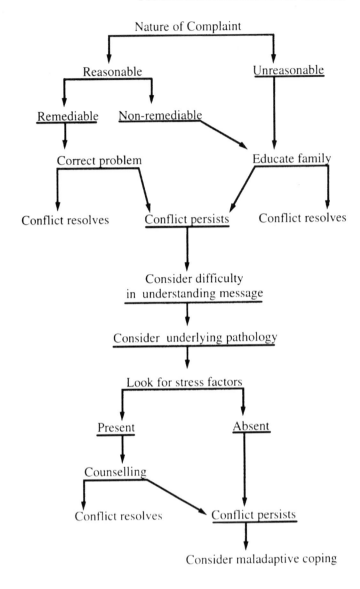

Figure 14.1. Management of conflict.

may reinforce the family's perception that the team failed to provide adequate care. Or, the family's demands may conflict with the team's value system. In that case, the staff must decide whether the issue is sufficiently vital not to compromise. On minor issues, it may be better for the patient if the staff gives in to family demands in order to preserve a therapeutic alliance with the family. On fundamental issues, conflict may be preferable. For example, letting the family give the patient a useless, or even potentially harmful, herbal remedy may be allowable in the interests of harmony; acceding to a family's request for active euthanasia would not.

Unrealistic demands have two causes. First, the family may genuinely be confused about what is possible. Alternatively, the demand may be a manifestation of poor coping. Initially assuming that there is a genuine misunderstanding and educating the family about what is possible is a useful strategy for managing conflict. Not only may this resolve the conflict, but spending time explaining issues to the family builds rapport. Indeed, the family's perception that they are being well informed is a major determinant of their level of satisfaction.[22] There are several caveats to this. First, there is a difference between the information given and the information received. The ability to absorb information is decreased by stress. Thus families may absorb only parts of the information given. Frequent repetition, as well as asking families what their understanding of the information is, may be helpful. Both the nature of the treatment and the reasons behind the management decision should be explained. Although it may be obvious to staff that blood-work and X-rays are necessary to adequately diagnose and treat symptoms, families may perceive these as unnecessarily invasive interventions. Second, intellectual understanding does not necessarily mean emotional understanding, and explanations must address both emotional and factual issues. This is particularly important when the family is responding viscerally to perceived suffering. This occurs commonly in agitated delirium, when families overestimate the degree of pain because of the marked increase in pain behaviors associated with the disinhibiting effects of delirium. Rather than disagreeing with the family's perception that the patient is in pain, it may be better to reframe the issue to an area where both parties can find agreement. Thus it may be better to acknowledge the family's perception that the patient is suffering, even though we may disagree about the cause that suffering, and to focus on explaining that treating the delirium will reduce the behavior of concern.

If conflict persists despite these efforts, or if multiple conflicts over different issues arise, poor coping should be considered. The degree to which families should be confronted with this possibility must be weighed individually. Families who cope through conflict usually lack insight into their own weaknesses and may react badly to the suggestion that they are the problem. For this reason, family stresses should be addressed only after the substance of the problem has been extensively addressed and the issue should be broached in as nonconfrontative manner as possible.

Style

As much as possible, discussions should be held in an atmosphere of calm. Adequate time should be allowed to hear the family's concerns and to answer their questions. Distractions should be minimized. Because conflict may be distressing for the patient, and families may not be willing to talk freely in front of the patient, these discussions should be held outside of the patient's room whenever possible. One limit to this may be a competent patient who wishes to be privy to all discussions concerning his care. Ideally, the entire multidisciplinary team should be involved. This distributes the responsibility for dealing with this family over more persons and may protect the individual staff member. It also increases the chances that there will be one team member with whom the family develops trust, and this person can then be used as a mediator. However, these conditions are not always immediately available and a balance must be struck between dealing with the problem expeditiously and waiting until ideal conditions are available.

Allowing the family to vent is a commonly used tactic that has several theoretical advantages. First, it channels the energy behind the conflict into an acceptable form. Second, the act of listening to the family helps reinforce that the staff is concerned. Third, empathic listening does not require extensive training. However, listening to venting drains both staff time and energy away from direct patient care—tasks that families themselves identify as more important than being given the chance to vent.[4] And venting does not address any of the underlying reasons for the conflict. The extent to which staff wish to use the discussion to probe for underlying stresses—that is, to move from a containment to a therapeutic role—must be individualized. Factors to be weighed in the decision include the training and resources of the staff to provide therapy, the willingness of the family to accept some responsibility for the conflict, and whether other, less intrusive, techniques are working.

Although it is tempting to avoid hostile families, it is crucial that care be continued. To do otherwise will merely re-enforce the family's perception that care is inadequate and perpetuate the conflict. An unpleasant family does not diminish the professional's duty of care towards the patient.

Format

Family conferences are a commonly used forum for dealing with conflict, but their efficacy has not been studied in comparison to individual discussions. There are several theoretical advantages to family conferences. First, assembling the team underlines that the complaints are being taken seriously. Second, it ensures that the entire team delivers a consistent message. Third, intrafamilial conflicts may become apparent, and a structure for dealing with the family can be established. But there are also several theoretical disadvantages to family conferences. First, conferences often cannot be convened quickly and this allows time for the conflict to increase. Second, conferences are very expensive in terms of staff resources, as many team members are usually asked to be present. Third, conferences convey a great deal of information at one sitting, particularly when each discipline comments on their findings. However, stress reduces the ability to register information, and families may retain more information if small amounts are presented at different times. If the family is particularly stressed, it may be better to confine the conference to just the areas of conflict and defer a comprehensive family conference for a less stressful period. Fourth, large groups can be intimidating. Although this show of strength can be useful with aggressive families, others may find it more difficult to openly discuss their concerns. The alternative, discussions involving one staff member only, can be set up quickly and, because fewer resources are used, can be repeated more frequently. Issues which may be difficult for the family to discuss in front of an audience can be dealt with more easily But multiple individual meetings make it easier for families to fractionate the team. Until there are more data on this issue, a combination of team and individual conferences should probably be used.

When Conflict Resolution Fails

If conflict persists despite all attempts at resolution, the team has three alternatives. First, they can give in to the family's demands, however unreasonable. Second, they can decide to live with ongoing conflict. Third, they can withdraw from providing care. Each option carries its own dilemmas. Capitulation to unreasonable demands, particularly in those cases in which the patient is unable to participate in the decision, may compromise the patient's well-being. Diverting resources to meet one family's demands may compromise other patients' care. This may not diminish the conflict, as families may feel rewarded, thus their behavior may be re-enforced. Living with the conflict can be disruptive both to staff morale and, if the conflict is public, to other patients. Before a health care team can withdraw from care, most ethical codes require that they arrange an equivalent source of care. However, given the paucity of palliative care services, there may not be an alternative program within the geographic area. One compromise may be to remove individual team members who are most involved with the conflict. This may be logistically impossible if the team is small and destructive of team morale. What solutions are available to the staff will depend in part on whether the patient is competent to help in the decision or whether the family is the surrogate decision-maker. If the patient is competent, then his wishes should supersede the family's. Thus, if the patient wishes to continue receiving care, then the staff should try to continue to do so. However, they may require that the patient put restraints on his family's behavior so that care can continue. When the family has become the surrogate decision-maker, particularly if they do not have legal guardianship, the situation is more problematic. Involvement of a separate mediator, such as a hospital ethics committee, may be required.

Directions for Future Research

Given the lack of research in this area, the scope for further research is broad and the question becomes which areas should be targeted first. A predictive model for conflict needs to be developed. At the Acute Palliative Care Unit in Edmonton, an assessment tool is being piloted to identify families at a high risk for maladaptive coping; however, this tool does not address conflict specifically. Nor is it known if targeted interventions toward the high-risk group will change outcomes. Staff and team characteristics which predispose to conflict have not been studied, and since there is theoretically more control over who is chosen as staff than there is over patient's families, studying this area may be the most constructive. However, there are two logistical problems with this area of study. First, it would require comparing services of similar acuities and family profiles, and finding comparable units is difficult. Second, any study would need to rely on staff identification of conflict. Since there is a stigma against admitting conflict, particularly if there are attributions of blame attached to identifying conflict,[23] accurate reporting would be difficult. Finally, the long-term impact of conflict is unknown. Most teams are familiar with the phenomenon of families who fight with the staff throughout the course of the illness and then send flowers. It may be that for some families, conflict is a beneficial process in working through their anger. And the drive to provide a level of care that will satisfy even the most impossible families may be a spur to improving patient care.

References

1. Kristjanson L, Ashcroft P. The family cancer journey. *Cancer Nurs* 1994; 17:3–15.
2. Emery B, Bruera E. Patterns of patient family/staff conflict on a palliative care unit: a 2 year analysis (Abstract). *J Palliat Care* 1990:53–54.
3. Kristjanson LJ. Indicators of quality of care from a family perspective. *J Palliat Care* 1986; 7:8–17.
4. Hull MM. Family needs and supportive nursing behaviours during terminal cancer: a review. *Oncol Nurs Forum* 1989; 16:787–792.
5. Stiles MK. The shining stranger: nurse–family spiritual relationship. *Cancer Nurs* 1990; 13:235–245.
6. Bruera E, Fainsinger R, Miller M, Kuehn N The assessment of pain intensity in patients with cognitive failure: a preliminary report. *J Pain Symptom Manage* 1992;7:267–270
7. Hepburn K, Reed R. Ethical and cultural issues with native American elders: end of life decision making. *Clin Geriatr Med* 1995;97–111.
8. Tong KL, Spicer BJ The Chinese palliative patient and family in North America: a cultural perspective. *J Palliat Care* 1994; 10:26–28.
9. Wellwood I, Dennis M, Warlow C. Patient's and career's satisfaction with acute stroke management. *Age Ageing* 1995; 24:419–425.
10. Kubler-Ross Elizabeth. *On Death and Dying.* New York: McMillan 1969.
11. Davis-Martin S. Perceived needs of families of long-term critical care patients a brief report. *Heart Lung* 1994; (6):515–518.
12. Grau L, Teresi J, Burton, B, Chandler B. Family members' perception of the quality of nursing home care. *Int J Geriatr Psychiatry* 1995; 10:787–796.

13. Baumgarten M, Hanley JA, Infante-Rivard C, Battista RN, Becker R, Gauthier S. Health of family members caring for elderly persns with dementia: a longitudinal study. *Ann Int Med* 1994; 120:126–132.

14. Eiser C, Havernans T, Eiser JP. Parent's attributions about childhood cancer: implications for relationships with medical staff. *Child Care Health Dev* 1995; 21:31–42.

15. Powell-Cope, GM. Family caregivers of people with AIDS: negotiating partnerships with professional health care providers. *Nurs Res* 43(6):324–330.

16. Powers RJ, Kutash IL. Stress and alcohol. *Int J Addict* 1995; 20(3):461–482.

17. Molley DW, Clarnette RM, Braun EA, Eisemann MR, Sneiderman B. Decision making in the incompetent elderly: the daughter from California syndrome. *J Am Geriatr Soc* 1991; 39(4):396–399.

18. Rudman D, Alverna L, Mattson D. A comparison of physically aggressive behaviour in two VA nursing homes. *Hosp Community Psychiatry* 1993; 44(6):571–573.

19. Beckman HB, Markatis KM, Suchman AL, Frankel RM The doctor-patient relationship and malpractice. Lesson from plaintiff depositions. *Arch Int Med* 1994; 154(12):1365–1370.

20. Peruselli C, Camporesi E, Colombo AM, Franceschi P, Legori T, Perri L. Satisfaction of patients and families with palliative home care. *J Palliat Care* 1994; 10(2):99.

21. Wilkinson JH. Assessment of patient satisfaction and hospice: a review and an investigation. *Hospice J* 1986; 2(4):69–94.

22. Kristjanson LJ. Quality of terminal care. Salient indicators identified by families. *J Palliat Care* 1989; 5:21–30.

23. Lusk SL. Violence experienced by nurses' aids in nursing homes: an exploratory study. *Am Assoc Occup Health Nurses J* 1992; 40(5):237–241.

Index

aberrant perception of pain, as neuropathic
  pain symptom, 8
accidents, in bereaved persons, 303
acetylcholine receptors, antidepressant reaction
  with, 44
aching pain, 4, 8
aciclovir, use for herpes zoster, 67
activity diary, for self-assessment of fatigue,
  197–198
acute myeloid leukemia, cell line from, 109
acute nonlymphocytic leukemia, weight loss in,
  93, 95
adaptibility, of families, 220–222
addictions, in cancer patient and family,
  236–237
Addisonian signs, from megestrol acetate, 134
Addison's disease, asthenia in, 172, 194, 195
adenylate cyclase, inhibition of, 102
adipose tissue, loss in cancer cachexia, 97, 102,
  103
adjuvant analgesics
  anticonvulsants as, 46–48
  antidepressants as, 43–46
  classes of and drugs as, 42–55
  principles guiding use of, 41–42
  use for neuropathic cancer pain, 3, 23, 41–62
adolescents
  cancer patient's effect on, 235
  Symptom Distress Scale applied to, 186
adriamycin, fatigue induced by, 190
afferent nerves, irritation of, 9
age, of caregiver, role in stress, 253, 254, 255,
  258, 260, 261, 264, 267, 272
aged persons. *See* elderly persons
agnostics, attitude toward death, 219
AIDS
  anorexia/cachexia in, drug therapy of, 133,
    135
  asthenia in, 172

caregiver stress in, 260, 261, 280, 286
  physiological conflict based on, 313–314
  postherpetic neuralgia in, 67
  as source of family-staff conflict, 317
akithesia, from serotonin reuptake inhibitors, 45
alcohol
  as neurolytic agent, 21
  use for spinal subarachnoid blocks, 71
  use in lumbosacral block, 72
  use in sympathetic blocks, 73
alcohol use and abuse
  by advanced cancer patients, 162, 233
  by caregivers, 248, 253, 272
  by grieving persons, 299, 303
allodynia
  etiology of, 9, 19
  from morphine, 79, 82
  from neuropathic pain, 63
  from sympathetically maintained pain, 69
alopecia, as drug side effect, 47
alpha-2-adrenergic agonists
  as adjuvant analgesics, 42, 43, 45, 49–50
  clinical guidelines for, 50
  mechanism of action, 49
  side effects of, 50
alpha-adrenoceptor response, increase in reflex
  sympathetic dystrophy, 9
alprazolam, as adjuvant analgesic, 44
American Society of Clinical Oncology, stress
  study of, 250–251
amino acids
  altered metabolism, in cancer cachexia, 103,
    104, 135, 178
  branched-chain, as appetite stimulants, 135
amitriptyline
  as adjuvant analgesic, 43, 45
  clinical guidelines for, 45
  use for neuropathic pain, 19, 31
  use for postherpetic neuralgia, 68